APLEY'S CONCISE SYSTEM OF
ORTHOPAEDICS
AND FRACTURES

WITHDRAWN

D1239560

This edition of the *Concise System* is dedicated to the memory of Alan Graham Apley, whose teaching has inspired us throughout the work

Library & Media Ctr.
Carroll Community College
1601 Washington Rd.
Westminster, MD 21157

APLEY'S CONCISE SYSTEM OF
ORTHOPAEDICS
AND FRACTURES

THIRD EDITION

Louis Solomon MB ChB MD FRCS FRCSEd
Emeritus Professor of Orthopaedic Surgery, University of Bristol

David Warwick MD BM DIMC EDHS FRCS FRCS(Orth)
Consultant Orthopaedic Surgeon, Southampton University Hospitals; and
Honorary Senior Lecturer, University of Southampton

Selvadurai Nayagam BSc MCh(Orth) FRCS(Orth)
Consultant Orthopaedic Surgeon, Royal Liverpool Children's Hospital
and Royal Liverpool University Hospital, Liverpool

Hodder Arnold

A MEMBER OF THE HODDER HEADLINE GROUP

First published in Great Britain in 1988 by Butterworth Heinemann
Revised reprint 1989
Reprinted 1991, 1992, 1993
Second edition 1994
Reprinted 1997 (twice), 1998, 1999, 2000 (twice), 2001, 2003
This third edition published in 2005 by
Arnold, a member of the Hodder Headline Group,
338 Euston Road, London NW1 3BH

http://www.hoddereducation.com

Distributed in the United States of America by
Oxford University Press Inc.,
198 Madison Avenue, New York, NY10016
Oxford is a registered trademark of Oxford University Press

© 2005 Edward Arnold

All rights reserved. No part of this publication may be reproduced or
transmitted in any form or by any means, electronically or mechanically,
including photocopying, recording or any information storage or retrieval
system, without either prior permission in writing from the publisher or a
licence permitting restricted copying. In the United Kingdom such licences
are issued by the Copyright Licensing Agency: 90 Tottenham Court Road,
London W1T 4LP.

Whilst the advice and information in this book are believed to be true and
accurate at the date of going to press, neither the author[s] nor the publisher
can accept any legal responsibility or liability for any errors or omissions
that may be made. In particular (but without limiting the generality of the
preceding disclaimer) every effort has been made to check drug dosages;
however, it is still possible that errors have been missed. Furthermore,
dosage schedules are constantly being revised and new side-effects
recognized. For these reasons the reader is strongly urged to consult the
drug companies' printed instructions before administering any of the drugs
recommended in this book.

British Library Cataloguing in Publication Data
A catalogue record for this book is available from the British Library

Library of Congress Cataloging-in-Publication Data
A catalog record for this book is available from the Library of Congress

ISBN-10: 0 340 80984 1
ISBN-13: 978 0 340 80984 6

2 3 4 5 6 7 8 9 10

Commissioning Editor: Joanna Koster
Development Editor: Sarah Burrows
Project Editor: Gavin Smith
Production Controller: Lindsay Smith
Cover Design: Amina Dudhia

Typeset in 10½ on 11 pt Garamond by Phoenix Photosetting, Chatham, Kent
Printed and bound in Italy

What do you think about this book? Or any other Arnold title?
Please visit our website: www.hoddereducation.com

CONTENTS

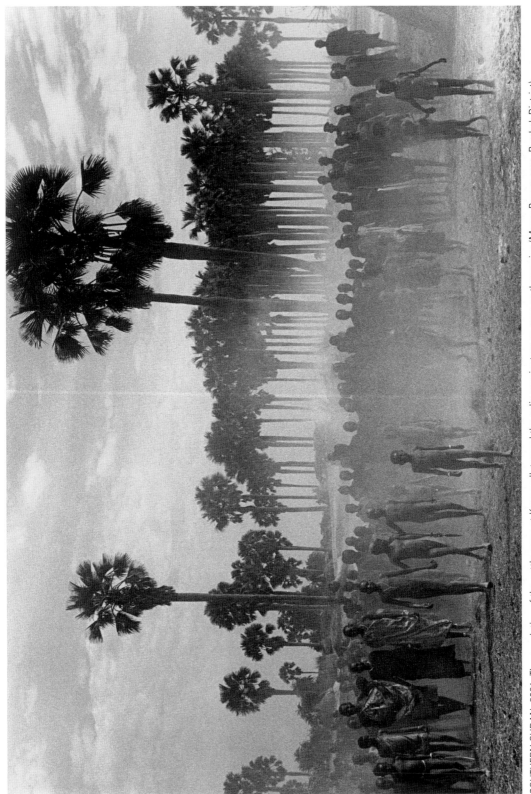

SOUTHERN SUDAN, 2001. The population of the cattle camp at Keny walk toward the polio vaccinators as soon as they arrive (Maper Payem area. Rumbek District).
© Sebastiao Selgado/Amazonas/nbpictures

PREFACE

When the Concise System of Orthopaedics and Fractures was conceived ten years ago, it was designed to answer the needs of advanced medical undergraduates, newly qualified doctors and especially surgeons-in-training who were still learning to master the principles and practices of orthopaedic surgery. It would exclude the extended descriptions and surgical detail of the larger, well-established Apley System of Orthopaedics and Fractures (now in its 8th edition) on which it was based. By following the same layout and order of subjects, it would be easy to refer to the larger edition where more detail was needed.

Within a year of its first appearance we were delighted to find that the Concise System appealed to a much wider range of readers than we had at first envisaged: trainees in other surgical specialties, experienced general practitioners, physiotherapists, occupational therapists and even – at the other end of the spectrum – practising orthopaedic consultants and teachers who wanted a reasonably short, up-to-date review of subjects with which they were already familiar.

While satisfying this wide readership, the new edition is only slightly longer than its predecessors; concise as it is, we have avoided any lapse into 'notebook' writing or 'telegraphese'. In a short volume covering one of the largest specialties in medicine, there must necessarily be omissions; nevertheless we have covered all the common – and some of the less common but important – conditions that might be encountered in an orthopaedic practice. Indeed, some readers have complained, of previous editions, that we have included too much; diseases such as poliomyelitis and tuberculosis, they say, are 'hardly ever seen nowadays'. Hardly ever in industrially advanced countries, perhaps, but we are deeply conscious of the suffering that these disorders still inflict on less privileged societies in the wider world; our frontispiece bears witness to their plight.

As before, the book is divided into three major sections: *General Orthopaedics*, which comprises the main categories of clinical examination, special investigations and the important musculoskeletal disorders such as infection, arthritis, metabolic bone disease, developmental abnormalities, tumours and neuromuscular conditions. This ends with a chapter on the principles of operative orthopaedics and other methods commonly used in treating patients with musculoskeletal complaints. The second section, *Regional Orthopaedics*, deals with the common conditions affecting each of the major joints and the spine. The final section, *Fractures and Joint Injuries*, covers the principles of skeletal trauma and the common fractures encountered in each region.

Each section is liberally illustrated. Most of the old black-and-white pictures of earlier editions have been replaced by coloured illustrations which lend an added degree of clarity. Alan Apley always believed that a good picture – especially a composite picture that tells a story – is worth a thousand words. Students have often told us that the pictures and their captions alone constitute a kind of 'quick-revision manual'.

Sadly, Alan Apley is no longer with us for the present edition. In rewriting the text we have paid silent homage to his engaging style and simplicity of expression. As principal co-author in the past, he would refuse to accept any sentence that sounded more erudite than the context required; even, in some cases, individual words that were not commonly used in everyday speech. He was proud to be known as someone whose preference was for four-letter words: *look, feel, move* became the Apley trademark for systematic clinical examination. If some quality of this great teacher is still recognisable in the present edition we shall be well satisfied.

L.S
D.J.W.
D.N.

ACKNOWLEDGEMENTS

The material for this edition of the Concise System is based mainly on that of the larger 'Apley's System of Orthopaedics and Fractures, 8th Edition', which was published in 2001. Detailed acknowledgements were set out in that volume. Here we would like to express, once more, our indebtedness and gratitude to those many colleagues who have encouraged and helped us to make this smaller edition a worthy successor to the 'Apley textbooks' which have been appearing for the last forty years.

New pictures for these recent editions were generously supplied by Mr John Albert, Mr John Dorgan, Mr Stephen Eisenstein, Mr Neeraj Garg, Mr Martin Gargan, Mr Mike Manning, Mr Ian Nelson, Mr Alistair Ross, Mr Evert Smith and Dr John Wakeley. Colleagues from abroad who have also added to this collection are Professor Kjeld Søballe of Aarhus University Hospital, Denmark and Professor Sidney Biddulph of the Johannesburg Hospital, South Africa.

We owe a special debt of gratitude to Mr Robin Denham for giving us free access to his unique Droxford collection of pictures and illustrations, many of which were produced (and reproduced) during the years when he worked with Alan Apley. We have used a number of these pictures in the present edition and we know that he was looking forward to seeing them in the book that bears Alan's name. Sadly he passed away only a few months before this edition appeared.

As before, most of the drawings are the work of Mr Peter Cox of Creative Design. New photographs, especially those showing methods of clinical examination, were produced by the Department of Medical Illustration at the Bristol Royal Infirmary. The manuscript was typed by Ms Carol Marks, a model of patience, efficiency and attention.

Joan Solomon kept a watchful eye on every aspect of the production of this book, urging us always to aim for perfection whatever the cost in time and effort. We owe her our deepest thanks.

Nina Solomon gave helpful professional advice and assistance in graphic design.

The most important contributors are, unfortunately, more difficult to identify. They are the patients who have allowed us to intrude upon their suffering and use their case histories, x-rays and photographs as illustrations. We cannot name them, for reasons of confidentiality, but we thank them most sincerely. Without their co-operation in the entire teaching enterprise, textbooks such as this would never see the light of day.

Finally, we want to acknowledge the students and trainees whose constant curiosity and healthy scepticism keep goading us to reach for the highest standards of both sense and sensibility.

L.S.
S.N.
D.J.W

1 General Orthopaedics

CHAPTER 1

DIAGNOSIS IN ORTHOPAEDICS

Information consists of differences that make a difference.
Gregory Bateson

Diagnosis is the identification of disease. It begins with the systematic gathering of information – from the patient's history, the physical examination, x-ray appearances and special investigations. It should, however, never be forgotten that every orthopaedic disorder is part of a larger whole – a patient who has a unique personality, a job and hobbies, a family and a home; all have a bearing upon, and are in turn affected by, the disorder and its treatment.

HISTORY

'Taking a history' is a misnomer. The patient tells a story; it is we the listeners who construct a history. The story may be maddeningly disorganized; the history has to be systematic. Carefully and patiently compiled, it can be every bit as informative as examination or laboratory tests.

As we record it, certain key words will inevitably stand out: *injury, pain, stiffness, swelling, deformity, instability, weakness, altered sensibility* and *loss of function*. Each symptom is pursued for more detail: we need to know when it began, whether suddenly or gradually, spontaneously or after some specific event; how it has changed or progressed; what makes it worse; what makes it better.

While listening, we consider whether the story fits some pattern that we recognize – for we are already thinking of a diagnosis. Every piece of information should be thought of as part of a larger picture which gradually unfolds in our understanding. The surgeon-philosopher Wilfred Trotter (1870–1939) put it well: '*Disease reveals itself in casual parentheses*'.

SYMPTOMS

Pain

Pain is the most common symptom. Its precise location is important, so ask the patient to point to where it hurts. But don't assume that the site of pain is always the site of pathology: often pain is 'referred'.

Referred pain

Pain arising in or near the skin is usually localized accurately. Pain arising in deep structures is more diffuse and is sometimes of unexpected distribution; thus, hip disease may manifest with pain in the knee (so might an obturator hernia!). This is not because sensory nerves connect the two sites: it is due to inability of the cerebral cortex to distinguish between sensory messages from embryologically related sites.

Stiffness

Stiffness may be generalized (typically in rheumatoid arthritis and ankylosing spondylitis) or localized to a particular joint. Patients often have difficulty distinguishing stiffness from painful movement; limited movement should never be assumed until verified by examination.

Ask when it occurs: regular early morning stiffness of many joints is one of the cardinal features of rheumatoid arthritis, whereas transient stiffness of one or two joints after periods of inactivity is typical of osteoarthritis.

Locking

This term is used to describe the sudden inability to complete a certain movement; it suggests a mechanical block, e.g. due to a loose body or a torn meniscus becoming trapped between the articular surfaces. Unfortunately, patients use the term for any painful limitation of movement; much more reliable is a history of 'unlocking', when the offending body suddenly moves out of the way.

Swelling

Swelling may be in the soft tissues, the joint or the bone; to the patient they are all the same. It is important to establish whether the swelling followed an injury, whether it appeared rapidly (probably a haematoma or a haemarthrosis) or slowly (soft tissue inflammation or a joint effusion), whether it is painful (acute inflammation, infection – or a tumour!) and whether it is constant or comes and goes.

Deformity

The common deformities are well described in terms such as round shoulders, spinal curvature, knock-knees, bow-legs, pigeon-toes and flat-feet. Some 'deformities' are merely variations of the normal (e.g. short stature or wide hips); others disappear spontaneously with growth (e.g. flat-feet or bandy-legs in an infant). However, if the deformity is progressive, it may be serious.

Weakness

Muscle weakness may be associated with any joint dysfunction. It may also suggest a more specific neurological disorder. Try to establish which movements are affected: this may give important clues to the site of the lesion.

Instability

The patient complains that the joint 'gives way' or 'jumps out'. If this happens repeatedly, it suggests ligamentous deficiency, recurrent subluxation or some internal derangement, such as a loose body.

Change in sensibility

Tingling or numbness signifies interference with nerve function – pressure from a neighbouring structure (e.g. a prolapsed intervertebral disc), local ischaemia (e.g. nerve entrapment in a fibro-osseous tunnel) or a peripheral neuropathy. It is important to establish its exact distribution; from this we can tell whether the fault lies in a peripheral nerve or in a nerve root.

Loss of function

Functional disability is more than the sum of individual symptoms and its expression depends upon the needs of the patient. The patient may say

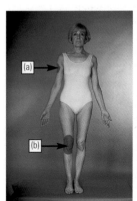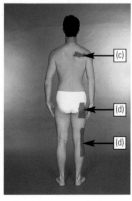

1.1 Referred pain Common sites of referred pain: (a) from the shoulder; (b) from the hip; (c) from the neck; (d) from the lumbar spine.

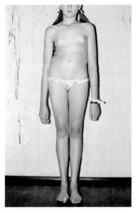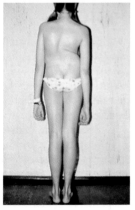

1.2 Deformity This young girl complained of a prominent right hip; the real deformity was scoliosis.

'I can't sit for long' rather than 'I have backache', or 'I can't put my socks on' rather than 'my hip is stiff'. Moreover, what to one patient is merely inconvenient may, to another, be incapacitating. Thus a lawyer or a teacher may readily tolerate a stiff knee provided it is painless and does not impair walking; but to a plumber the same disorder might spell economic disaster.

PREVIOUS DISORDERS

Patients should always be asked about previous accidents, illnesses, operations and drug therapy. They may give vital clues to the present disorder.

FAMILY HISTORY

Patients often wonder (and worry) about inheriting a disease or passing it on to their children. To the doctor, information about musculoskeletal disorders in the patient's family may help with both diagnosis and counselling.

SOCIAL BACKGROUND

No history is complete without enquiry about the patient's background: details about work, travel, recreation, home circumstances and the level of support from family and friends. These always impinge on the assessment of disability; occasionally a particular activity (at work, on the sports' field or in the kitchen) is responsible for the entire condition.

EXAMINATION

In *A Case of Identity*, Sherlock Holmes has the following conversation with Dr Watson:

Watson: You appeared to read a good deal upon [your client] which was quite invisible to me.
Holmes: Not invisible but unnoticed, Watson.

Some disorders can be diagnosed at a glance: who would mistake the facies of acromegaly or the hand deformities of rheumatoid arthritis for anything else? Nevertheless, even in these cases a systematic approach is rewarding: it keeps reinforcing the habit and the patients feel that they have been properly attended to.

The examination actually begins from the moment we set eyes on the patient. We observe his or her general appearance, posture and gait. Are they walking freely or do they use a stick? Are they in pain? Do their movements look natural? Can you spot any distinctive features immediately? A characteristic facies? A spinal curvature? A short

limb? Any type of asymmetry? They may have a tell-tale gait suggesting a painful hip, an unstable knee or a foot-drop. The clues are endless and the game is played by everyone (qualified or lay) at each new encounter throughout life. In the clinical setting the assessment needs to be more focused.

When we proceed to the structured examination, the patient must be suitably undressed: no mere rolling up of a trouser leg is sufficient. If one limb is affected, both must be exposed so that they can be compared.

Classic approach to examination	
Look:	*skin*
	shape
	position
Feel:	*skin*
	soft tissues
	bones and joints
Move:	*active*
	passive
	abnormal

We examine first the good limb, then the bad. The student is often inclined to rush in with both hands – a temptation which must be resisted. Only by proceeding in a purposeful, orderly way can we avoid missing important signs. The system we normally use is simple but comprehensive: first we LOOK, then we FEEL, then we MOVE. Obviously, though, the sequence may sometimes have to be changed because a patient is in pain or severely disabled: you would not try to 'move' a limb with a suspected fracture when an x-ray can provide the answer. Furthermore, resuscitation will always take priority, and in severely injured patients the detailed local examination may have to be curtailed or deferred.

■ **Look**
  – First at the skin: for scars, colour changes and abnormal creases.
  – Then at the shape: is there swelling, wasting or a lump? Is a normally straight bone bent?
  – And then the position: many joint disorders and nerve lesions have characteristic deformities.

■ **Feel**
  – The skin: is it warm or cold, moist or dry, and is sensation normal?

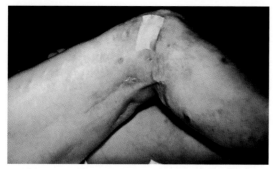

1.3 Look Scars often give clues to the previous history. The faded scar on this patient's thigh is an old operation wound – internal fixation of a femoral fracture. The other scars are due to postoperative infection; one of the sinuses is still draining.

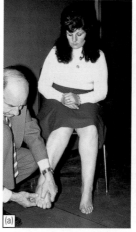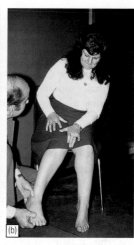

1.4 Feeling for tenderness (a) The wrong way – there is no need to look at your fingers, you should know where they are. (b) It is much more informative to look at the patient's face!

- The bones and joints: are the outlines normal? Is the synovium thickened? Is there excessive fluid in the joint?
- Tenderness: if you know precisely *where* the trouble is, you're halfway to knowing *what* it is.

■ **Move**
- *Active movement:* ask the patient to move the joint, and test for power.
- *Passive movement:* here it is the examiner who moves the joint in each anatomical plane. The range of movement should be expressed in degrees, starting with zero, which is the neutral or anatomical position of the joint. Note whether movement is painful, and whether it is associated with crepitus.

- *Abnormal movement:* is the joint unstable? You may be able to tell by shifting or angulating the joint (without causing pain) out of its normal plane of movement.
- *Special manoeuvres:* special tests for conditions such as joint stability are described in the relevant chapters.

NEUROLOGICAL EXAMINATION

If the symptoms include weakness or inco-ordination or a change in sensibility, or if they point to any disorder of the neck or back, a

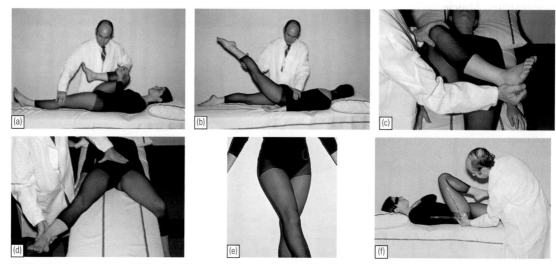
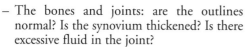

1.5 Testing for movement (a) Flexion, (b) extension, (c) rotation, (d) abduction, (e) adduction. The range of movement can be estimated by eye or measured accurately using a goniometer (f).

complete neurological examination of the related part is mandatory.

Once again we follow a systematic routine, first looking at the *general appearance,* then assessing *motor function* (muscle tone, power and reflexes) and finally testing for *sensory function* (both skin sensibility and deep sensibility).

Appearance

Some neurological disorders result in postures that are so characteristic as to be almost diagnostic, e.g. the claw hand of an ulnar nerve lesion or a drop-wrist due to radial nerve palsy. Usually, however, it is when the patient moves that we can best appreciate the type and extent of motor disorder, e.g. the 'spastic' movement of cerebral palsy, and the flaccid posture of a lower motor neuron lesion.

Concentrating on the affected part, we look for trophic changes that signify loss of sensibility: the smooth, hairless skin that seems to be stretched too tight; atrophy of the fingertips and the nails; scars that tell of accidental burns; and ulcers that refuse to heal. Muscle wasting is rapidly assessed by comparing the two limbs.

Tone and power

Tone in individual muscle groups is tested by moving the nearby joint to stretch the muscle. Increased tone (spasticity) is characteristic of upper motor neuron disorders such as cerebral palsy and stroke. It must not be confused with rigidity (the 'lead-pipe' or 'cogwheel' effect), which is seen in Parkinson's disease. Decreased tone (flaccidity) is found in lower motor neuron lesions such as poliomyelitis. Muscle power is diminished in all three states; it is important to recognize that a 'spastic' muscle may still be weak.

Testing for power is not as easy as it sounds; the difficulty is to make ourselves understood. The simplest way is to place the limb in the 'test' position, then ask the patient to hold it there as firmly as possible and resist any attempt to undo that position. The normal limb is examined first, then the affected limb, and the two are compared. Finer muscle actions, such as those of the thumb and fingers, may be reproduced by first demonstrating the movement yourself. We can also assess the patient's ability to perform complicated movements by asking him or her to perform specific tasks such as gripping a rod, holding a pen, doing up a button or picking up a pin. The power of movement is usually graded on the Medical Research Council scale shown in the box.

Muscle power: Medical Research Council grading
Grade 0 – *no movement*
Grade 1 – *only a flicker of movement*
Grade 2 – *movement with gravity eliminated*
Grade 3 – *movement against gravity*
Grade 4 – *movement against resistance*
Grade 5 – *normal power*

Tendon reflexes

A deep tendon reflex is elicited by rapidly stretching the tendon near its insertion. A sharp tap with the tendon hammer does this well, but all too often this is performed with a flourish and with such force that the finer gradations of response are missed. It is better to employ a series of taps, starting with the most forceful and reducing the force with each successive tap until there is no response. Comparing the two sides in this way, we can pick up fine differences showing that a reflex is 'diminished' rather than 'absent'. In the upper limb we test biceps, triceps and brachioradialis; and in the lower limb the patellar ligament and Achilles tendon.

The tendon reflexes are monosynaptic segmental reflexes; that is, the reflex pathway takes a 'short cut' through the spinal cord at the segmental level. Depression or absence of the reflex signifies interruption at some point along this pathway. It is a reliable pointer to the segmental level of dysfunction. An unusually brisk reflex, on the other hand, is characteristic of an upper motor neuron disorder (e.g. cerebral palsy, a stroke or injury to the spinal cord); the lower motor neuron is released from the normal central inhibition and there is an exaggerated response to tendon stimulation.

Superficial reflexes

The superficial reflexes are elicited by stroking the skin at various sites to produce a specific muscle contraction; the best known are the abdominal (T7–T12), cremasteric (L1, 2) and anal (S4, 5) reflexes. These are corticospinal (upper motor neuron) reflexes. Absence of the reflex indicates an upper motor neuron lesion (usually in the spinal cord) above that level.

The plantar reflex

Forceful stroking of the sole normally produces flexion of the toes (or no response at all). An extensor response (the big toe extends while the others remain in flexion) is characteristic of upper motor neuron disorders. This is the *Babinski sign* – a type of withdrawal reflex which is present in young infants and which normally disappears after the age of 18 months.

Sensibility

Sensibility to touch and to pinprick may be increased *(hyperaesthesia)* or unpleasant *(dysaesthesia)* in certain irritative nerve lesions. More often, though, it is diminished *(hypoaesthesia)* or absent *(anaesthesia)*, signifying pressure on or interruption of a peripheral nerve, a nerve root or the sensory pathways in the spinal cord. The area of sensory change can be mapped out on the skin and compared with the known segmental or dermatomal pattern of innervation. If the abnormality is well defined, it is an easy matter to establish the level of the lesion, even if the precise cause remains unknown.

Brisk percussion along the course of an injured nerve may elicit a tingling sensation in the distal distribution of the nerve *(Tinel's sign)*. The point of hypersensitivity marks the site of abnormal nerve sprouting: if it progresses distally at successive visits, this signifies regeneration; if it remains unchanged, this suggests a local neuroma.

Tests for *temperature recognition* and *two-point discrimination* (the ability to recognize two touch-points a few millimetres apart) are sometimes used in the assessment of peripheral nerve disorders.

Deep sensibility can be examined in several ways. In the *vibration test,* a sounded tuning-fork is placed over a peripheral bony point (e.g. the medial malleolus or the head of the ulna); the patient is asked if he or she can feel the vibrations and to say when they disappear. By comparing the two sides, differences can be noted. *Position sense* is tested by asking the patient to find certain points on the body with the eyes closed – for example, touching the tip of the nose with the forefinger. *The sense of joint posture* is tested by grasping the big toe and placing it in different positions of flexion and extension. The patient is asked to say whether it is 'up' or 'down'. *Stereognosis* – the ability to recognize shape and texture by feel alone – is tested by giving the patient (whose eyes are closed) a variety of familiar objects to hold and asking him or her to name each object.

The pathways for deep sensibility run in the posterior columns of the spinal cord. Disturbances are, therefore, found in peripheral neuropathies and in spinal cord lesions such as posterior column injuries or tabes dorsalis. The sense of balance is also carried in the posterior columns. This can be tested by asking the patient to stand upright with his or her eyes closed; excessive body sway is abnormal *(Romberg's sign)*.

Cortical and cerebellar function

A staggering gait may imply drunkenness, an unstable knee or a disorder of the spinal cord or cerebellum. If there is no musculoskeletal abnormality to account for the sign, a full examination of the central nervous system will be necessary.

EXAMINING INFANTS AND CHILDREN

Paediatric practice requires special skills. You may have no first-hand account of the symptoms; a baby screaming with pain will tell you very little, and over-anxious parents will probably tell you too much. When examining the child, you should be flexible. If he or she is moving a particular joint, take your opportunity to examine movement then and there. You will learn much more by adopting methods of play than by applying a rigid system of examination. And leave any test for tenderness until last!

Infants and small children

The baby should be undressed, in a warm room, and placed on the examining couch. Look carefully for birthmarks, deformities and abnormal movements – or absence of movement. If there is no urgency or distress, take time to examine the head and neck, including facial features which may be characteristic of specific dysplastic syndromes. The back and limbs are then examined for abnormalities of position or shape. Examining for joint movement can be difficult. Active movements can often be stimulated by gently stroking the limb. When testing for passive mobility, be careful to avoid frightening or hurting the child.

In the neonate, and throughout the first 2 years of life, examination of the hips is mandatory, even if the child appears to be normal. This is to avoid missing the subtle signs of developmental dysplasia of the hips (DDH) at the early stage when treatment is most effective.

It is also important to assess the child's general development by testing for the normal milestones which are expected to appear during the first 2 years of life (see box).

Normal developmental milestones	
Newborn:	Grasp reflex present
	Morrow reflex present
3–6 months:	Holds head up unsupported
6–9 months:	Able to sit up
9–12 months:	Crawling and standing up
9–18 months:	Walking
18–24 months:	Running

Older children

Most children can be examined in the same way as adults, though with different emphasis on particular physical features. Posture and gait are very important; subtle deviations from the norm may herald the appearance of serious abnormalities such as scoliosis or neuromuscular disorders, while more obvious 'deformities' such as knock-knees and bow-legs may be no more than transient stages in normal development – similarly with mild degrees of 'flat-feet' and 'pigeon-toes'. More complex variations in posture and gait patterns, when the child sits and walks with the knees turned inwards (medially rotated) or outwards (laterally rotated), are usually due to anteversion or retroversion of the femoral necks, sometimes associated with compensatory rotational 'deformities' of the femora and tibiae. Seldom need anything be done about this; the condition usually improves as the child approaches puberty and only if the gait is very awkward would one consider performing corrective osteotomies of the femora.

COMMON CLINICAL PROBLEMS

DEFORMITY

Most deformities are easily spotted; some escape attention, especially if they are bilateral and symmetrical, and some 'deformities' are merely variations of the normal. *Shortness of stature* may be normal, but sometimes it is part of a generalized deformity; try to establish whether it is proportionate or whether there is a disproportionate shortness of the limbs or trunk. *If one limb is deformed,* it is important to establish whether the fault is in the bone or in the joint. The more common deformities have special names.

Varus and valgus

It may seem pedantic to replace 'bow-legs' and 'knock-knees' with 'genu varum' and 'genu valgum', but comparable colloquialisms are not available for deformities of the elbow, hip or big toe; and, besides, the formality is justified by the need for clarity and consistency. Varus means that the part distal to the joint is displaced towards the midline, valgus away from it.

Kyphosis and lordosis

Seen from the side, the spine has a series of curves – convex posteriorly in the dorsal region (kyphosis), and convex anteriorly in the cervical and lumbar regions (lordosis). Excessive curvature constitutes a kyphotic or lordotic deformity.

Scoliosis

Seen from behind, the spine is straight. Any curvature in this (coronal) plane is called scoliosis.

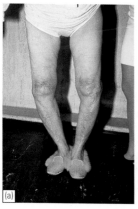 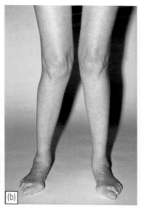 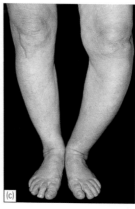

1.6 Varus and valgus
(a) Varus knees due to osteoarthritis; (b) valgus deformity in rheumatoid arthritis. (c) Another varus knee? No – the deformity here is in the tibia, due to Paget's disease.

'Fixed' deformity of a joint

This does not mean that the joint is unable to move: it means that one particular movement cannot be completed. Thus, the knee may flex fully but not extend fully – at the limit of its extension it is still 'fixed' in a certain amount of flexion. In the spine a fixed deformity is called a *structural deformity*; this differs from a *postural deformity*, which the patient can, if properly instructed, correct by his or her own muscular effort.

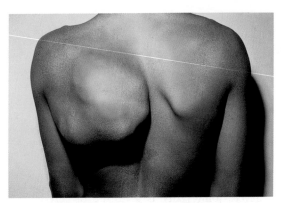

1.7 Bony lumps This young man developed a large, lobulated tumour on his scapula, typical of chrondosarcoma.

Six causes of bone deformity
1. Congenital disorders
2. Rickets or osteomalacia
3. Bone dysplasia
4. Physeal injury
5. Fracture malunion
6. Paget's disease

Six causes of joint deformity
1. Skin contracture (e.g. burn)
2. Fascial contracture (e.g. Dupuytren's)
3. Muscle contracture (e.g. Volkmann's)
4. Muscle imbalance
5. Joint instability
6. Joint destruction

BONY LUMPS

A bony lump may be due to faulty development, injury, inflammation or a tumour. Although x-ray examination is essential, the clinical features can be highly informative.

Size

A large lump attached to bone, or a lump which is getting bigger, is nearly always a tumour.

Site

A lump near a joint is most likely to be a tumour (benign or malignant); a lump in the shaft may be fracture callus, inflammatory new bone or a tumour.

Shape

A benign tumour has a well-defined margin; malignant tumours, inflammatory lumps and callus have a vague edge.

Consistency

A benign bone tumour feels hard; malignant tumours often give the impression that they can be indented.

Tenderness

Lumps due to active inflammation, recent callus or a rapidly growing sarcoma are tender.

Multiplicity

Multiple bony lumps are uncommon: they occur in hereditary multiple exostosis and in Ollier's disease.

STIFF JOINTS

It is convenient to distinguish three grades of joint stiffness.

All movements absent

Surgical fusion of a joint is called arthrodesis; pathological fusion is called ankylosis. Acute suppurative arthritis typically ends in bony ankylosis; tuberculous arthritis often heals by fibrosis and causes fibrous ankylosis.

All movements limited

Restriction of movement in all directions is characteristic of non-infective arthritis and is usually due to synovial swelling or capsular fibrosis.

One or two movements limited

Limitation of movement in some directions with full movement in others suggests a mechanical block or joint contracture.

LAX JOINTS

Generalized joint hypermobility occurs in about 5 per cent of people and is familial. Hypermobile joints are not necessarily unstable – as witness the controlled performances of acrobats – but they do have a tendency to recurrent dislocation (e.g. of the shoulder or patella).

Severe joint laxity is a feature of certain rare connective tissue disorders such as Marfan's syndrome and osteogenesis imperfecta.

DIAGNOSTIC IMAGING

PLAIN FILM RADIOGRAPHY

Despite the remarkable technical advances of recent years, plain film x-ray examination remains the most useful method of diagnostic imaging.

The radiographic image

Radiographic images are produced by the attenuation of x-rays as they pass through intervening tissues before striking an appropriately sensitized plate or film. The more dense and impenetrable the tissue, the greater the attenuation and therefore the more blank, or white, the image in the film. Thus, a metal implant appears intensely white, bone less so and soft tissues in varying shades of grey depending on their 'density'. Cartilage, which causes little attenuation, appears as a dark area between adjacent bone ends.

It is important to appreciate that these are two-dimensional images. Thus, if one image (say that of a bullet) is seen to be superimposed upon another (say that of a bone), it is impossible to tell whether the bullet is lying in front of the bone, behind the bone or inside the bone – unless you have another view of the area taken from a different angle. For this reason we always ask for at least two views projected at right angles to each other.

How to read an x-ray

Although 'radiograph' is more correct, the term 'x-ray' (or 'x-ray film') has become entrenched by usage. The process of 'reading an x-ray' should be as methodical as clinical examination. It is seductively easy to be led astray by some flagrant anomaly; systematic study is the only safeguard against missing other important signs.

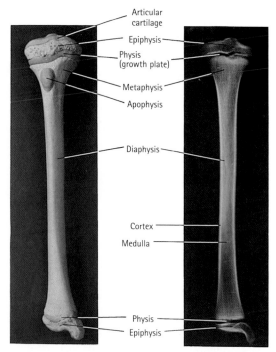

1.8 The radiographic image X-ray of an anatomical specimen to show the appearance of various parts of the bone in the x-ray image.

Start with a general orientation: identify the part, the particular view and, if possible, the type of patient; try to visualize the living person, the age, build and sex. Then examine, in sequence, the soft tissues, the bones, the joints.

Soft tissues

Unless examined early, these are liable to be forgotten. Look for variations in shape (swelling or wasting) and variations of density (e.g. calcification).

Bones

Look for deformity or local irregularities; examine the cortices for areas of destruction or new-bone formation; then look for areas of reduced density (osteoporosis or destruction), or increased density (sclerosis). Remember that 'vacant' areas are not necessarily spaces or cysts: any tissue that is radiolucent may look 'cystic'.

Joints

The radiographic 'joint' consists of the articulating bones and the 'space' between them. The 'joint space' is, of course, illusory; it is occupied by radiolucent articular cartilage. Look for narrowing of this space, which signifies loss of cartilage

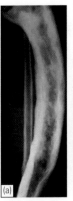
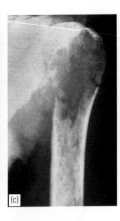
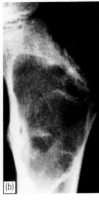
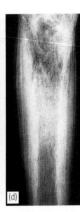

1.9 X-rays – important features to look for (a) *General shape and appearance*: in this case the cortices are thickened and the bone is bent (Paget's disease). (b,c) *Interior density*: a vacant area may represent a true cyst (b), or radiolucent material infiltrating the bone, like the metastatic tumour in (c). *Periosteal reaction*: typically seen in healing fractures, bone infection and malignant bone tumours – as in this example of Ewing's sarcoma (d).

thickness, and examine the bone ends for flattening, erosion, cavitation or sclerosis – all features of arthritis. The joint margins may show osteophytes (typical of osteoarthritis) or erosions (typical of rheumatoid arthritis). Similarly, intervertebral disc 'spaces' are not gaps in the vertebral column; you must imagine the fibrous discs which occupy those 'spaces', and if a 'disc space' is abnormally flattened or narrowed, it means that the intervertebral disc has collapsed.

OTHER X-RAY TECHNIQUES
Contrast radiography
Injected radio-opaque liquids may be used to outline cavities during x-ray examination (air or gas can be used in the same way). Common examples are sinography (outlining a sinus), arthrography (outlining a joint) and myelography (outlining the spinal theca).

Tomography
Tomography provides an image 'focused' on a selected plane and may show changes that are obscured by the overlapping images (produced by the surrounding tissues) in conventional x-ray films. It is particularly useful for detecting changes in the spine.

Computed tomography (CT)
This method is capable of recording bone and soft-tissue outlines in cross-section. It is particularly useful for showing detailed fracture patterns, for displaying the shape of the spinal canal and for mapping the spread of tumours into the soft tissues. The computed data can also be reconstructed as a three-dimensional image. A disadvantage of CT is the relatively high radiation exposure. It should, therefore, be used with discretion.

Radionuclide scanning
A bone-seeking radioisotope compound – usually ^{99m}technetium methylene diphosphonate (^{99m}Tc-HDP) – is injected intravenously and its presence in the tissues is recorded with a gamma camera or rectilinear scanner. Increased uptake during the blood phase (immediately after injection) signifies

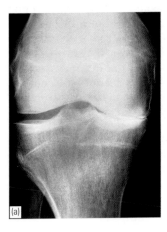
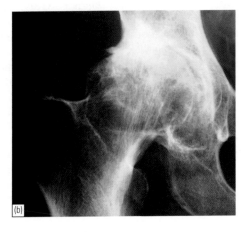

1.10 Joint x-rays (a) Loss of articular cartilage in the medial compartment of this knee has resulted in the joint 'space' being markedly reduced in width. (b) In this hip the superior joint 'space' is virtually obliterated and there are juxta-articular cysts with reactive sclerosis – typical features of osteoarthritis.

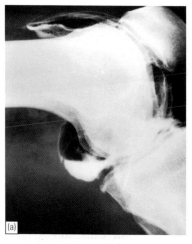

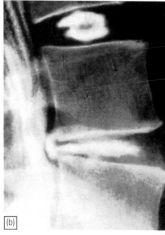

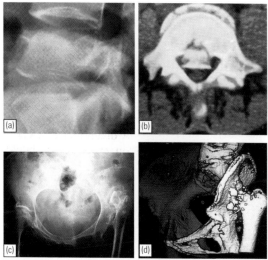

1.11 Contrast radiography (a) Contrast arthrography of the knee. Note the small popliteal herniation. (b) Discography is sometimes useful. Compare the degenerate intervertebral disc (lower level) with the normal disc (upper level).

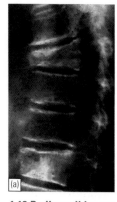

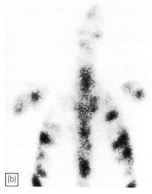

1.13 Radionuclide scanning (a) The plain x-ray showed a pathological fracture, probably through a metastatic tumour. (b) The bone scan revealed generalized secondaries, here involving the spine and ribs.

1.12 Computed tomography (CT) The plain x-ray (a) shows a fracture of the vertebral body but one cannot tell precisely how the bone fragments are displaced. The CT (b) shows clearly that they are dangerously close to the cauda equina. (c) Congenital hip dislocation, defined more clearly by (d) three-dimensional CT reconstruction.

a hyperaemia; activity during the bone phase (about 3 hours later) suggests new-bone formation. This information is valuable in the diagnosis of stress fractures (which often do not show on x-ray), bone infection and bone tumours.

MAGNETIC RESONANCE IMAGING (MRI)

Unlike x-ray imaging, MRI relies upon radiofrequency emissions from atoms and molecules in tissues exposed to a static magnetic field. It does not involve ionizing radiation. The images produced by these signals are similar to those of CT scans, but with even better contrast resolution and more refined differentiation of tissues.

Tissues containing abundant hydrogen (fat, cancellous bone and marrow) emit high-intensity signals and produce the brightest images; those containing little hydrogen (cortical bone, ligament, tendon and air) appear black; intermediate in the grey scale are cartilage, spinal canal and muscle. By adjusting various parameters,

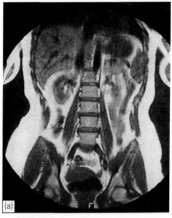 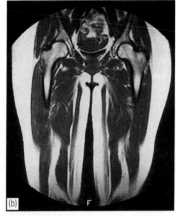 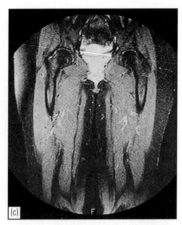

1.14 Magnetic resonance imaging (MRI) (a,b) T_1-weighted and (c) STIR (short tau inversion recovery) sequences of the torso and thigh areas, showing the contrasting definition and brightness of the various structures and tissues.

different tissues and organs can be displayed with extraordinary clarity. Bone tumours can be shown in their transverse and longitudinal extent, and extraosseous spread can be accurately assessed. Moreover, there is the potential for characterizing the actual tissue, thus allowing a pathological as well as an anatomical diagnosis.

Other areas of usefulness are in the early diagnosis of bone ischaemia and necrosis, the investigation of backache and spinal disorders, and the elucidation of cartilage and ligament injuries. In the knee, MRI is as accurate as arthroscopy in diagnosing meniscal tears and cruciate ligament injuries. It is also useful for diagnosing rotator cuff tears and labral injuries in the shoulder and ligament injuries around the ankle.

As MRI is so versatile, and free of the risks of ionizing radiation, it is tempting to over-indulge its use. It is well to remember that it is still only one diagnostic method among many.

DIAGNOSTIC ULTRASOUND

High-frequency sound waves, generated by a transducer, can penetrate several centimetres into the soft tissues; as they pass through the tissue interfaces, some of these waves are reflected back (like echoes) to the transducer, where they are registered as electrical signals and displayed as images on a screen or plate. With modern equipment, tissues of varying density can be 'imaged' in gradations of grey that allow reasonable definition of the anatomy. Real-time display on a monitor gives a dynamic image, which is more useful than the usual static images on transparent plates. One big advantage of this

technique is that the equipment is simple and portable and can be used almost anywhere. Another is that it produces no harmful side-effects.

As a result of the marked echogenic contrast between cystic and solid masses, ultrasonography is particularly useful for identifying hidden 'cystic' lesions such as haematomas, abscesses, popliteal cysts and arterial aneurysms. It is also capable of detecting intra-articular fluid.

One of the most useful applications is in screening newborn babies for developmental dysplasia of the hip, where the anatomical outlines can be identified even though they are entirely cartilaginous.

BONE BIOPSY

Bone biopsy is often the only means of establishing a diagnosis or distinguishing between local conditions that closely resemble one another, e.g. an area of bone destruction that could be due to a compression fracture, a bone tumour or infection. Even if it is obvious that the lesion is a tumour, we need to know what type of tumour, whether benign or malignant, primary or metastatic. Radical surgery should never be undertaken for a suspected neoplasm without first confirming the diagnosis histologically. In bone infection, the biopsy permits not only histological proof of acute inflammation but also bacteriological typing of the organism and tests for antibiotic sensitivity.

Open or closed?

Open biopsy is the most reliable way of obtaining a suitable sample of tissue, but it has several drawbacks: (1) it requires an operation, with the attendant risks of anaesthesia and infection; (2) tissue planes are opened up, predisposing to spread of infection or tumour; and (3) the incision may interfere with subsequent plans for tumour excision.

A carefully performed *closed biopsy*, using a needle or trephine, is the procedure of choice except when the lesion cannot be accurately localized or when the tissue consistency is such that a sufficient sample cannot be obtained.

Precautions

1 The biopsy site and approach should be carefully planned with the aid of x-rays or other imaging techniques.

2 If there is any possibility of the lesion being malignant, the approach should be sited so that the wound and biopsy track can be excised if later radical surgery proves to be necessary.

3 The procedure should be carried out in an operating theatre, under anaesthesia (local or general) and with full aseptic technique.

4 For deep-seated lesions, fluoroscopic control of the needle insertion is essential.

5 The appropriate size of biopsy needle or cutting trephine should be selected.

6 A knowledge of the local anatomy and of the likely consistency of the lesion is important. Large blood vessels and nerves must be avoided; potentially vascular tumours may bleed profusely and the means to control haemorrhage should be readily to hand. More than one surgeon has set out to aspirate an 'abscess' only to plunge a wide-bore needle into an aneurysm!

7 Clear instructions should be given to ensure that the tissue obtained at the biopsy is suitably processed. If infection is suspected, the material should go into a culture tube and be sent to the laboratory as soon as possible. A smear may also be useful. Whole tissue is transferred to a jar containing formalin, without damaging the specimen or losing any material. Aspirated blood should be allowed to clot and can then be preserved in formalin for later paraffin embedding and sectioning. Tissue thought to contain crystals should not be placed in formalin as this may destroy the crystals; it should either be kept unaltered for immediate examination or stored in saline.

8 No matter how careful the biopsy, there is always the risk that the tissue will be too scanty or too unrepresentative for accurate diagnosis. Close consultation with the radiologist and pathologist beforehand will minimize this possibility. In the best hands, needle biopsy has an accuracy rate of more than 95 per cent.

ELECTRODIAGNOSIS

Nerve and muscle function can be studied by electrical methods. Two types of investigation are employed: nerve conduction and electromyography.

Nerve conduction

The time interval between stimulation of a motor nerve and muscle contraction can be measured accurately. If the test is repeated at two points a fixed distance apart along the nerve, the *conduction velocity* between these points can be determined. Normal values are about 40–60 m/s. Sensory nerve conduction can be measured in a similar way.

Conduction velocity is slowed in peripheral nerve damage or compression, and the site of the lesion can be established by taking measurements in different segments of the nerve.

If the nerve is divided, there is no response to stimulation of the nerve (and an abnormal response to galvanic stimulation of the muscle – the *'reaction of degeneration'*). By plotting the voltage against the duration of stimulus necessary to produce contraction, a *strength/duration curve* can be obtained, which reflects the degree of muscle innervation after nerve injury. Serial examinations will show whether recovery is taking place.

Electromyography

Electromyography does not involve electrical stimulation. Instead, an electrode in the muscle is used to record motor unit activity at rest and

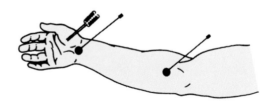

1.15 Electrodiagnosis Electrodes at different levels are used to stimulate the nerve, and the contraction signal is picked up in an appropriate distal muscle. If the distance between the electrodes is measured and the time interval from stimulation to muscle contraction is recorded, conduction velocity can be calculated.

during attempts to contract the muscle. Normally there is no electrical activity at rest, but on voluntary contraction, characteristic oscilloscopic patterns appear. Changes in these patterns can identify certain neuropathic and myopathic disorders. After nerve injury there may be typical *denervation potentials,* and with recovery equally typical *re-innervation potentials.*

CHAPTER 2

INFECTION

Micro-organisms may reach the bones and joints via the *bloodstream* from a distant site, or by *direct invasion* from a skin puncture, operation or open fracture. Depending on the type of organism, the site of infection and the host response, the result may be a *pyogenic osteomyelitis* or *arthritis,* a chronic *granulomatous reaction* (classically seen in tuberculosis), or an *indolent response to an unusual organism* (e.g. a fungal infection).

Acute pyogenic infections are characterized by the formation of pus – a concentration of defunct leucocytes, dead and dying bacteria and tissue debris – which is often localized in an abscess. Pressure builds up within the abscess and infection may then extend directly along the tissue planes. It may also spread further afield via lymphatics (causing lymphangitis and lymphadenopathy) or via the bloodstream (bacteraemia and septicaemia). The accompanying systemic reaction is due to the release of bacterial enzymes and endotoxins as well as cellular breakdown products from the host tissues.

Chronic infection may follow acute infection or, depending on the type of organism and the host reaction, it may be 'chronic' from the start. It usually involves the formation of granulation tissue (a combination of fibroblastic and vascular proliferation) leading to fibrosis. Some organisms provoke a non-pyogenic reaction involving the formation of cellular granulomas which consist largely of lymphocytes, modified macrophages and multinucleated giant cells; this is seen most typically in tuberculosis. Systemic effects are less acute but may ultimately be very debilitating, with lymphadenopathy, splenomegaly and tissue wasting.

The *host response* is crucial in determining the course of the disease. Resistance is likely to be depressed in the very young and the very old, in states of malnutrition or immunosuppression, and in certain diseases such as diabetes.

Local factors also are important. Damaged muscle is a favourable substrate for certain organisms, and the presence of foreign material may interfere with the phagocytic response to invading bacteria. Bone, which consists of a collection of rigid compartments, is more susceptible than soft tissues to pressure build-up, vascular damage and cell death. The honeycomb of inaccessible spaces also makes it very difficult to eradicate infection once it is established.

The *principles of treatment* are: (1) to provide analgesia and general supportive measures; (2) to rest the affected part; (3) to initiate antibiotic treatment or chemotherapy; and (4) to undertake surgical eradication of pus and necrotic tissue.

ACUTE HAEMATOGENOUS OSTEOMYELITIS

Acute osteomyelitis almost invariably occurs in children; when adults are affected it may be because of compromised host resistance due to debilitation, disease or drugs (e.g. immuno-

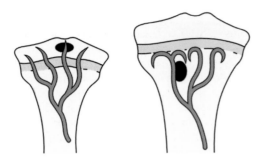

2.1 Acute osteomyelitis – pathogenesis In babies infection may settle near the very end of the bone; joint infection and growth disturbance are common sequelae in untreated cases. In older children, the physis (growth plate) acts as a barrier to spread from the metaphysis to the epiphysis.

suppressive therapy). The causal organism is usually *Staphylococcus aureus,* less often *Streptococcus pyogenes* or *Strep. pneumoniae.* In young children, *Haemophilus influenzae* is not uncommon. Patients with sickle-cell anaemia are prone to develop salmonella bone infections. Unusual organisms are also found in heroin addicts.

The bloodstream is invaded, perhaps from a minor skin abrasion, a boil or – in the newborn – from an infected umbilical cord. In adults the source of infection may be an arterial line or a dirty needle and syringe. The organisms usually settle in the metaphysis at the growing end of a long bone, possibly because the hairpin arrangement of capillaries slows down the rate of blood flow. In young infants the epiphysis may be involved. In adults, haematogenous infection is more common in the vertebrae than in the long bones.

Pathology

Inflammation

The earliest change is an acute inflammatory reaction. The intraosseous pressure rises, causing intense pain and obstruction of blood flow.

Suppuration

By the second day, pus appears in the medulla and forces its way along the Volkmann canals to the surface, where it forms a subperiosteal abscess. It then spreads along the shaft, to re-enter the bone at another level, or bursts out into the soft tissues. In infants, infection often extends into the epiphysis and thence into the joint. In older children the physis is a barrier to direct spread, but

where the metaphysis is partly intracapsular (e.g. at the hip, shoulder or elbow), pus may discharge through the periosteum into the joint. Vertebral infection may spread across the intervertebral disc to an adjacent vertebral body.

Necrosis

The rising intraosseous pressure, vascular stasis, infective thrombosis and periosteal stripping increasingly compromise the blood supply; by the end of a week there is usually evidence of necrosis. Pieces of bone may separate as sequestra which act as foreign-body irritants, causing persistent discharge through a sinus until they escape or are removed. However, the larger sequestra remain entombed in cavities of bone.

New-bone formation

New bone forms from the deep layer of the periosteum. With time, the new bone thickens to form an involucrum enclosing the infected tissue and sequestra. If the infection persists, pus may discharge through perforations (cloacae) in the involucrum and track by sinuses to the skin surface; the condition is now established as a chronic osteomyelitis.

Resolution

If infection is controlled and intraosseous pressure released, the bone will heal, though it may remain thickened.

Clinical features

The patient, usually a child, presents with pain, malaise and a fever; in neglected cases toxaemia may be marked. Sometimes a history of a preceding skin lesion, an injury or a sore throat may be obtained.

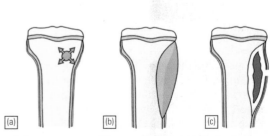

2.2 Acute osteomyelitis – pathology (a) Infection in the metaphysis spreads towards the surface to form (b) a subperiosteal abscess. (c) Bone may die and become encased in periosteal new bone as a sequestrum. The encasing involucrum is sometimes perforated by sinuses.

The limb is held still and there is acute 'fingertip' tenderness near one of the larger joints. Even the gentlest manipulation is painful and joint movement is restricted. Local redness, swelling, warmth and oedema are later signs and signify the presence of pus.

In infants, and especially in the newborn, the constitutional disturbance can be misleadingly mild; the baby simply fails to thrive and is drowsy but irritable. Suspicion should be aroused by a history of birth difficulties or umbilical artery catheterization. There may be metaphyseal tenderness and resistance to joint movement. Always look for other sites – multiple infections are not uncommon.

In adults, the commonest site of haematogenous infection is the spine. Suspicious features are backache and a mild fever, possibly following a urological procedure. It may take weeks for x-ray signs to appear, and even then the diagnosis may need to be confirmed by fine-needle aspiration and bacteriological culture.

Imaging

For the first 10 days, *x-rays* show no abnormality. However, *radio-isotope scans* may show increased activity – a non-specific sign of acute inflammation. By the end of the second week there may be early radiographic signs of rarefaction of the metaphysis and periosteal new-bone formation. Later still, if treatment is delayed or ineffectual, the bone may appear increasingly ragged. With healing there is sclerosis and thickening of the cortex. Sometimes sequestra are seen, separated from the surrounding bone.

MRI may help to distinguish between bone and soft-tissue infection.

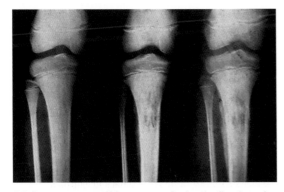

2.3 Acute osteomyelitis – x-rays During the first 2 weeks the x-ray looks normal; later the bone may look mottled and there are increasing signs of periosteal new-bone formation.

Investigations

There is usually a leucocytosis and the blood culture may be positive. However, the most certain way to confirm the clinical diagnosis is to aspirate pus from the subperiosteal abscess or the adjacent joint. Even if no pus is found, a smear of the aspirate is examined immediately for cells and organisms. A sample is also sent for bacteriological examination and tests for sensitivity to antibiotics.

Complications

Spread

Infection may spread to the joint (septic arthritis) or to other bones (metastatic osteomyelitis).

Growth disturbance

If the physis is damaged, there may later be shortening or deformity.

Persistent infection

Treatment must be prompt and effective. 'Too little too late' may result in chronic osteomyelitis.

Treatment

Antibiotics

Blood and, if possible, aspiration samples are sent immediately for culture, but the prompt administration of antibiotics is so vital that the result is not awaited. Initially the choice of antibiotics is based on the findings from direct examination of the aspirate and a 'best guess' at the most likely pathogen; a more appropriate drug can be substituted once the organism is identified and its antibiotic sensitivity is known.

Older children and previously fit adults, who probably have a staphylococcal infection, are started on intravenous flucloxacillin (a penicillinase-resistant penicillin) and fusidic acid; the antibiotic may have to be changed when the results of sensitivity tests are known. This is continued until there is clinical and laboratory evidence of improvement (usually for 1 or 2 weeks) and is then followed by oral antibiotics for another 3–6 weeks. If methicillin-resistant *Staphylococcus aureus* (MRSA) appears, vancomycin is the antibiotic of choice.

Children under 4 years have a high incidence of haemophilus infection. In this group, and in any case in which Gram-negative organisms are seen in the smear, it is advisable to start with one of the third-generation cephalosporins.

Heroin addicts and immuno-compromised patients often have unusual infections and may need more specific antibiotic treatment.

Analgesics

Osteomyelitis is extremely painful; adequate and repeated analgesics must be given.

Splintage

Complete bed-rest is essential. A splint is desirable but should not conceal the affected area.

Drainage

If antibiotics are given early, drainage may not be necessary. If a subperiosteal abscess can be detected (overlying oedema is a useful sign), or if pyrexia and local tenderness persist for more than 24 hours after treatment with adequate antibiotics, the pus should be let out; this will also allow the organism to be identified. About 30 per cent of patients with confirmed osteomyelitis are likely to need an operation.

Follow-up

Once the infection has subsided, movements are encouraged; however, the patient has to use crutches for a few weeks. Outpatient follow-up is important, to ensure that there is no recurrence of infection.

SUBACUTE HAEMATOGENOUS OSTEOMYELITIS

Osteomyelitis may present in a relatively mild form, presumably because the organism is less virulent or the patient more resistant. The distal femur and the proximal and distal tibia are the favourite sites. The patient is usually a child or adolescent who has had pain near one of the large joints for several weeks. The typical x-ray picture is of a small, oval cavity surrounded by sclerotic bone – the classic *Brodie's abscess* – but sometimes the lesion is more diffuse. A small abscess is easily mistaken for an osteoid osteoma and the diagnosis may be made only when the lesion is explored. If the condition is troublesome, the abscess is opened under antibiotic cover.

CHRONIC OSTEOMYELITIS

This used to be a common sequel to acute haematogenous osteomyelitis; nowadays it more frequently follows an open fracture or operation.

An area of bone has been destroyed by the acute infection, leaving sequestra surrounded by dense sclerosed bone. The imprisoned sequestra provoke a chronic seropurulent discharge which escapes through a sinus. Bacteria may remain dormant for

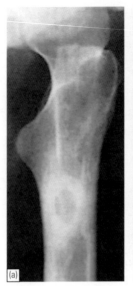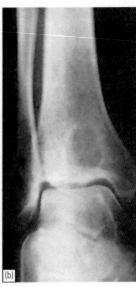

2.4 Subacute osteomyelitis (a) The classic Brodie's abscess looks like a small walled-off cavity in the bone with little or no periosteal reaction. (b) Sometimes the area of rarefaction is more diffuse and there may be cortical erosion and periosteal reaction.

years, giving rise to recurrent flares of acute infection. The usual suspects are *Staph. aureus*, *Escherichia coli*, *Staph. pyogenes*, *Proteus* and *Pseudomonas;* in the presence of surgical implants, *Staph. epidermidis* is the commonest pathogen.

Clinical features

Following acute bone infection, the patient returns with recurrent bouts of pain, redness and tenderness at the affected site. Classic signs are healed and discharging sinuses and x-ray features of bone rarefaction surrounded by dense sclerosis and cortical thickening; within this area of bone there may be an obvious sequestrum. A sinogram may help to localize a particular focus of infection, and bone scans are useful in revealing hidden foci of inflammatory activity.

Treatment

Treatment depends on the frequency of relapsing flare-ups; if seldom, it can be conservative. A sinus may be painless and need a dressing simply to protect the clothing; a flare often settles with a few days' rest, although if an abscess presents it should be incised. Antibiotics are often used, though most fail to penetrate the barrier of fibrous tissue plus bone sclerosis. Sequestrectomy should be performed only if a sequestrum is radiologically visible and surgically accessible.

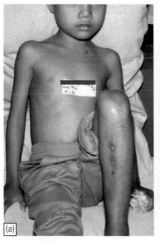
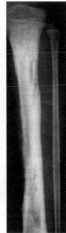
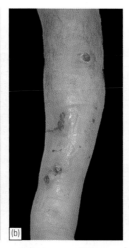
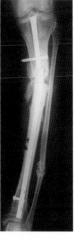

2.5 Chronic osteomyelitis Chronic osteomyelitis may follow acute. The young boy in (a) presented with draining sinuses at the site of a previous acute infection. The x-ray shows densely sclerotic bone. (b) In adults, chronic osteomyelitis is usually a sequel to open trauma or operation.

In refractory or frequently recurring cases, it may be possible to excise the infected and/or devitalized segment of bone and then close the gap by the *Ilizarov method* of 'transporting' a viable segment from the remaining diaphysis. This is especially useful if infection is associated with an ununited fracture (see page 126).

Aftercare

Success is difficult to measure: a minute focus of infection might escape the therapeutic onslaught, only to flare into full-blown osteomyelitis many years later. Prognosis should always be guarded; local trauma must be avoided and any recurrence of symptoms, however slight, should be taken seriously and investigated. The watchword is 'cautious optimism' – a 'probable cure' is better than no cure at all.

POST-TRAUMATIC INFECTION

An open fracture may become infected; this is the usual cause of osteomyelitis in adults. Many different organisms are involved but *Staphylococcus aureus* is the most common offender.

The patient is feverish and develops pain and swelling over the fracture site; the wound is inflamed and there may be a seropurulent discharge. Blood tests show a leucocytosis and an increased sedimentation rate. A wound swab should be examined and cultured for organisms.

The essence of treatment is prophylaxis: thorough debridement of open fractures, stabilization of the fracture, antibiotics and early definitive closure of exposed bone surfaces (see page 289).

For established infection, regular wound dressing is required. Loose or ineffectual implants should be removed; stable implants can often be left undisturbed until the fracture has united. If the fracture is unfixed and unstable, an external fixator can be applied.

It is wise to collaborate at all times with a plastic surgeon.

POSTOPERATIVE INFECTION

Postoperative infection is not uncommon: the incidence in general hospitals is 3–5 per cent. Predisposing factors are debility, chronic disease (e.g. rheumatoid arthritis), previous infection, corticosteroid therapy, difficult or long operations, haematoma formation, wound tension and tight dressings or plasters. There is also an increased risk with the use of foreign material such as metal implants and acrylic cement.

Prophylaxis is the key to management: the cleanest possible surgical environment, a meticulous technique, careful haemostasis and suction drainage. In all high-risk situations, prophylactic antibiotics are essential.

Treatment is more or less the same as for post-traumatic infection. However, intractable infection following joint replacement usually calls for removal of the prosthetic implants, local and systemic antibiotic treatment and revision of the arthroplasty.

 There are no euphemisms for wound infection. If the wound *looks* infected, it probably *is* infected.

ACUTE SUPPURATIVE ARTHRITIS

Cause and pathology

The causal organism is usually *Staphylococcus aureus;* in children under the age of 3 years *Haemophilus influenzae* is fairly common. The joint is invaded through a penetrating wound, by eruption of a bone abscess or by blood spread from a distant site. As infection spreads through the joint, articular cartilage is destroyed. Pus may burst out of the joint to form abscesses and sinuses. Later, with healing, the raw articular surfaces may adhere, producing fibrous or bony ankylosis.

Clinical features

Typical features are acute pain and swelling in a single large joint – commonly the hip in children and the knee in adults. However, any joint can be affected. The patient becomes ill, with a rapid pulse and swinging fever. The white cell count is raised and blood culture may be positive.

Many of the local signs can be elicited only in superficial joints. The skin looks red, the joint is held flexed and it is swollen. There is superficial warmth, diffuse tenderness and fluctuation. All movements are grossly restricted and often completely abolished by pain and spasm (pseudoparesis).

In *newborn infants* the emphasis is on septicaemia rather than joint pain. The baby is irritable and refuses to feed; there is a rapid pulse and sometimes a fever. Infection is usually suspected, but it could be anywhere! The joints should be carefully felt and moved to elicit the local signs of warmth, tenderness and resistance to movement. The umbilical cord should be examined for a source of infection. An inflamed intravenous infusion site should always excite suspicion.

 Paralysis or pseudoparalysis? If the baby is distressed and won't move his/her leg, think of hip infection.

Imaging

X-rays may show soft-tissue swelling, widening of the joint space (due to the effusion) and periarticular osteoporosis during the first 2 weeks of bacterial arthritis. Later, when the articular cartilage is attacked, the 'joint space' is narrowed. In advanced cases there are signs of bone destruction. *Radionuclide imaging* and *MRI* are helpful for detecting signs in difficult sites such as the sternoclavicular and sacroiliac joints.

Investigations

The diagnosis can usually be confirmed by joint aspiration and immediate microbiological investigation of the fluid. Blood cultures also may be positive, though only in about 50 per cent of proven cases. Non-specific features of acute inflammation – leucocytosis, raised erythrocyte sedimentation rate (ESR) and C-reactive protein – are suggestive but not diagnostic.

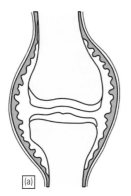 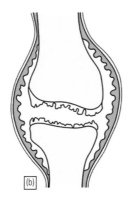 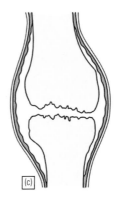 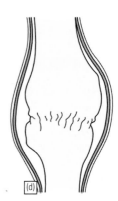

2.6 Acute suppurative arthritis – pathology In the early stage (a), there is an acute synovitis with a purulent joint effusion. (b) Soon the articular cartilage is attacked by bacterial and cellular enzymes. If the infection is not arrested, the cartilage may be completely destroyed (c). Healing then leads to bony ankylosis (d).

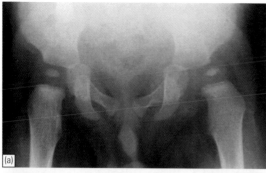

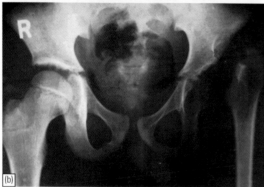

2.7 Suppurative arthritis – x-ray (a) In this child the left hip is subluxated and the soft tissues are swollen. (b) If the infection persists untreated, the cartilaginous epiphysis may be entirely destroyed, leaving a permanent pseudarthrosis (Tom Smith's dislocation).

Diagnosis

Osteomyelitis near a joint may be indistinguishable from septic arthritis; the safest is to assume that both are present.

An *acute haemarthrosis,* either post-traumatic or due to a haemophilic bleed, can closely resemble infection. The history is helpful and joint aspiration will resolve any doubt.

Transient synovitis (irritable joint) in children (see page 212) causes symptoms and signs which are less acute, but there is always the fear that this is the beginning of an infection.

Gout and pseudogout in adults can be indistinguishable from joint infection and cellulitis. Aspirated fluid may look turbid, but the presence of urate or pyrophosphate crystals will confirm the diagnosis.

Complications

Dislocation
A tense effusion may cause dislocation.

Epiphyseal destruction
In neglected infants, the largely cartilaginous epiphysis may be destroyed, leaving an unstable pseudarthrosis *(Tom Smith's dislocation).*

Growth disturbance
Physeal damage may result in shortening or deformity.

Ankylosis
If articular cartilage is eroded, healing may lead to ankylosis.

Treatment

The first priority is to aspirate the joint and examine the fluid. Treatment is then started without further delay and follows the same lines as for acute osteomyelitis.

Antibiotics
Intravenous antibiotics should be started as soon as joint fluid and blood samples have been taken for culture. If Gram-positive organisms are identified, flucloxacillin is suitable. If in doubt, a third-generation cephalosporin will cover both Gram-positive and Gram-negative organisms. Once the bacterial sensitivity is known, the appropriate drug is substituted. Intravenous administration is continued for several weeks and is followed by oral antibiotics for a further 2 or 3 weeks.

Splintage
The joint must be rested, either on a splint or in a widely split plaster. At the hip, the joint should be held abducted and 30 degrees flexed.

Drainage
Under anaesthesia, pus is drained and the joint washed out. This is best done by open operation, but in a superficial joint it can be achieved by repeated needle aspiration and irrigation or, in the case of the knee, by arthroscopy.

Once the patient's general condition is good and the joint is no longer inflamed, gentle and gradually increasing movements are encouraged. However, if articular cartilage has been destroyed, the aim is to keep the joint immobile in the optimum position while ankylosis is awaited.

SEPTIC BURSITIS

Bursal infection is common, especially in the olecranon bursa at the back of the elbow and the prepatellar bursa, both of which are vulnerable to local pressure and skin trauma. Olecranon bursitis is also seen in patients with rheumatoid arthritis or gout.

The condition usually starts as a non-septic bursitis which is then infected by an overlying skin abrasion or puncture. The common organism is *Staph. aureus.*

Pain, swelling and redness – sometimes extending well beyond the boundaries of the bursa itself – are typical features. The diagnosis is confirmed by aspirating the bursal fluid and submitting it for microscopic and bacteriological examination.

Treatment consists of local rest or splintage and intravenous administration of flucloxacillin (or a more appropriate antibiotic as dictated by sensitivity tests). If pus has formed, it must be released, preferably by open drainage. Intractable infection, or recurrent septic bursitis, may need prolonged antibiotic treatment and operative bursectomy.

TUBERCULOSIS

Tuberculosis is on the increase; bones or joints are affected in about 5 per cent of patients. *Mycobacterium tuberculosis* has a predilection for the vertebral bodies and the large synovial joints.

Where pulmonary tuberculosis is endemic, skeletal tuberculosis is seen mainly in children and young adults. In non-endemic areas the disease usually appears in patients with chronic debilitating disorders or reduced immune defence mechanisms (e.g. acquired immunodeficiency syndrome, AIDS).

Pathology

Infection reaches the skeleton by haematogenous seeding from the lung or intestine. There is a chronic inflammatory reaction, characteristically leading to granuloma formation and caseation. Spread into soft tissues leads to a subacute abscess (the so-called 'cold abscess'), which may track along tissue planes and 'point' somewhere quite remote from the original site of bone infection. Infected material may discharge through the skin leaving a chronic sinus. Secondary pyogenic infection may follow.

Vertebral tuberculosis usually begins in the anterior part of the vertebral body near the intervertebral disc. After progressive bone destruction, the infection spreads across the disc into an adjacent vertebral body. The two vertebrae may collapse forwards, causing a sharp angulation, or gibbus, in the affected segment – usually in the lower thoracic or lumbar spine.

Joint tuberculosis may start either in the synovium or in a nearby metaphysis, from where it spreads across the physis, through the articular surface into the synovial cavity. Either way, the presenting picture is of a chronic monoarthritis affecting a large joint (usually the hip or knee, less often the shoulder or ankle). If the condition is not arrested, the articular surfaces will be destroyed. Healing is by fibrosis, resulting in a tight 'fibrous ankylosis' of the joint.

Clinical features

The patient complains of pain and (in a superficial joint) swelling. Muscle wasting is characteristic and synovial thickening is often striking. Movements are limited in all directions. As articular erosion progresses, the joint becomes stiff and severely deformed; in late cases there may be a sinus.

In tuberculosis of the spine, pain may be deceptively slight. Consequently the patient may

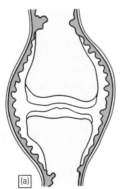 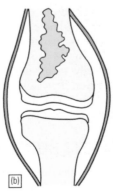 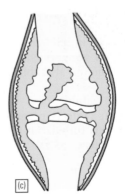 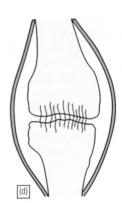

2.8 Tuberculous arthritis – pathology The disease may begin as synovitis (a) or osteomyelitis (b). From either, it can extend to become a true arthritis (c); not all the cartilage is destroyed, and healing is usually by fibrous ankylosis (d).

not present until there is a visible abscess or until collapse causes a localized kyphosis (gibbus). Occasionally the presenting feature is weakness or loss of sensibility in the lower limbs. In areas where treatment is delayed or non-existent, this may progress to paralysis (Pott's paraplegia).

X-rays

X-rays show soft-tissue swelling and rarefaction of the bone. In the early stages the joint space is retained, but later there is narrowing and irregularity, with bone erosion on both sides of the joint. Cystic lesions may appear in the bone.

Tuberculous spondylitis may appear as localized bone erosion and collapse across an intervertebral disc space. Always look for soft-tissue traces of a paravertebral abscess.

Diagnosis

Except in areas where tuberculosis is common, diagnosis is often delayed simply because the disease is not suspected. In many respects it resembles *rheumatoid arthritis*. Features suggesting tuberculosis, and calling for more active investigation, are a long history, involvement of only one joint, marked synovial thickening, marked muscle wasting and periarticular osteoporosis.

In patients with spinal tuberculosis, *metastatic bone disease, multiple myeloma, sarcoidosis* and other *unusual infections* must be excluded.

The ESR is usually raised and the Mantoux test is positive.

Synovial biopsy for histological examination and culture is often necessary.

Treatment

The mainstay of treatment is anti-tuberculous chemotherapy, using a combination of drugs (e.g. rifampicin and isoniazid) for 6 months or more. Resistance to isoniazid may call for additional treatment with pyrazinamide and streptomycin or ethambutol. If chemotherapy is started early, the joint may heal and function be completely restored.

Local measures include rest, traction and – occasionally – operation. Splintage should be continued for several months, by which time it is usually clear whether the joint has been saved. If the articular surfaces are destroyed, the joint is immobilized until all signs of disease activity have disappeared. If the disease remains quiescent, arthrodesis – or joint replacement – may be considered.

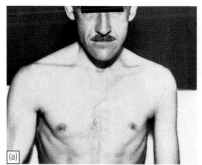
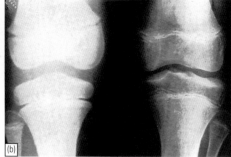
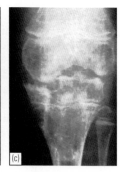

2.9 Tuberculosis – clinical and x-ray features (a) Generalized wasting used to be a common feature of all forms of tuberculosis. Nowadays, skeletal tuberculosis occurs in deceptively healthy-looking individuals. An early feature is periarticular osteoporosis due to synovitis – the left knee in (b). This often resolves with treatment, but if cartilage and bone are destroyed (c), healing occurs by fibrosis and the joint retains a 'jog' of painful movement.

These are a group of conditions which cause chronic pain, swelling and tenderness of joints and tendon sheaths. Although characterized by a persistent arthritis, they are essentially systemic diseases affecting connective tissues throughout the body.

RHEUMATOID ARTHRITIS

Rheumatoid arthritis affects about 3 per cent of the population, women three times more often than men. It usually starts in the fourth or fifth decade.

Cause

The cause is unknown, but it is believed that some antigen – possibly a virus – sets off a chain of events culminating in a chronic inflammatory disorder in which abnormal immunological reactions are prominent. These include the production of antibodies (both IgG and IgM) to the body's own IgG. Such 'autoantibodies' appear as serum rheumatoid factors in 80 per cent of patients with rheumatoid arthritis, and they can also be demonstrated in the synovium.

The abnormal immune response may be genetically predetermined, for patients with rheumatoid arthritis show increased frequencies of HLA-DR4.

Pathology

Although tissues throughout the body are affected, the brunt of the attack falls on synovium. The pathological changes, if unchecked, proceed in three stages.

Stage 1: synovitis

Synovial membrane becomes inflamed and thickened, giving rise to a cell-rich effusion. Although painful and swollen, the joints and tendons are still intact and the disorder is potentially reversible.

Stage 2: destruction

Persistent inflammation causes tissue destruction. Articular cartilage is eroded and tendon fibres may rupture.

Stage 3: deformity

The combination of articular destruction, capsular stretching and tendon rupture leads to progressive instability and deformity.

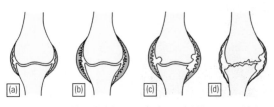

3.1 Rheumatoid arthritis – pathology (a) The normal joint. (b) Stage 1 – synovitis and joint swelling. (c) Stage 2 – early joint destruction with periarticular erosions. (d) Stage 3 – advanced joint destruction and deformity.

Extra-articular features

The most characteristic extra-articular lesion is the *rheumatoid nodule,* a small granuloma occurring under the skin (especially over bony prominences), on tendons, in the sclera and in viscera. Other systemic features are *lymphadenopathy, vasculitis, muscle weakness* and *visceral disease* affecting the lungs, heart, kidneys, brain and gastrointestinal tract.

Clinical features

The usual pattern is the insidious emergence of a symmetrical polyarthritis affecting mainly the hands and feet, together with early-morning stiffness and a general lack of well-being.

During *stage 1 (synovitis)* there is typically swelling, increased warmth and tenderness of the proximal finger joints and the wrists, as well as of the tendon sheaths around these joints. Later the disease may 'spread' to the elbows, shoulders, knees, ankles and feet. Occasionally the condition begins in one of the larger joints.

In *stage 2 (destruction)* joint movements are limited and isolated tendon ruptures appear. Subcutaneous nodules may be felt over the olecranon process; although they occur in only 25 per cent of patients, they are pathognomonic of rheumatoid arthritis.

In *stage 3 (deformity)* the diagnosis is obvious at a glance. Fingers are deviated ulnarwards, often with subluxation or dislocation of the metacarpophalangeal joints; elbows cannot be straightened and the shoulders have lost abduction; knees may be swollen and held in flexion and valgus; the toes are clawed and there are painful callosities under the metatarsal heads. Muscle wasting is often severe. About a third of all patients develop pain and stiffness in the cervical spine.

In long-standing cases there may be vasculitis and peripheral neuropathy. Marked visceral disease is rare.

X-rays

In *stage 1* x-rays show only soft-tissue swelling and periarticular osteoporosis. In *stage 2* there is narrowing of the 'joint space' and marginal bony erosions, especially around the wrists and the proximal joints of the hands and feet. In *stage 3* articular destruction and joint deformity are obvious.

⚠ **Erosive arthritis in a single joint: check for rheumatoid arthritis and tuberculosis (?synovial biopsy).**

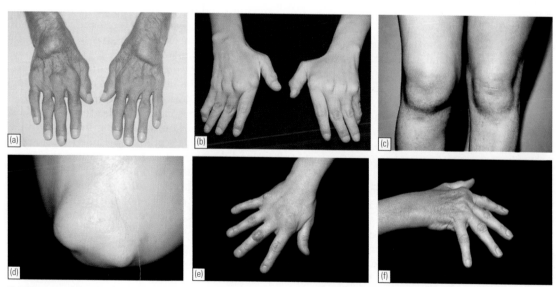

3.2 Rheumatoid arthritis – clinical features (a) Early features of swelling and stiffness of the proximal finger joints and the wrists. (b) The late hand deformities are so characteristic as to be almost pathognomonic. (c) Occasionally rheumatoid disease starts with synovitis of a single large joint (in this case the right knee). Extra-articular features include subcutaneous nodules (d,e) and tendon ruptures (f).

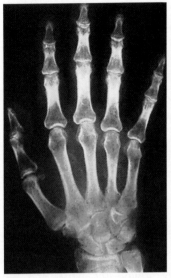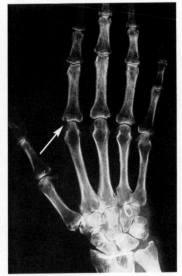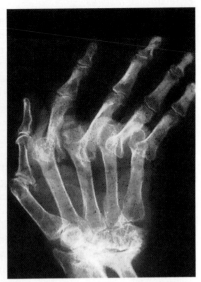

3.3 Rheumatoid arthritis – x-ray changes The progress of disease is well shown in this patient's x-rays. First, there was only soft-tissue swelling and periarticular osteoporosis; later, juxta-articular erosions appeared (arrow); ultimately, the joints became unstable and deformed.

Investigations

In active phases the erythrocyte sedimentation rate (ESR) is raised and C-reactive protein is present. Serological tests for rheumatoid factor are positive in 80 per cent of patients; sometimes antinuclear factors also are present.

Diagnosis

The minimal criteria for diagnosing rheumatoid arthritis are: (1) bilateral, symmetrical polyarthritis (2) involving the proximal joints of the hands or feet, (3) present for at least 6 weeks. If, in addition, there are subcutaneous nodules or periarticular erosions on x-ray, the diagnosis is certain. *A positive test for rheumatoid factor in the absence of the above features is not sufficient to diagnose rheumatoid arthritis, nor does a negative test exclude the diagnosis if all the other features are present.* The chief value of the rheumatoid factor tests is in assessing prognosis: high titres herald more serious disease.

In the differential diagnosis of polyarthritis, several disorders must be considered.

Seronegative polyarthritis is a feature of a number of conditions vaguely related to rheumatoid arthritis: psoriatic arthritis, juvenile chronic arthritis (Still's disease), systemic lupus erythematosus and other connective tissue diseases.

Ankylosing spondylitis may involve the peripheral joints, but it is primarily a disease of the sacroiliac and intervertebral joints, causing back pain and progressive stiffness.

Reiter's disease affects the large joints and the lumbosacral spine. There is a history of urethritis or colitis and often also conjunctivitis.

Polyarticular gout affects large and small joints, and tophi on fingers and toes may be mistaken for rheumatoid nodules.

Polyarticular osteoarthritis affects the distal interphalangeal joints and causes nodular swellings with radiologically obvious osteophytes.

Polymyalgia rheumatica occurs mostly in middle-aged or elderly women, causing marked stiffness and weakness after inactivity. Pain is most severe around the pectoral and pelvic girdles; tenderness is in muscles rather than joints. The ESR is almost always high. This is a form of giant-cell arteritis and carries the risk of temporal arteritis resulting in blindness. Corticosteroids provide rapid and dramatic relief of all symptoms.

 Swollen finger joints: proximal joints = inflammatory arthritis, distal joints = osteoarthritis.

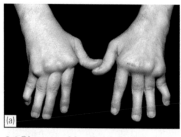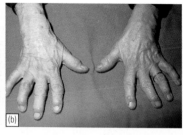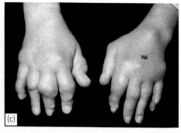

3.4 Rheumatoid arthritis – differential diagnosis All three patients presented with painful swollen fingers. In (a) mainly the proximal joints were affected (rheumatoid arthritis); in (b) the distal joints were the worst (Heberden's osteoarthritis); in (c) there were asymmetrical nodular swellings around the joints (gouty tophi).

Course

In 80 per cent of patients rheumatoid arthritis follows a periodic course, with intermittent 'flares' during which symptoms and signs of inflammation are more severe. With time, these attacks occur less frequently and the disease may become almost quiescent; by then, however, the joints are often permanently damaged.

In 5 per cent of cases there is relentless progression of the disease, with increasing inflammatory activity, joint destruction, muscle wasting and visceral involvement.

In 10 per cent – usually men over the age of 55 – symptoms start explosively but, rather paradoxically, the condition tends to subside and follows a relatively mild course.

In the fortunate few, the condition settles after the first or second attack and does not recur.

Complications

Infection

Patients with rheumatoid arthritis – and even more so those on corticosteroid therapy – are susceptible to infection. Sudden clinical deterioration, or increased pain in a single joint, should alert one to the possibility of septic arthritis and the need for joint aspiration.

Tendon rupture

Nodular infiltration may lead to tendon rupture. This is seen most often at the wrist, where it contributes significantly to the development of characteristic rheumatoid deformities (Fig. 3.2f).

Joint rupture

Occasionally the joint lining ruptures and synovial contents spill into the soft tissues. Treatment is directed at the underlying synovitis – i.e. splintage and injection of the joint, with synovectomy as a second resort.

Secondary osteoarthritis

Articular cartilage erosion may leave the joint so damaged that, even if the rheumatoid disease subsides or is kept under control, the end stage will be very similar to advanced osteoarthritis.

Treatment

There is no cure for rheumatoid arthritis. This must be explained to the patient, who also needs to be reassured that it is not necessarily a crippling disease, that much can be done to alleviate symptoms and delay progression, and that there is every chance of a useful and active life despite some functional limitations.

Principles of treatment
Control the synovitis
Prevent deformity
Reconstruct
Rehabilitate

Management is guided by five principles:

1. stop the synovitis,
2. keep the joints moving,
3. prevent deformity,
4. reconstruct,
5. rehabilitate.

A multidisciplinary approach is needed from the beginning: ideally, the therapeutic team should include a rheumatologist, orthopaedic surgeon, physiotherapist, occupational therapist, orthotist and social worker. Their deployment and priorities will vary according to the stage of the disease. The following scheme should meet the needs of most patients.

At the onset of the disease both the patient and the doctor will be uncertain about the likely rate of progress. Treatment is mainly palliative and supportive: the control of pain and stiffness with non-steroidal anti-inflammatory drugs (NSAIDs), maintaining muscle tone and joint mobility by a balanced programme of exercise, and general advice on coping with the activities of daily living.

During the early phase of established rheumatoid arthritis (the first 6–12 months) the main problem is the control of synovitis. NSAIDs may have to be stepped up and, if the pain, swelling, stiffness and joint tenderness are not alleviated, may need to be supplemented by the introduction of low-dosage corticosteroids (5–7.5 mg prednisolone daily) and 'second-line' drugs such as gold or penicillamine.

Systemic corticosteroids, once feared because of their side-effects, have been shown to be effective at low dosage in delaying the onset of articular erosion and slowing disease progression. If they are used, it should be during the early active phase of rheumatoid arthritis, for up to 2 years. During that time, the 'second-line' drugs, which take a long time to start acting, can be introduced and then continued (if necessary) when corticosteroid treatment is tailed off.

Additional measures include the injection of long-acting corticosteroid preparations into inflamed joints and tendon sheaths. It is sometimes feared that such injections may themselves cause damage to articular cartilage or tendons. However, there is little evidence that they are harmful, provided they are used sparingly and with full precautions against infection.

Physiotherapy is still important, but so is rest – one of the oldest methods of treating inflammation. During an acute flare-up, the patient may benefit from a few weeks' rest; gentle active and passive exercises are kept up and care should be taken to prevent postural deformities. Sometimes a week or two of continuous splintage (e.g. for the knees or wrists) is all that is needed; night splints can be used intermittently at any stage of the disease.

During the phase of progressive erosive arthritis (1–5 years) the combination of muscle weakness, joint instability and tendon rupture may lead to progressive deformity. By now the patient will probably be on long-term treatment with one of the 'second-line' drugs such as gold, penicillamine or methotrexate. However, these drugs cannot restore what has already been destroyed, and local counteractive measures become increasingly important. Preventive splintage and orthotic devices may delay the march of events. If these fail

to restore and maintain function, operative treatment is indicated. At first this consists mainly of soft-tissue procedures (synovectomy, tendon repair or replacement and joint stabilization); in some cases osteotomy may be more appropriate.

In late rheumatoid disease (5–20 years) severe joint destruction, fixed deformity and loss of function are clear indications for reconstructive surgery. Arthrodesis, osteotomy and arthroplasty all have their place and are considered in the appropriate chapters. However, it should be recognized that patients who are no longer suffering the pain of active synovitis and who are content with a limited pattern of life may not want or need heroic surgery merely to improve their anatomy. Careful assessment for occupational therapy, the provision of mechanical aids and adjustments to their home environment may be much more useful.

ANKYLOSING SPONDYLITIS

Like rheumatoid arthritis, this is a generalized chronic inflammatory disease – but its effects are seen mainly in the spine and sacroiliac joints. It is characterized by pain and stiffness of the back, with variable involvement of the hips and shoulders and (more rarely) the peripheral joints. Its prevalence is about 0.2 per cent in Western Europe, but is much lower in Japanese and Negroid peoples. Males are affected more frequently than females (estimates vary from 2:1 to 10:1) and the usual age at onset is between 15 and 25 years.

Cause

The disease tends to run in families; close relatives may have either classic ankylosing spondylitis or one of the other 'spondarthritides', such as Reiter's disease, psoriatic arthritis or enteropathic arthritis. The fact that all these conditions are associated with a particular tissue type, the HLA-B27, suggests a common genetic predisposition; the specific clinical syndrome is probably triggered by some recent event – often genitourinary or bowel infection.

Pathology

There are three characteristic lesions:

1. *synovitis* of diarthrodial joints;
2. *inflammation at the fibro-osseous junctions* of syndesmotic joints, tendons and ligaments (enthesopathy);
3. *ossification* across the peripheries of the intervertebral discs.

The disease starts as an inflammation of the sacroiliac and vertebral joints and ligaments. Sometimes the hips and shoulders also are affected, and very occasionally the peripheral joints.

Pathological changes follow a fairly constant sequence: inflammation – granulation tissue formation – erosion of articular cartilage or bone – replacement by fibrous tissue – ossification of the fibrous tissue – ankylosis.

If many vertebrae are involved, the spine may become absolutely rigid. If the costovertebral joints are involved, respiratory excursion is diminished.

Clinical features

Most patients are young men who complain of persistent backache and stiffness, often worse in the early morning or after inactivity. About 10 per cent have pain in peripheral joints.

The most typical sign is stiffness of the spine. All movements are diminished, but loss of extension is both the earliest and the most severe. The 'wall test' is useful: if a healthy person stands with his back to a wall, his heels, buttocks, scapulae and occiput can all touch the wall simultaneously; if extension is seriously diminished, this is

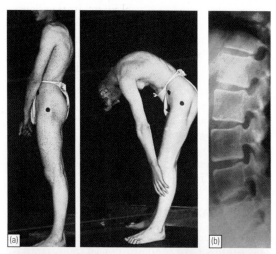

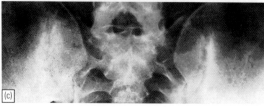

3.5 Ankylosing spondylitis – early The early features are (a) a stiff spine, (b) squaring of the lumbar vertebrae and (c) bilateral sacroiliac joint erosion.

impossible. In advanced cases the entire spine may be rigid ('poker back') and chest expansion is decreased to well below the normal 7 cm.

If the hips are involved, they also may go on to complete ankylosis.

Occasionally, peripheral joints are swollen and tender. Some patients complain of painful heels and have tenderness at the insertion of the tendo Achilles.

Extraskeletal manifestations include general fatigue and loss of weight, ocular inflammation, aortic valve disease, carditis and pulmonary fibrosis.

X-rays

The cardinal sign is fuzziness or frank erosion of the sacroiliac joints. Later these joints become sclerosed and, eventually, completely ankylosed.

Ossification across the intervertebral discs produces bony bridges (syndesmophytes) spanning the gaps between adjacent vertebral bodies. Bridging at several levels gives the appearance of a 'bamboo spine'.

Peripheral joints may show erosive arthritis resembling that of rheumatoid arthritis.

Investigations

The ESR is usually elevated during active phases of the disease. HLA-B27 is present in 90 per cent of cases.

Diagnosis

Diagnosis is easy in patients who present with chronic back pain and spinal rigidity. However, in more than 10 per cent of cases the disease starts in a peripheral joint and it may be several years before the true diagnosis reveals itself. Atypical onset is more common in women. A history of ankylosing spondylitis in a relative is strongly suggestive.

There are three syndromes in particular which may cause confusion.

Other seronegative spondarthritides

These are a group of conditions which are related to ankylosing spondylitis and may, in fact, share a genetic and pathogenetic background. They are described in the next section of this chapter.

Ankylosing hyperostosis (Forestier's disease)

This is a radiological teaser. Clinical features are non-existent or mild, but x-rays (taken for other complaints) show widespread ossification of ligaments and tendon insertions. The inexperienced clinician may mistake these appearances for those of ankylosing spondylitis,

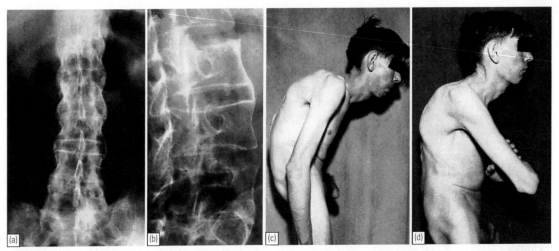

3.6 Ankylosing spondylitis – late (a,b) Bony bridges (syndesmophytes) between the vertebral bodies convert the spine into a rigid column ('bamboo spine'); note that the sacroiliac joints have fused. If the resulting deformity is marked (c), it may need correction by spinal osteotomy. After osteotomy, this patient's back is still rigid but his posture and function are vastly improved (d).

but the absence of symptoms and signs of an inflammatory disorder should suggest the correct diagnosis.

Mechanical back pain

Low back pain in young adults is usually attributed to one of many 'mechanical' conditions, including muscle strain, facet joint dysfunction and discogenic disorders. Ankylosing spondylitis should be kept in mind, lest the diagnosis be missed merely for lack of thinking about it.

Treatment

There is no specific treatment. Pain may be controlled by analgesics and NSAIDs; above all, the patient must be encouraged to exercise and keep moving. Postural training can prevent serious deformity; if ankylosis is inevitable, let it at least be in good position.

Stiffness of the hips can be treated by joint replacement, although this seldom provides more than moderate mobility. Severe flexion deformity of the spine may be reduced by vertebral osteotomy.

SERONEGATIVE SPONDARTHRITIS

A number of conditions usually associated with seronegative polyarthritis (i.e. without serum rheumatoid factors) may show changes in the spine and sacroiliac joints indistinguishable from those of ankylosing spondylitis. The best defined of these conditions are *psoriatic arthritis, Reiter's disease* and the arthritis that sometimes accompanies *ulcerative colitis* or *Crohn's disease*; together with classic *ankylosing spondylitis*, they are often grouped as the 'seronegative spondarthritides'.

The exact relationship between these disorders is unknown, but they share certain important features:

1. the characteristic spondylitis and sacroiliitis occur in all of them;
2. they are all associated with HLA-B27;
3. they show familial aggregation;
4. there is considerable overlap within families, some members having one disorder and close relatives another.

PSORIATIC ARTHRITIS

About 4 per cent of patients with chronic polyarthritis have psoriasis; not all, however, have psoriatic arthritis, which is a distinct entity and not simply 'rheumatoid arthritis plus psoriasis'. Unlike rheumatoid arthritis, psoriatic arthritis affects men and women equally and tends to run in families. The arthritis is not as clearly symmetrical as in rheumatoid arthritis and – in marked contrast to the latter – it occurs mainly in the interphalangeal joints of the fingers and toes. Bone destruction may be so severe that the digits are completely flail or badly deformed ('arthritis

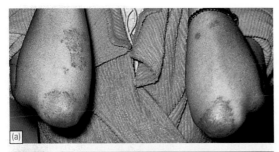

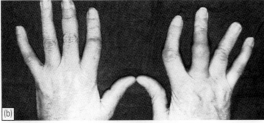

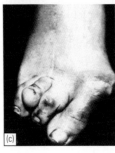
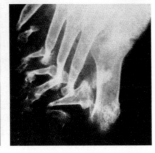

3.7 Psoriatic arthritis (a) Psoriasis of the elbows and forearms; (b) typical finger deformities; (c) the small joints of the hands and feet may suffer a particularly severe form of destructive arthritis (*arthritis mutilans*).

mutilans'). About a quarter of the patients develop sacroiliac and vertebral changes like those of ankylosing spondylitis. HLA-B27 occurs in about 60 per cent of those with overt sacroiliitis.

General treatment aims at controlling the skin disorder with topical preparations, and alleviating

joint symptoms with NSAIDs. In resistant forms of arthritis, immunosuppressive agents have proved effective.

Local treatment consists of judicious splintage to prevent undue deformity, and surgery for unstable joints.

REITER'S DISEASE AND REACTIVE ARTHRITIS

'Classic' Reiter's disease is a clinical triad: polyarthritis, conjunctivitis and non-specific urethritis. However, the term is now used more loosely for a *reactive arthritis* associated with non-specific urogenital or bowel infection. It is probably the most common type of large-joint polyarthritis in young men. Familial aggregation, overlap with other forms of seronegative spondarthritis in first-degree relatives and an increased frequency of HLA-B27 in all these disorders point to a genetic predisposition. *Lymphogranuloma venereum* and *Chlamydia trachomatis* have been implicated as urogenital infective agents, but arthritis also occurs with bowel infection due to *Shigella, Salmonella* or *Yersinia enterocolitica.*

The joints themselves are not infected; the synovitis is the end stage of an abnormal immune response to infection elsewhere or to its products.

Clinical features

Reiter's disease affects mainly large joints, especially the knee and ankle. Often it starts as an acute arthritis with marked effusion suggesting gout or a mechanical derangement. Tenosynovitis and plantar fasciitis are common. Backache and stiffness, due to sacroiliitis and spondylitis, occur in the majority of patients at some stage. Although the disease is said to be self-limiting, 80 per cent of patients continue to have symptoms for many years.

Typically there is a history of *urethritis, prostatitis, cervicitis* or *diarrhoea*. Ocular lesions include *conjunctivitis, episcleritis* and *uveitis.*

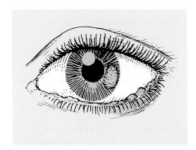
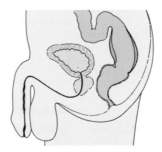
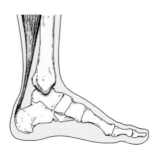

3.8 Reiter's syndrome – the classic 'Reiter's triad' consists of conjunctivitis, urethritis (sometimes colitis) and arthritis. Tenderness of the tendo Achilles and the plantar fascia is also common.

X-rays are at first normal, but after many months may show an erosive arthritis. Sacroiliac and vertebral changes are similar to those of ankylosing spondylitis.

Special investigations

Tests for HLA-B27 are positive in 75 per cent of patients with sacroiliitis. The ESR may be high in the active phase. The causative organism can sometimes be isolated from urethral fluids or faeces, and tests for antibodies may be positive.

Diagnosis

If the condition affects only one or two joints, it is usually mistaken for gout or infective arthritis. Examination of the synovial fluid for organisms and crystals will help to exclude these disorders.

Treatment

General treatment is indicated for active urogenital or bowel infection; a short course of antibiotics is usually sufficient, but for *Chlamydia* tetracycline daily for 6 months is recommended.

Local treatment is non-specific and palliative: rest and splintage if arthritis is severe, and then prolonged administration of anti-inflammatory agents while waiting for spontaneous remission.

JUVENILE CHRONIC ARTHRITIS (STILL'S DISEASE)

Juvenile chronic arthritis (JCA) is the preferred term for non-infective inflammatory joint disease of more than 3 months' duration in children under 16 years. It embraces a group of disorders, in all of which pain, swelling and stiffness of the joints are common features.

The prevalence is about 1 per 1000 children, and boys and girls are affected with equal frequency.

The cause is probably similar to that of rheumatoid disease: an abnormal immune response to some antigen in children with a particular genetic predisposition. However, rheumatoid factor is usually absent.

Clinical features

Juvenile chronic arthritis occurs in several characteristic forms.

Systemic JCA

This, the classic Still's disease, is usually seen below the age of 3 years. It starts with intermittent fever, rashes and malaise; there may also be lymphadenopathy, splenomegaly and hepato-megaly. Joint swelling occurs some weeks or months after the onset; fortunately, it usually resolves when the systemic illness subsides, but it may go on to progressive arthritis. Rheumatoid factor tests are negative.

Pauciarticular JCA

This is by far the commonest form of JCA. It usually occurs below the age of 6 years and is more common in girls. Only a few joints are involved and there is no systemic illness. The child presents with pain and swelling of medium-sized joints (knees, ankles, elbows and wrists); rheumatoid factor tests are negative. A serious complication is chronic iridocyclitis, which occurs in about 50 per cent.

Polyarticular seropositive JCA

This is usually seen in older children – mainly girls – and it resembles classic rheumatoid arthritis, with multiple small-joint involvement, progressive articular destruction and positive tests for rheumatoid factor. The term 'juvenile rheumatoid arthritis' can be used for this group.

Seronegative spondarthritis

In older children – usually boys – the condition may take the form of sacroiliitis and spondylitis; hips and knees are sometimes involved as well. Tests for HLA-B27 are often positive and this should probably be regarded as 'juvenile ankylosing spondylitis'.

Complications

Stiffness

Although most patients recover good function, some permanent loss of movement is common.

Growth defects

There is general retardation of growth, sometimes aggravated by prolonged corticosteroid therapy.

Iridocyclitis

This is most common in pauciarticular disease; untreated, it may lead to blindness.

Amyloidosis

In children with long-standing active disease there is a serious risk of amyloidosis, which may be fatal.

Treatment

General treatment is similar to that of rheumatoid arthritis. Corticosteroids should be used only for severe systemic disease and chronic iridocyclitis unresponsive to topical therapy.

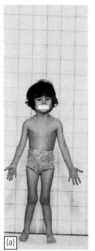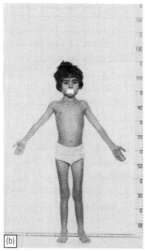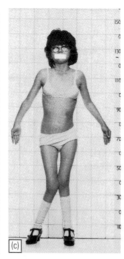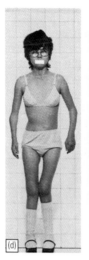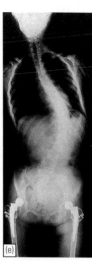

3.9 Juvenile chronic arthritis This young girl developed juvenile chronic arthritis when she was 5 years old. Here we see her at 6, 9 and 14 years of age (a–c). The arthritis became inactive, leaving her with a knee deformity, which was treated by osteotomy (d). (e) X-ray of another girl who required hip replacements at the age of 14 years and, later, surgical correction of her scoliosis.

Local treatment aims to prevent stiffness and deformity. Night splints are useful for the wrists, hands, knees and ankles; prone lying for some period each day may prevent flexion contracture of the hips. Between periods of splinting, active exercises are encouraged.

Fixed deformities may need correction by serial plasters; when progress is no longer being made, joint capsulotomy may help.

For painful, eroded joints, operation is indicated. Useful procedures include custom-designed arthroplasties of the hip and knee (even in children), and arthrodesis of the wrist or ankle.

Outcome

Fortunately, most children with JCA recover from the arthritis and are left with only moderate deformity and limitation of function. However, 5–10 per cent (and especially those with juvenile rheumatoid arthritis) are severely crippled and require treatment throughout life.

A significant number of children with JCA (about 3 per cent) still die – usually as a result of renal failure due to amyloidosis, or following overwhelming infection.

THE SYSTEMIC CONNECTIVE TISSUE DISEASES

'Systemic connective tissue disease' is a collective term for a group of closely related conditions that have features which overlap with those of rheumatoid disease. Like rheumatoid arthritis, these are 'autoimmune disorders', probably triggered by viral infection in genetically predisposed individuals.

Systemic lupus erythematosus is the best known. It occurs mainly in young females and may be difficult to differentiate from rheumatoid arthritis. Although joint pain is usual, it is often overshadowed by systemic symptoms such as malaise, anorexia, weight loss and fever. Characteristic clinical features are skin rashes (especially the 'butterfly rash' of the face), Raynaud's phenomenon, peripheral vasculitis, splenomegaly, and disorders of the kidney, heart, lung, eyes and central nervous system. Anaemia, leucopenia and elevation of the ESR are common. Tests for antinuclear factor are always positive.

Corticosteroids are indicated for severe systemic disease and may have to be continued for life. Progressive joint deformity is unusual and the arthritis can almost always be controlled by anti-inflammatory drugs, physiotherapy and intermittent splintage.

A curious complication of systemic lupus is avascular necrosis (usually of the femoral head). This may be due in part to the corticosteroid treatment, but the disease itself seems to predispose to bone ischaemia.

FIBROMYALGIA

Fibromyalgia is not so much a diagnosis as a descriptive term for a condition in which patients complain of pain and tenderness in the muscles and other soft tissues around the back of the neck and shoulders and across the lower part of the back and the upper parts of the buttocks. What sets the condition apart from other 'rheumatic' diseases is the complete absence of demonstrable pathological changes in the affected tissues. Indeed, it is often difficult to give credence to the patient's complaints, an attitude which is encouraged by the fact that similar symptoms are encountered in some patients who have suffered trivial injuries in a variety of accidents; a significant number also develop psychological depression and anxiety.

The criteria for making the diagnosis were put forward by the American College of Rheumatology in 1990. These included symptoms of widespread pain in all four quadrants of the body, together with at least nine pairs of designated 'tender points' on physical examination. In practice, however, the diagnosis is often made in patients with much more localized symptoms and signs, and it is now quite common to attach this label to almost any condition associated with myofascial pain where no specific underlying disorder can be identified.

The cause of fibromyalgia remains unknown; no pathology has been found in the 'tender spots'. It has been suggested that this is an abnormality of 'sensory processing', which is perhaps another way of saying that the sufferers have a 'low pain threshold'; in fact they often do display increased sensitivity to pain in other parts of the body. There are also suggestions that the condition is related to stress responses which can be activated by sudden accidents or traumatic life events. This does not mean that such patients will necessarily show other features of psychological dysfunction, and the condition cannot be excluded merely by psychological testing.

In mild cases, treatment can be limited to keeping up muscle tone and general fitness (hence the advice to have physiotherapy and then continue with daily exercises on their own), perhaps together with injections into the painful areas simply to reduce the level of discomfort. Patients with more persistent and more disturbing symptoms may benefit from various types of psychotherapy.

CHAPTER 4

GOUT AND PSEUDOGOUT

The crystal deposition disorders are a group of conditions characterized by the presence of crystals in and around the joints, bursae and tendons. Three clinical conditions in particular are associated with this phenomenon:

- gout – urate crystal deposition disorder,
- pseudogout – calcium pyrophosphate dihydrate (CPPD) deposition disease,
- calcium hydroxyapatite (HA) deposition disorders.

Characteristically, in each of the three conditions, crystal deposition has three distinct consequences: (1) it may be *totally inert and asymptomatic;* (2) it may induce *an acute inflammatory reaction;* or (3) it may result in *slow destruction* of the affected tissues.

GOUT

This is a disorder of purine metabolism characterized by hyperuricaemia, deposition of monosodium urate monohydrate crystals in joints and periarticular tissues, and recurrent attacks of acute synovitis. Late changes include cartilage degeneration, renal dysfunction and uric acid kidney stones.

The clinical disorder was known to Hippocrates and its association with hyperuricaemia was recognized well over 100 years ago. The prevalence of symptomatic gout varies from 1 to more than 10 per 1000, depending on the race, sex and age of the population studied. It is much commoner in Caucasian than in Black African peoples; it is more widespread in men than in women (the ratio may be as high as 20:1) and it is rarely seen before the menopause in females.

Although the risk of developing clinical features of gout increases with increasing levels of serum uric acid, only a fraction of those with hyperuricaemia develop symptoms. However, 'hyperuricaemia' and 'gout' are generally regarded as aspects of the same disorder.

Pathology

Hyperuricaemia

Nucleic acid and purine metabolism normally proceeds, through complex pathways, to the production of hypoxanthine and xanthine; the final breakdown to uric acid is catalysed by the enzyme xanthine oxidase. Monosodium urate appears in ionic form in all the body fluids; about 70 per cent is derived from endogenous purine metabolism and 30 per cent from purine-rich foods in the diet. It is excreted (as uric acid) mainly by the kidneys and partly in the gut.

Serum uric acid concentration varies considerably and some populations (for example New Zealand Maoris) have much higher levels than others. The term 'hyperuricaemia' is therefore generally reserved for individuals with a serum urate concentration which is significantly higher than that of the population to which they belong (more than two standard deviations above the mean); this is about 0.42 mmol/L for men and 0.35 mmol/L for women in Western Caucasian peoples. By this definition, about 5 per cent of men and less than 1 per cent of women have hyperuricaemia; the majority suffer no pathological consequences and they remain asymptomatic throughout life.

Gout

Urate crystals are deposited in minute clumps in connective tissue, including articular cartilage; the commonest sites are the small joints of the hands and feet. For months, perhaps years, they remain inert. Then, possibly as a result of local trauma, the needle-like crystals are dispersed into the joint and the surrounding tissues, where they excite an acute inflammatory reaction.

With the passage of time, urate deposits may build up in joints, periarticular tissues, tendons and bursae; common sites are around the metatarsophalangeal joints of the big toes, the Achilles tendons, the olecranon bursae and the pinnae of the ears. These clumps of chalky material, or tophi, vary in size from less than 1 mm to several centimetres in diameter. They may ulcerate through the skin or destroy cartilage and periarticular bone.

Urate calculi appear in the urine, and crystal deposition in the kidney parenchyma may cause renal failure.

Classification

Gout is often classified into 'primary' and 'secondary' forms. *Primary gout* (95 per cent) occurs in the absence of any obvious cause and may be due to constitutional under-excretion (the vast majority) or over-production of urate. *Secondary gout* (5 per cent) results from prolonged hyperuricaemia due to acquired disorders such as myeloproliferative diseases, administration of diuretics or renal failure.

This division is somewhat artificial; people with an initial tendency to 'primary' hyperuricaemia may develop gout only when secondary factors are introduced – for example obesity and alcohol abuse, or treatment with diuretics or salicylates, which increase tubular reabsorption of uric acid.

Clinical features

Patients are usually men over the age of 30 years. Often there is a family history of gout.

The acute attack

The sudden onset of severe joint pain which lasts for a week or two is typical of acute gout. This is usually spontaneous but may be precipitated by minor trauma, operation, unaccustomed exercise or alcohol. The commonest sites are the metatarsophalangeal joint of the big toe, the ankle

and finger joints, and the olecranon bursa. The skin looks red and shiny and there is considerable swelling. The joint feels hot and extremely tender, suggesting a cellulitis or septic arthritis. Sometimes the only feature is acute pain and tenderness in the heel or the sole of the foot.

Hyperuricaemia is present at some stage, although not necessarily during an acute attack. The diagnosis can be established beyond doubt by finding the characteristic birefringent crystals in the synovial fluid.

Chronic gout

Recurrent acute attacks may eventually merge into polyarticular gout. Tophi may appear around

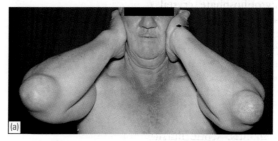

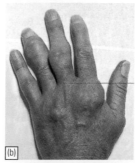 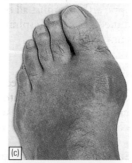

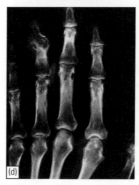 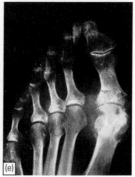

4.1 Gout (a) This man is the typical 'gouty type', with his rubicund face, large olecranon bursae and small subcutaneous tophi over the elbows. (b,c) Tophaceous gout affecting the hands and feet; the swollen big toe joint is particularly characteristic. (d,e) X-rays showing the juxta-articular defects due to the tophi.

joints, over the olecranon and in the pinna of the ear. A large tophus can ulcerate and discharge its chalky material. Joint erosion causes chronic pain, stiffness and deformity. Renal lesions include calculi and parenchymal disease.

X-rays

During the acute attack, x-rays show only soft-tissue swelling. Chronic gout may show asymmetrical, punched-out 'cysts' in the juxta-articular bone, joint-space narrowing and secondary osteoarthritis.

Differential diagnosis

Pseudogout

Pyrophosphate crystal deposition may cause an acute arthritis indistinguishable from gout – except that it tends to affect large rather than small joints and is somewhat more common in women than in men. Articular calcification may show on x-ray. Demonstrating the crystals in synovial fluid establishes the diagnosis.

Infection

Cellulitis, septic bursitis, an infected bunion or septic arthritis must all be excluded, if necessary by immediate joint aspiration and examination of synovial fluid.

Rheumatoid arthritis

Polyarticular gout affecting the fingers may be mistaken for rheumatoid arthritis, and elbow tophi for rheumatoid nodules. In difficult cases, biopsy will establish the diagnosis.

Treatment

The acute attack should be treated by resting the joint and giving large doses of a non-steroidal anti-inflammatory agent. In severe cases, colchicine may be helpful.

Between attacks, attention should be given to simple measures such as losing weight, cutting out alcohol and eliminating diuretics. Interval therapy is indicated if attacks recur at frequent intervals, if there are tophi or if renal function is impaired. Asymptomatic hyperuricaemia does not call for treatment. Uricosuric drugs (probenecid or sulphinpyrazone) can be used if renal function is normal. Allopurinol, a xanthine oxidase inhibitor, is usually preferred. *These drugs should never be started during an acute attack, and they should always be covered by an anti-inflammatory preparation or colchicine,* otherwise they may actually precipitate an acute attack.

 An acutely inflamed joint in an adult: check for haemarthrosis, sepsis, gout and pseudogout. Aspirate and look for blood, pus and crystals.

CALCIUM PYROPHOSPHATE DIHYDRATE DEPOSITION

Calcium pyrophosphate dihydrate deposition encompasses three overlapping conditions: (1) *chondrocalcinosis* – the appearance of calcific material in articular cartilage and menisci; (2) *pseudogout* – a crystal-induced synovitis; and (3) *chronic pyrophosphate arthropathy* – a type of degenerative joint disease.

Pathology

Pyrophosphate is probably generated in abnormal cartilage by enzyme activity at chondrocyte surfaces; it combines with calcium ions in the matrix, where crystal nucleation occurs on collagen fibres. The crystals grow into microscopic 'tophi' which appear in the cartilage matrix and in fibrocartilaginous structures such as the menisci of the knee and the intervertebral discs.

From time to time, CPPD crystals are extruded into the joint, where they excite an inflammatory reaction similar to gout.

Clinical features

The clinical disorder takes several forms, all of them appearing with increasing frequency in relation to age. Most of the patients are women over the age of 60 years.

Asymptomatic chondrocalcinosis

Calcification of the menisci is common in elderly people and is usually asymptomatic. When it is seen in association with osteoarthritis, this does not necessarily imply cause and effect: both are common in elderly people and they are bound to be seen together in some patients. X-rays may reveal chondrocalcinosis in other asymptomatic joints. Chondrocalcinosis in patients under 50 years of age should suggest the possibility of an underlying metabolic disease or a familial disorder.

Acute synovitis (pseudogout)

The patient, typically a middle-aged woman, complains of acute pain and swelling in one of the larger joints – usually the knee. Sometimes the attack is precipitated by a minor illness or operation. The joint is tense and inflamed, though usually not as acutely as in gout. Untreated, the condition lasts for a few weeks and then subsides spontaneously. *X-rays* may show signs of chondrocalcinosis, and the diagnosis can be confirmed by finding *positive birefringent crystals* in the synovial fluid.

Chronic pyrophosphate arthropathy

The patient, usually an elderly woman, presents with polyarticular 'osteoarthritis' affecting the larger joints (hips, knees) and – more helpfully – unusual joints, such as the ankles, shoulders, elbows and wrists, where osteoarthritis is seldom seen. This is often diagnosed as 'generalized osteoarthritis' but the x-ray features are distinctive. Sometimes alternating bouts of acute synovitis and chronic arthritis may mimic rheumatoid disease. Occasionally, joint destruction is so marked as to suggest neuropathic joint disease.

Diagnosis

Pseudogout must be distinguished from other acute inflammatory disorders such as gout and infection. Diagnosis rests on identifying the characteristic crystals in synovial fluid.

Chronic pyrophosphate arthropathy can resemble other types of polyarticular arthritis and will come into the differential diagnosis of rheumatoid arthritis and polyarticular osteoarthritis (see page 43).

Treatment

The treatment of pseudogout is similar to that of classic gout: rest, non-steroidal anti-inflammatory

Gout and pseudogout	
Gout	**Pseudogout**
Smaller joints	Larger joints
Pain intense	Pain moderate
Joint inflamed	Joint swollen
Gouty tophi	Chondrocalcinosis
Hyperuricaemia	Uric acid normal
Urate crystals	Calcium pyrophosphate crystals

drugs, joint aspiration and intra-articular injection of corticosteroid. Chronic pyrophosphate arthropathy is treated like osteoarthritis.

CALCIUM HYDROXYAPATITE DEPOSITION DISORDERS

Minute deposits of hydroxyapatite crystals in periarticular soft tissues may give rise to an acute, painful reaction; this is seen most commonly in tendons around the shoulder. Treatment is by systemic non-steroidal anti-inflammatory drugs or by topical injection of corticosteroids.

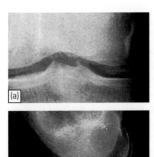
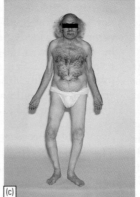
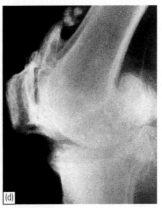

4.2 Pyrophosphate arthropathy (a,b) Chondrocalcinosis (calcification of articular cartilage and menisci) in the knee. (c) This middle-aged man presented with osteoarthritis in several large joints, including the elbow and ankle, where osteoarthritis is uncommon. (d) A characteristic feature is patellofemoral arthritis associated with large, trailing osteophytes.

CHAPTER 5

OSTEOARTHRITIS AND RELATED DISORDERS

OSTEOARTHRITIS

Osteoarthritis is a chronic joint disorder in which there is progressive softening and disintegration of articular cartilage accompanied by new growth of cartilage and bone at the joint margins (osteophytes) and capsular fibrosis. It is defined as primary when no cause is obvious, and secondary when it follows a demonstrable abnormality.

Cause

The most obvious thing about osteoarthritis is that it increases in frequency with age. This does not mean that it is an expression of senescence: it simply shows that osteoarthritis takes many years to develop. To be sure, cartilage ageing does occur, resulting in splitting and flaking of the surface, but these changes are not progressive and they do not cause symptomatic arthritis.

Osteoarthritis results from a disparity between the stress applied to articular cartilage and the ability of the cartilage to withstand that stress. This could be due to one or a combination of two processes: (1) *weakening of the articular cartilage* (possibly due to genetic defects in type II collagen or to enzymatic activity in certain inflammatory disorders such as rheumatoid disease), and (2) *increased mechanical stress in some part of the articular surface.* Increased stress may be produced either by excessive impact loading or by reduction of the articular contact area in conditions causing joint incongruity. This would explain why an incongruent or an unstable joint almost inevitably develops osteoarthritis. Theoretically, defects in the subchondral bone also may lead to stress concentration at particular sites.

The subsequent sequence of changes is still disputed, but at an early stage there appears to be damage to the cartilage collagen network and loss of proteoglycans from the matrix, giving rise to deformation and gradual structural disintegration.

Pathology

The cardinal features are: (1) progressive loss of cartilage thickness; (2) subarticular cyst formation

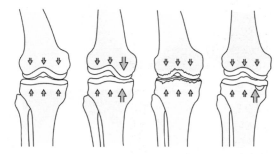

5.1 Osteoarthritis – pathogenesis In a normal joint (a), the loading forces are evenly distributed. Cartilage damage results from (b) increased stress on some part of the articular surface, (c) a preceding inflammatory disorder which weakens the cartilage and renders it unable to bear even normal loads, or (d) abnormality of the subarticular bone which alters its ability to support the cartilage appropriately.

and sclerosis; (3) remodelling of the bone ends and osteophyte formation; (4) synovial irritation; and (5) capsular fibrosis.

The earliest morphological change is softening of the articular cartilage. The normally smooth and glistening surface becomes frayed, or fibrillated, and eventually it is worn away to expose the underlying bone.

The subarticular bone reacts to these changes in several ways. In the area of greatest stress, cysts form, around which the trabeculae become thickened or sclerotic. There is vascular congestion and the intraosseous pressure rises. Meanwhile, as the disease progresses, cartilage in peripheral, unstressed areas proliferates and ossifies, producing bony outgrowths (osteophytes). This remodelling process restores a measure of congruity to the increasingly malopposed joint surfaces. It is clear, therefore, that osteoarthritis is not a purely degenerative disorder, and the term 'degenerative arthritis' – which is often used as a synonym for osteoarthritis – is a misnomer. Osteoarthritis is a dynamic phenomenon showing interacting features of both destruction and repair.

Although osteoarthritis is not primarily an inflammatory disease, shedding of fragments from the fibrillated articular cartilage, as well as release of enzymes from damaged cells, may give rise to a low-grade synovitis. In the late stages, capsular fibrosis is common and may account for joint stiffness.

The cause of pain is problematic; articular cartilage and synovium have no nerve supply, but the capsule is sensitive to stretching and the bone is sensitive to changes in pressure. Pain, therefore, may be due to both capsular fibrosis and vascular congestion of the subarticular bone.

Clinical features

Patients usually present after middle age, although it is likely that cartilage changes start 10 or even 20 years before that. Sometimes – especially in younger patients – there is a history of some preceding joint disorder or injury.

Pain starts insidiously and increases slowly over months or years. It is aggravated by exertion and relieved by rest, although, with time, relief is less and less complete. Stiffness, characteristically, is worst after periods of rest. Typically, symptoms follow an intermittent course, with periods of remission sometimes lasting for months. Swelling, deformity, loss of mobility and muscle wasting are features of advanced disease. Ultimately the joint may become unstable.

In contrast to inflammatory joint disease, osteoarthritis is not associated with any systemic manifestations.

X-rays

The characteristic changes are: (1) narrowing of the joint 'space', due to cartilage depletion; (2) subarticular cyst formation and sclerosis; and

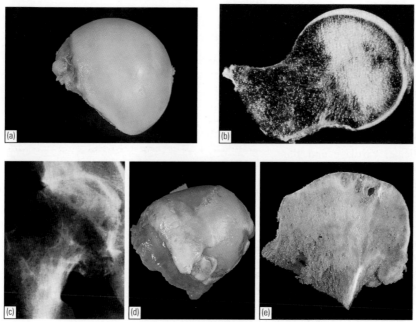

5.2 Osteoarthritis – pathology (a) Normal ageing causes slight degeneration of the articular surface, but the coronal section (b) shows that the cartilage thickness is well preserved. By contrast, in progressive osteoarthritis, the weight-bearing area suffers increasing damage: the x-ray (c) shows that the superolateral joint space (cartilage) has virtually disappeared and there are cysts in the underlying bone. In the femoral head specimen (d), the superior surface is completely denuded of cartilage and there are large osteophytes around the periphery. In the coronal section (e), the subarticular cysts are clearly revealed.

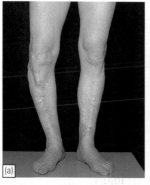
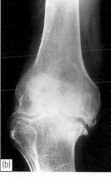

5.3 Osteoarthritis – clinical and x-ray (a) Varus deformity of the right knee due to osteoarthritis. (b) The x-ray shows the classic features: disappearance of the joint 'space', subarticular sclerosis and osteophyte formation at the margins of the joint.

(3) osteophyte formation. Initially the first two features are restricted to the major load-bearing part of the joint, but in late cases the entire joint is affected. Evidence of previous disorders (congenital defects, old fractures, rheumatoid arthritis) may be present.

 Osteoarthritis is not simply 'wear-and-tear'. Always look for an underlying cause.

Clinical variants of osteoarthritis

Although the features of osteoarthritis in any particular joint are fairly consistent, the overall pattern of involvement shows variations which define a number of sub-groups.

Monoarticular and pauciarticular osteoarthritis

In its 'classic' form, osteoarthritis presents with pain and dysfunction in one or two of the large weight-bearing joints. There may be an obvious underlying abnormality: acetabular dysplasia, old Perthes' disease or slipped epiphysis, long-standing joint deformity, a previous fracture or damage to ligaments or menisci. In many cases, however, the abnormality is so subtle that one may question whether the osteoarthritis is 'primary' or 'secondary'.

Polyarticular (generalized) osteoarthritis

This is far and away the most common form of osteoarthritis, though most of the patients never consult an orthopaedic surgeon. The typical patient is a middle-aged woman who presents with pain, swelling and stiffness of the finger joints. The first carpometacarpal and the big toe metatarsophalangeal joints, or the knees and lumbar facet joints, may be affected as well.

The changes are most obvious in the hands. The interphalangeal joints become swollen and tender, and in the early stages they often appear to be inflamed. Over a period of years, osteophytes and soft-tissue swelling produce a characteristic knobbly appearance of the distal interphalangeal joints (Heberden's nodes) and, less often, the proximal interphalangeal joints (Bouchard's nodes); pain may disappear, but stiffness and deformity can be disturbing. Some patients present with painful knees or backache and the knobbly fingers are noticed only in passing.

Osteoarthritis in unusual sites

Osteoarthritis is uncommon in the shoulder, elbow, wrist and ankle. If any of these joints is affected, one should suspect a previous abnormality – congenital or traumatic – or an associated generalized disease such as a crystal arthropathy (see page 40).

Treatment

Early

There are three principles in the treatment of early osteoarthritis: (1) relieve pain; (2) increase movement; (3) reduce load.

Pain relief is achieved by analgesics and non-steroidal anti-inflammatory drugs (NSAIDs). Rest periods and modification of activities may also be necessary. NSAIDs are powerful prostaglandin

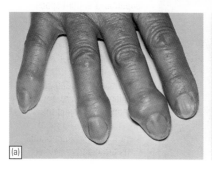
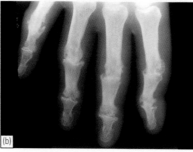

5.4 Osteoarthritis – Heberden's nodes This type of polyarticular osteoarthritis affects about 70 per cent of women over the age of 60 years. The clinical picture is easily distinguishable from that of rheumatoid arthritis – in osteoarthritis it is the terminal joints that are most severely affected.

inhibitors which reduce the vascular congestion in the subchondral bone. Unfortunately, they have a serious drawback: they cause gastrointestinal irritation, and in some patients this leads to ulceration and bleeding. NSAIDs should be used only under medical supervision.

Joint mobility can often be improved by physiotherapy; even a small increase in range and power will reduce pain and improve function.

Load reduction can be achieved by using a walking stick, wearing soft-soled shoes, avoiding prolonged, stressful activity and by weight reduction. Physiotherapists and occupational therapists will give useful advice on how to modify daily activities and improve the work environment so as to reduce exposure to painful joint loading.

Treatment of osteoarthritis
Conservative
▪ Relieve pain
▪ Reduce load
▪ Improve mobility
Operative
▪ Osteotomy
▪ Arthroplasty
▪ Arthrodesis

Intermediate

If symptoms increase despite conservative treatment, some form of operative treatment may be needed. This will usually be a 'holding' procedure, especially in younger patients who are not yet ready for a joint replacement. For osteoarthritis of the knee, joint debridement (removal of interfering osteophytes, cartilage tags and loose bodies) can be performed arthroscopically. For both the hip and the knee, a realignment osteotomy may be considered, but it must be done while the joint is still stable and mobile. Pain relief is often dramatic and is ascribed to (a) vascular decompression of the subchondral bone, and (b) redistribution of loading forces towards less damaged parts of the joint.

Late

The indications for radical surgery are unrelieved pain and progressive disability. For patients over the age of 60, *arthroplasty* (usually total joint replacement) is the operation of choice. In younger patients, the physical demands are much greater and there is an increased risk that the arthroplasty will have to be revised within the patient's natural life-span. *Arthrodesis* is occasionally indicated if stiffness is not a drawback.

> ⚠ **Enquire about lifestyle before advocating surgery. The patient may be happier without an operation.**

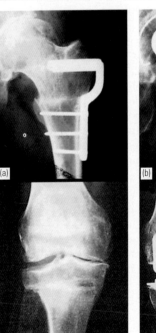 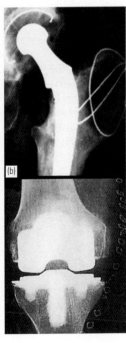 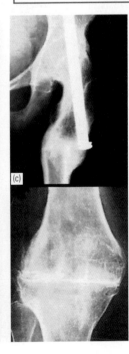

5.5 Osteoarthritis – operative treatment The basic operations are (a) osteotomy, (b) arthroplasty and (c) arthrodesis. X-ray appearances in the hip and knee are illustrated here.

NEUROPATHIC ARTHRITIS (CHARCOT'S DISEASE)

Neuropathic arthritis is a rapidly progressive degeneration in a joint which lacks position sense and protective pain sensation. In the lower limb it is associated with tabes dorsalis, cauda equina lesions, peripheral neuropathies (especially diabetic) and congenital indifference to pain; in the upper limbs it is usually due to syringomyelia.

Pathology

The joint disorder is a rapidly progressive form of osteoarthritis. There is marked destruction of articular cartilage and the underlying bone, and microscopic spicules of bone become embedded in the synovium. Ligaments and capsule are lax and at the joint periphery there is florid new-bone formation.

Clinical features

The patient complains of instability, swelling and deformity; the symptoms may progress rapidly.

The appearance of the joint suggests that movement would be agonising and yet it is often painless. The paradox is diagnostic.

Swelling and deformity are marked, yet there is no warmth or tenderness. Fluid is greatly increased and bits of bone can be felt everywhere. All movements are increased, and the joint is unstable yet painless.

The underlying neurological disorder should be sought.

X-rays

The joint may be subluxed or dislocated; gross bone destruction is obvious and there are irregular calcified masses in the capsule.

Treatment

The underlying condition may need treatment, but the affected joints cannot recover. They should, if necessary, be splinted. Arthrodesis is sometimes needed; joint replacement is not advisable.

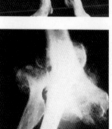
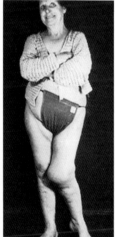
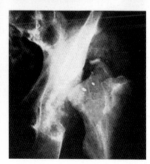

5.6 Charcot's disease This patient with Charcot's disease developed neuropathic arthritis in her left knee. Her happy expression contrasts sharply with the gross joint destruction. Other joints also can be affected by neuropathic disorders, as seen here in x-rays of the elbow and hip.

HAEMOPHILIC ARTHROPATHY

Of the various bleeding disorders, two are associated with recurrent haemarthroses and progressive joint destruction: classic haemophilia, in which there is a deficiency of clotting factor VIII; and Christmas disease, due to deficiency of factor IX. These are rare X-linked recessive disorders manifesting in males but carried by females.

When plasma-clotting factor levels fall below 40 per cent, there is a risk of prolonged bleeding after injury or operation; with levels below 5 per cent, spontaneous bleeding occurs.

Acute bleeding into a joint

With trivial injury, a joint may rapidly fill with blood. Pain, warmth, boggy swelling, tenderness and limited movement are the outstanding features. The resemblance to inflammatory arthritis is striking but the history is diagnostic.

Treatment

The appropriate purified clotting factor must be given intravenously. If this is not available, cryoprecipitate or fresh-frozen plasma will do. Aspiration is avoided unless distension is severe or there is a strong suspicion of infection. A removable splint provides comfort, but once the acute episode has passed, movement is encouraged.

Acute bleeding into muscles

A painful swelling appears in the arm or leg. There is a danger of a compartment syndrome and Volkmann's ischaemia, but decompression is unwise and ineffectual.

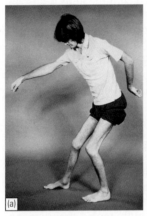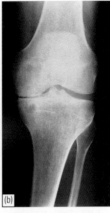

5.7 Haemophilic arthritis (a) This young man has developed contractures of the knees and ankles following repeated bleeds. (b) X-ray of the knee shows features of an erosive arthritis.

Treatment

Treatment is by splintage and early factor replacement, followed by physiotherapy. Later, operation may be needed to correct any resulting joint deformity.

Joint degeneration

This, the sequel to repeated bleeding, usually begins before the age of 15. Chronic synovitis is followed by cartilage degeneration. An affected joint shows wasting and fixed deformity not unlike a tuberculous or rheumatoid joint. X-rays show periarticular osteoporosis and progressive joint erosion.

Treatment

Progressive degeneration is preventable by controlling bleeds, encouraging movement and counteracting joint deformity. Operative treatment (including joint replacement) is feasible but must be covered by factor replacement. It is important to screen patients for hepatitis B virus and human immunodeficiency virus (HIV) antibodies, as their presence demands special precautions during operation.

CHAPTER 6

OSTEONECROSIS AND OSTEOCHONDRITIS

Osteonecrosis – or bone death – is due either to impaired blood supply or to severe cell damage. *Osteochondritis* is a poorly defined (and badly named) condition in which bone damage and necrosis follow trauma to articular surfaces.

OSTEONECROSIS (AVASCULAR NECROSIS)

The prototypical example of avascular necrosis (AVN) is aseptic death of a large segment of the femoral head following fracture of the femoral neck and severance of the local blood supply. It is now recognized that aseptic osteonecrosis occurs at a number of other sites, due either to local injury or to non-traumatic conditions (including high-dosage corticosteroid administration and alcohol abuse) which result in ischaemia of a substantial segment of bone.

Sites most susceptible are the femoral head, femoral condyles, head of humerus and proximal poles of scaphoid and talus. What they have in common is that they lie at the outskirts of the bone's main vascular supply and are largely enclosed by articular cartilage, which is itself avascular and which restricts the area for entry of other, local blood vessels. Furthermore, at some of these sites the subarticular trabeculae are sustained largely by endarterioles with limited arterial connections.

Another factor which needs to be taken into account is that the vascular sinusoids which

Conditions associated with non-traumatic osteonecrosis	
Hypercortisolaemia Cortisone administration Cushing's disease	**Marrow infiltration** Gaucher's disease Malignant disease
Hyperlipidaemia Alcohol abuse	**Infection** Septic arthritis
Haemoglobinopathy Sickle-cell disease	**Other** Perthes' disease Systemic lupus erythematosus Clotting disorders
Capillary occlusion Dysbaric osteonecrosis	

nourish the marrow and bone cells, unlike arterial capillaries, have no adventitial layer and their patency is determined by the volume and pressure of the surrounding marrow tissue, which itself is encased in unyielding bone. The system functions essentially as a closed compartment within which one element can expand only at the expense of the others. Local changes such as vascular stasis, haemorrhage or marrow swelling can, therefore, rapidly spiral to a vicious circle of capillary occlusion, ischaemia, reactive oedema or inflammation, marrow swelling, increased intraosseous pressure and further ischaemia.

The process described above can be initiated in at least four different ways: (1) severance of the local blood supply; (2) venous stasis and retrograde arteriolar stoppage; (3) intravascular thrombosis; and (4) compression of capillaries and sinusoids by marrow swelling. *Ischaemia, in the majority of cases, is due to a combination of several of these factors.*

Pathology

Dead bone is structurally and radiographically indistinguishable from live bone. However, lacking a blood supply, it does not undergo renewal, and after a limited period of repetitive stress it collapses. The changes develop in four overlapping stages.

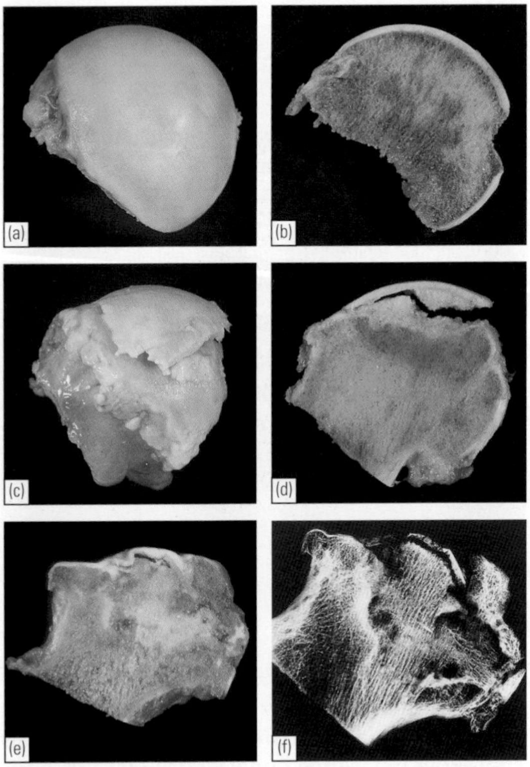

6.1 Osteonecrosis – pathology Three femoral head specimens showing different stages of pathology. (a,b) Normal femoral head with intact articular cartilage; the coronal section (b) shows the structurally perfect articular cartilage and vascularized subarticular bone. In the head with osteonecrosis (c), the articular cartilage is lifted off, and the coronal section in (d) shows that this is due to a subarticular fracture through a necrotic segment in the dome of the femoral head. In the latest stage there is marked cartilage and bone destruction, shown here in coronal section through the femoral head specimen (e) and a fine detail x-ray (f).

Stage 1: bone death without structural change

Within 48 hours after infarction there is marrow necrosis and cell death. However, for weeks or even months the bone may show no alteration in macroscopic appearance.

Stage 2: repair and early structural failure

Some days or weeks after infarction, the surrounding, living bone shows a vascular reaction; new bone is laid down upon the dead trabeculae and the increase in bone mass shows on the x-ray as exaggerated density. Despite this active repair, small fractures begin to appear in the dead bone.

Stage 3: major structural failure

The necrotic portion starts to crumble and the bone outline becomes distorted.

Stage 4: articular destruction

Cartilage, being nourished mainly by synovial fluid, is preserved even in advanced osteonecrosis. However, severe distortion of the surface eventually leads to cartilage breakdown and secondary osteoarthritis.

Clinical features

By the time the patient presents, the lesion is often well advanced. Pain is the usual complaint; it is felt near a joint and is accompanied by stiffness. Local tenderness may be present and the nearby joint may be swollen. Movements are usually restricted.

Imaging

X-ray

The distinctive x-ray feature of AVN is a subarticular segment of increased bone density. This is not because dead bone is more radio-opaque than living bone: it is due to reactive new-bone formation in the surrounding living tissue which increases the total mass of calcified bone. Other changes are subarticular fracturing and, in many cases, bone collapse.

MRI

The drawback in relying on x-ray examination is that changes appear only after several months. The only reliable method of picking up the early signs of osteonecrosis is by MRI (see Figure 6.2b).

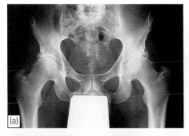
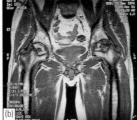
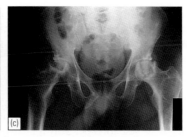
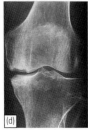
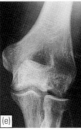

6.2 Osteonecrosis – imaging The cardinal x-ray feature is increased bone density in the weight-bearing part of the joint. In the early stages this may be equivocal (a), but marked changes are already visible in the MRI (b). A year later, these features are clearly reflected in the plain x-ray (c). In this case, similar changes appeared in the medial femoral condyle (d) and the capitulum (e).

Radionuclide scanning

Radioscintigraphy may show diminished activity in the avascular segment; more often one sees increased activity owing to the vascular reaction in the surrounding bone.

Diagnosis of the underlying disorder

In many cases of osteonecrosis, an underlying disorder will be obvious from the history: a known episode of trauma, an occupation such as deep-sea diving or working under compressed air, a family background of Gaucher's disease or sickle-cell disease.

There may be a record of high-dosage corticosteroid administration, for example after renal transplantation, where the drug is used for immunosuppression. However, smaller doses (e.g. as short-term treatment for asthma or as an adjunct in neurosurgical emergencies) can also be dangerous in patients with other risk factors. Combinations of drugs (e.g. corticosteroids and azathioprine, or corticosteroids after a period of alcohol abuse) also can be potent causes of osteonecrosis; occasionally corticosteroids have been given without the patient's knowledge.

 Unexplained necrosis: check for alcohol abuse. Don't just ask – do blood tests for alcohol-related changes.

Treatment

If possible, the cause should be eliminated. In stages 1 and 2, bone collapse can sometimes be prevented by a combination of weight-relief, splintage and (in some cases associated with venous stasis and marrow oedema) surgical decompression of the bone. Once bone collapse has occurred (stage 3), a realignment osteotomy, by transferring stress to an undamaged area, may relieve pain and prevent further bone distortion. In stage 4 the treatment is the same as for osteoarthritis. This protocol refers to the lower limb; in the upper limb, often no treatment is needed.

SPECIFIC TYPES OF AVASCULAR NECROSIS

Post-traumatic

A fracture or dislocation may interrupt the local blood supply. Although bone death is immediate, the diagnosis is usually made only when the x-ray shows increased density in the surrounding bone. The most common sites are (1) the femoral head, (2) the carpal bones and (3) the talus.

Treatment

The patient may require no treatment; however, if pain and disability are severe, the avascular portion may be replaced or removed, or the adjacent joint may be fused.

Sickle-cell disease

This is a genetic disorder, limited to people of Central and West African Negro descent. Red cells containing abnormal haemoglobin (HbS) become distorted and sickle shaped; this is especially likely to occur with hypoxia (e.g. under anaesthesia or in extreme cold). Clumping of the sickle-shaped cells causes diminished capillary flow and repeated episodes of pain ('bone crises') or, if more severe, ischaemic necrosis. Almost any bone may be involved and there is a tendency for the infarcts to become infected, sometimes with unusual organisms such as *Salmonella*.

X-ray

The tubular bones (including the phalanges) may show irregular endosteal destruction and medullary sclerosis, together with periosteal new-bone formation. Not only does this resemble osteomyelitis, but also true infection is often superimposed on the infarct. In children, femoral head necrosis could be mistaken for Perthes' disease.

Treatment

Acute episodes are treated by rest and analgesics, followed by physiotherapy to minimize stiffness. Established necrosis is treated according to the principles on page 49, but with the emphasis on conservatism. Anaesthesia carries serious risks and may even precipitate vascular occlusion in the central nervous system, lungs or kidneys; moreover, the chances of postoperative infection are high.

Caisson disease

Decompression sickness (caisson disease) and osteonecrosis are important causes of disability in deep-sea divers and compressed-air workers building tunnels or underwater structures. Under increased air pressure, the blood and other tissues (especially fat) become supersaturated with nitrogen; if decompression is too rapid, the gas is released as bubbles, which cause local tissue damage and generalized embolic phenomena. The symptoms of decompression sickness are pain near the joints ('the bends'), breathing difficulty and vertigo ('the staggers'). In the most acute cases there can be circulatory and respiratory collapse, severe neurological changes, coma and death. Bone necrosis may be due to capillary obstruction by gas bubbles and changes in marrow fat.

The patient complains of pain and loss of joint movement, but many lesions remain silent and are found only on routine x-ray examination.

Management

The aim is prevention; the incidence of osteonecrosis is proportional to the working pressure, the length of exposure, the rate of decompression and the number of exposures. Strict enforcement of suitable working schedules has reduced the risks considerably. The treatment of established lesions follows the principles already outlined.

Gaucher's disease (see page 81)

This familial disease occurs predominantly in Ashkenazi Jews. Deficiency of the specific enzyme causes an abnormal accumulation of glucocerebroside in the reticuloendothelial system. The effects are seen chiefly in the liver, spleen and bone marrow, where the large, polyhedral 'Gaucher cells' accumulate.

Bone complications are common and osteonecrosis is among the worst of them. The hip is most frequently affected, but lesions also appear in the distal femur, talus and head of humerus. Bone ischaemia is usually attributed to the increase in medullary cell volume and capillary compression.

Symptoms may occur at any age; the patient complains of pain around one of the larger joints and movements may be restricted. There is a tendency for the Gaucher deposits to become infected and the patient may present with septicaemia. A diagnostic, though inconstant, finding is a raised serum acid phosphatase level.

X-ray

A special feature (due to replacement of myeloid tissue by Gaucher cells) is expansion of the tubular bones, especially the distal femur, producing a flask-like appearance. Osteonecrosis of the femoral head is common.

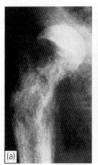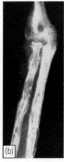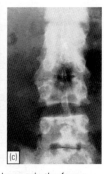

6.3 Sickle-cell disease (a) Typical changes in the femur due to marrow hyperplasia, with bone infarction and necrosis of the femoral head. (b) Infarctions of tubular bones may resemble osteomyelitis. (c) The spine also may be involved.

Treatment

The general disorder can now be treated by enzyme replacement. Management of the osteonecrosis follows the principles outlined on page 49. If joint replacement is contemplated, antibiotic cover is essential.

Drug-induced necrosis

Corticosteroids in high dosage may give rise to 'spontaneous' osteonecrosis; thus the condition is fairly common in renal transplant patients on immunosuppressive corticosteroids. Alcohol abuse is another potent cause. Both conditions result in widespread fatty changes and marrow infarction, which may be the cause of the bone necrosis. The sites usually affected are the femoral head, femoral condyles and the head of the humerus.

Pain may be present for many months before x-rays show any abnormality. MRI is the only reliable way of making an early diagnosis; typical changes are often discovered in asymptomatic joints.

Treatment

Early changes, if not actually reversible, can be prevented from extending by stopping the cortisone or alcohol. Analgesics, weight-relief and physiotherapy are often all that is required. Decompression of the affected bone by drilling may relieve symptoms and even prevent progressive changes in very early cases. If the joint surface has collapsed, reconstructive surgery is required.

OSTEOCHONDRITIS (OSTEOCHONDROSIS)

The term 'osteochondritis' is applied to a group of conditions in which there is compression, fragmentation or separation of a small segment of bone, usually at the bone end and involving the attached articular surface. The affected portion of bone shows many of the features of ischaemic necrosis, including increased vascularity and reactive sclerosis in the surrounding bone. These conditions occur in children and adolescents, often during phases of rapid growth and increased physical activity. Segmental ischaemia may be caused by trauma or repetitive stress.

Three types of osteochondritis are identified: 'shearing', 'crushing' and 'pulling'.

SHEARING OSTEOCHONDRITIS (OSTEOCHONDRITIS DISSECANS)

A small segment of articular cartilage and the subjacent bone may separate (dissect) as an avascular fragment. The cause is almost certainly repeated minor trauma producing an osteochondral fracture of a convex joint surface.

The condition occurs mainly in young adults, usually male. The knee is much the most common joint to be affected. The patient presents with intermittent pain, swelling and joint effusion. If the necrotic fragment becomes completely detached, it may cause locking or giving way.

Imaging

X-rays need to show the affected articular surface in tangential projection. The dissecting fragment is defined by a radiolucent line of demarcation. When it separates, the resulting 'crater' may be obvious. So might the loose body in the joint! However, these are comparatively late changes; the early features are best shown by *MRI*.

Treatment

If the fragment is in position, treatment consists of weight-relief and restriction of activity. In children, complete healing may occur, although it takes up to 2 years. If the fragment becomes detached and causes symptoms, it should be fixed back in position or completely removed.

CRUSHING OSTEOCHONDRITIS

This is seen mainly in adolescence. The characteristic feature is an apparently spontaneous

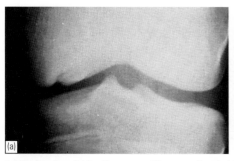 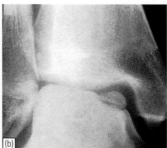 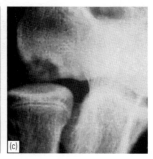

6.4 Osteochondritis dissecans The osteochondral fragment usually remains in place at the articular surface. The most common sites are (a) the medial femoral condyle, (b) the talus and (c) the capitulum.

necrosis of the ossific nucleus in a long-bone epiphysis or one of the cuboidal bones of the wrist or foot.

Pain and limitation of joint movement are the usual complaints. Tenderness is sharply localized. X-rays show increased density, accompanied in the later stages by collapse of the necrotic segment.

The common examples of crushing osteochondritis have, by long tradition, acquired eponymous labels: Freiberg's disease of a metatarsal head; Köhler's disease of the navicular; Kienböck's disease of the carpal lunate; and Panner's disease of the capitulum.

Treatment

This is usually conservative: analgesics and splintage until the symptoms settle down.

However, osteochondritis of the lunate may need operative treatment (see page 164).

PULLING OSTEOCHONDRITIS (TRACTION APOPHYSITIS)

Excessive pull by a large tendon may damage the unfused apophysis to which it is attached; this occurs typically at two sites: the tibial tuberosity *(Osgood–Schlatter's disease)* and the calcaneal apophysis *(Sever's disease)*. The traumatized apophysis becomes painful and tender. With rest, the symptoms invariably settle down. Though these conditions are usually classified with other types of osteochondritis, the common feature of locally increased bone density is probably a reparative reaction to slight trauma rather than bone necrosis.

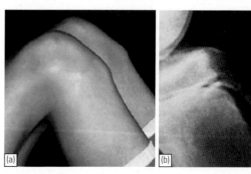

6.6 Osgood–Schlatter's disease This is a traction lesion due to excessively vigorous pull of the patellar ligament on the tibial apophysis. This young football player presented with painful bumps just below the knees (a). The x-ray (b) shows slight displacement of the as yet unfused tibial apophysis.

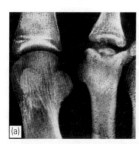 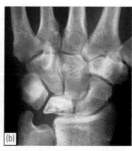

6.5 Crushing osteochondritis (a) Freiberg's disease of the head of the second metatarsal bone. (b) Kienböck's disease of the lunate.

CHAPTER 7

METABOLIC AND ENDOCRINE DISORDERS

Bones have obvious mechanical functions: they support and protect the soft tissues, transmit load and muscular force from one part of the body to another, and mediate movement and locomotion.

Bone as a tissue has an equally important role as a mineral reservoir which helps to regulate the composition – and in particular the calcium ion concentration – of the extracellular fluid. For all its solidity, bone is in a continuous state of flux, its internal shape and structure changing from moment to moment in concert with the normal variations in mechanical function and mineral exchange. All modulations in bone structure and composition are brought about by cellular activity, which is regulated by hormones and local factors; these agents, in turn, are controlled by alterations in mineral ion concentrations. The metabolic bone disorders are conditions in which generalized skeletal abnormalities result from disruption of this complex interactive system.

A short review of bone physiology may be helpful, not alone as an introduction to metabolic bone disorders, but also to assist in the understanding of other concepts in musculoskeletal pathology.

BONE AND BONES

BONE COMPOSITION AND STRUCTURE

Bone consists of a largely collagenous matrix which is impregnated with mineral salts and populated by cells – osteoclasts (concerned with bone resorption), osteoblasts (for bone formation) and osteocytes (resting bone cells which may have a function in communicating information about local stresses and strains to the other bone cells).

Newly formed bone tissue, which is unmineralized, is called *osteoid* and is usually seen only where active new-bone formation is taking place. Normally this soon becomes mineralized, but the immature tissue is somewhat disorganized, with collagen fibres arranged haphazardly and cells having no specific orientation; in this state it is called *woven bone.*

The mature tissue is *lamellar bone,* in which the collagen fibres are arranged parallel to each other to form multiple layers (or laminae) with the osteocytes lying between the lamellae. Almost half the bone volume is mineral matter – mainly calcium and phosphate in the form of *crystalline hydroxyapatite* – which is laid down in osteoid at the calcification front. The proportions of calcium and phosphate are constant and the molecule is firmly bound to collagen.

Lamellar bone exists in two structurally different forms: *compact (cortical) bone* and *cancellous (trabecular) bone.*

Compact bone is dense and strong and is found where support matters most: the outer walls of all bones, but especially the shafts of tubular bones, and the subchondral plates supporting articular

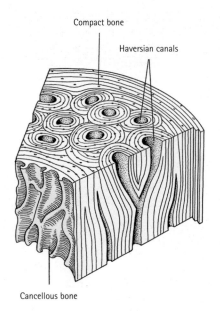

Compact bone

Haversian canals

Cancellous bone

7.1 Bone structure This picture represents a wedge taken from the cortex of a long bone. It shows the basic elements of compact bone: densely packed osteons, each made up of concentric layers of bone and osteocytes around a central haversian canal which contains the vessels; outer laminae of subperiosteal bone; and similar laminae on the interior surface (endosteum) merging into a lattice of cancellous bone.

cartilage. It is made up of compact units – *haversian systems* or *osteons* – each of which consists of a central canal (the *haversian canal*) containing blood vessels, lymphatics and nerves, surrounded by closely packed, more or less concentric lamellae of bone. Seen in three dimensions, the haversian canals are long, branching channels connecting extensively with each other and with the endosteal and periosteal surfaces by smaller channels called *Volkmann canals.*

Cancellous (trabecular) bone has a honeycomb appearance; it makes up the interior meshwork of all bones and is particularly well developed in the ends of the tubular bones and the vertebral bodies. Three-dimensionally the trabecular sheets are interconnected (like a honeycomb) and arranged according to the mechanical needs of the structure, the thickest and strongest along trajectories of compressive stress and the thinnest in the planes of tensile stress.

Cancellous bone is obviously more porous than cortical bone. Though it makes up only one-quarter of the total skeletal mass, the trabeculae provide two-thirds of the total bone surface. It is easy to understand why the effects of metabolic disorders are usually seen first in trabecular bone.

Fully formed bones are covered (except at the articular ends) by a tough *periosteal membrane,* the deepest layer of which consists of potentially bone-forming cells. The inner, endosteal, surfaces are irregular and lined by a fine *endosteal membrane* in close contact with the marrow spaces.

Bone has a rich *blood supply.* Vessels in the haversian canals form an anastomotic network between the medullary and periosteal blood supply. Blood flow in this capillary network is normally centrifugal – from the medullary cavity outwards – and it has long been held that the cortex is supplied entirely from this source. However, it seems likely that at least the outermost layers of the cortex are normally also supplied by periosteal vessels, and if the medullary vessels are blocked or destroyed, the periosteal circulation can take over entirely and the direction of blood flow is reversed. In cancellous bone, the spaces between the trabeculae contain marrow, fat and fine sinusoidal vessels that course through the tissue nourishing both marrow and bone.

BONE GROWTH, MODELLING AND REMODELLING

During growth the bone increases in size and changes in shape. At the epiphyseal growth plate (physis) new bone is added by endochondral ossification, while on the surface bone is added by subperiosteal appositional ossification. The medullary cavity is expanded by endosteal resorption and the bulbous bone ends are continuously re-formed and sculpted into shape by alternating bone resorption and formation – a process known as *bone modelling.*

The same process continues throughout adult life, except now it is directed not at the modelling of a particular shape but at the constant *remodelling* of existing bone. This serves a crucial purpose in the preservation of skeletal structure: 'old bone' is continually replaced by 'new bone', and in this way the skeleton is protected from stress failure due to repetitive loading. Besides, the maintenance of calcium homeostasis requires a constant turnover of the mineral deposits that would otherwise stay locked in bone.

At each *remodelling site,* work proceeds in an orderly and unvarying sequence: osteoclasts gather on a free bone surface and excavate a cavity; they disappear and, after a period of quiescence, are replaced by osteoblasts which proceed to fill in the excavation with new bone. Each cycle of bone

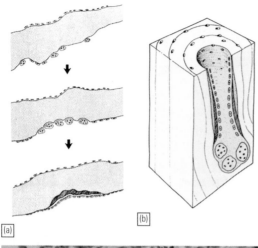

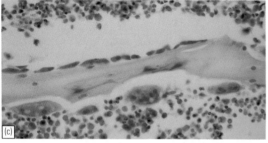

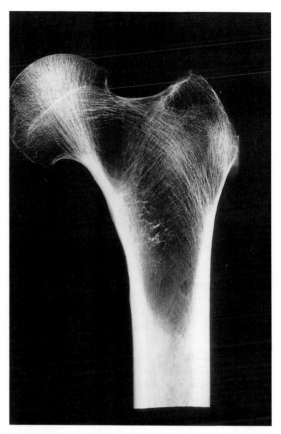

7.2 Bone remodelling (a) Open trabecular surfaces are first excavated by osteoclasts and then lined and filled in again by a following train of osteoblasts. (b) In compact bone the osteoclasts burrow deeply into the existing bone, with the osteoblasts following close behind to re-line the cavity with new bone. (c) Histological section showing a trabecula lined on one surface by excavating osteoclasts and on the other surface by a string of much smaller osteoblasts. This process gradually reshapes the bone.

7.3 Wolff's Law Wolff's Law is beautifully demonstrated in the trabecular pattern at the upper end of the femur. The thickest trabeculae are arranged along the trajectories of greatest stress.

This natural adaptation of bone structure to functional demands is known as *Wolff's Law.*

AGE-RELATED CHANGES IN BONE

During childhood and adolescence the entire bone increases in size and changes somewhat in shape. However, although the bones become bigger, the tissue of which they are made remains comparatively light and porous.

Between adolescence and 35 years of age the haversian canals and spaces between trabeculae are gradually filled in and the cortices increase in thickness, i.e. the bones become heavier and stronger. Bone mass increases at the rate of about 3 per cent per year, and during the third decade each individual attains a state of *peak bone mass.*

From 35 to about 50 years there is a slow but inexorable loss of bone; haversian spaces enlarge, trabeculae become thinner, the endosteal surface is resorbed and the medullary space expands – i.e.

turnover takes from 4 to 6 months. The annual rate of turnover is about 4 per cent for cortical bone and 25 per cent for trabecular bone.

During bone remodelling, resorption and formation are *coupled,* the one ineluctably following the other. This ensures that, on average, a balance is maintained, though at any moment and at any particular site one or other process may predominate.

In the long term, change is inevitable. During the first half of life, formation slightly exceeds resorption and bone mass increases; in later years, resorption exceeds formation and bone mass steadily declines. Throughout life, however, bone also adapts to the stresses imposed upon it, and at any particular site cortical and trabecular thickness will be greatest in the trajectories of highest stress.

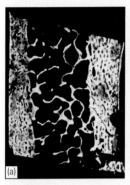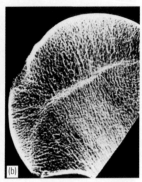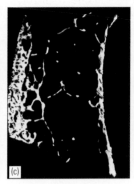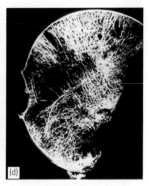

7.4 Age-related changes in bone These fine-detail x-rays of iliac crest biopsies and femoral head slices show the marked contrast between trabecular density in a healthy 40-year-old woman (a,b) and one of 75 years (c,d).

year by year, the bones become slightly more porous. The diminution in bone mass proceeds at a rate of about 0.3 per cent per year in men and 0.5 per cent per year in women up to the menopause.

From the onset of the menopause and for the next 10 years the rate of bone loss in women accelerates to about 3 per cent per year, occurring predominantly in trabecular bone. This steady depletion is due mainly to excessive resorption – osteoclastic activity seeming to be released from the restraining influence of gonadal hormone. (Similar changes are seen in younger women about 5 years after oophorectomy.) About 30 per cent of white women will lose bone to the extent of developing post-menopausal osteoporosis. For reasons that are not fully understood, the degree of bone depletion is less marked in Negroid than in Caucasoid peoples.

From the age of 65 or 70 years the rate of bone loss gradually tails off and by the age of 75 years it is about 0.5 per cent per year. This later phase of depletion is due mainly to diminishing osteoblastic activity.

Men are affected in a similar manner, but the phase of rapid bone loss occurs about15 years later than in women, at the climacteric.

BONE MASS AND BONE STRENGTH

Bone mass refers to the actual amount of osseous tissue in any unit volume of bone, which is made up of osseous tissue and variable numbers and sizes of spaces filled with soft tissue. Throughout life, and regardless of whether bone mass increases or decreases, the degree of mineralization in normal people varies very little from age to age or from one person to another. With advancing years, as the bones become more porous, there is a gradual loss of bone strength; but, curiously, the loss of

strength is out of proportion to the decrease in mass. This can be explained in a number of ways: (a) in addition to the *diminution in bone mass* there is also a *loss of structural connectivity* between the trabecular plates, and (b) in old age the *decrease in bone cell activity* makes for a slow remodelling rate, so that old bone takes longer to be replaced and microtrauma to be repaired. As a consequence, ageing is inevitably accompanied by an increasing likelihood of fracture.

REGULATION OF BONE TURNOVER AND MINERAL EXCHANGE

Most of the body's calcium and phosphate is tightly packed in bone and can be released only by resorption of the entire tissue – a slow process. The rapidly exchangeable component is in the extracellular fluid, where its concentration depends mainly on intestinal absorption and renal excretion; transient alterations in serum levels are accommodated quickly by changes in renal tubular reabsorption.

The control of calcium is much more critical than that of phosphate; thus, in persistent calcium deficiency, the extracellular calcium ion concentration is maintained by drawing on bone, whereas phosphate deficiency simply leads to lowered serum phosphate concentration. The regulation of calcium exchange is therefore linked inescapably to that of bone formation and resorption. The complex balance between calcium exchange and bone remodelling is controlled by an array of systemic and local factors.

Calcium

Calcium is essential for normal cell function and physiological processes such as nerve conduction and muscle contraction. The normal concentration in plasma and extracellular fluid is 8.8–10.4 mg/dL (2.2–2.6 mmol/L). Much of this is bound to protein; about half is ionized and effective in cell metabolism and the regulation of calcium homoeostasis.

The recommended daily intake of calcium is 800–1000 mg (20–25 mmol), and ideally this should be increased to 1500 mg during pregnancy and lactation. About 50 per cent of the dietary calcium is absorbed (mainly in the upper gut), but much of that is secreted back into the bowel and only about 200 mg (5 mmol) enters the circulation.

Calcium absorption is mediated by vitamin D metabolites and inhibited by excessive intake of phosphates (common in soft drinks), oxalates (found in tea and coffee), phytates (chapatti flour) and fats, as well as by the administration of corticosteroids; it is also reduced in malabsorption disorders of the bowel.

Urinary excretion varies between 100 and 200 mg (2.5 and 5 mmol) per 24 hours; if calcium intake is reduced, urinary excretion is adjusted by increasing tubular reabsorption. If calcium concentration is persistently reduced, calcium is drawn from the skeleton by increased bone resorption. These compensatory shifts in intestinal absorption, renal excretion and bone remodelling are regulated by parathyroid hormone (PTH) and vitamin D metabolites.

Phosphorus

Phosphorus is needed for many important metabolic processes. Plasma concentration – almost entirely in the form of ionized inorganic phosphates – is 2.8–4.0 mg/dL (0.9–1.3 mmol/L). It is abundantly available in the diet and is absorbed in the small intestine, more or less in proportion to the amount ingested; however, absorption is reduced in the presence of antacids such as aluminium hydroxide, which binds phosphorus in the gut.

Phosphate excretion is extremely efficient, but 90 per cent is reabsorbed in the proximal tubules. Tubular reabsorption is decreased (and overall excretion increased) by PTH.

Vitamin D

Vitamin D, through its active metabolites, is principally concerned with calcium absorption and transport and (acting together with PTH) bone remodelling. Target organs are the small intestine and bone.

Naturally occurring vitamin D_3 (cholecalciferol) is derived from two sources: directly from the diet and indirectly by the action of ultraviolet light on

7.5 Vitamin D metabolism The active vitamin D metabolites are derived either from the diet or by conversion of precursors when the skin is exposed to sunlight. The inactive 'vitamin' is hydroxylated, first in the liver and then in the kidney, to form the active metabolites 25-HCC and 1,25-DHCC.

the precursor 7-dihydrocholesterol in the skin. The normal requirement is about 400 IU (international units) per day. In most countries this is obtained mainly from exposure to sunlight.

Vitamin D itself is inactive. Conversion to active metabolites takes place first in the liver by 25-hydroxylation to form *25-hydroxycholecalciferol (25-HCC)*, and then in the kidneys by further hydroxylation (mediated by PTH) to *1,25-dihydroxycholecalciferol (1,25-DHCC)*.

The terminal metabolite 1,25-DHCC (calcitriol) and – to a lesser extent – 25-HCC act on the *lining cells of the small intestine*, stimulating the absorption of calcium and phosphate. *In bone* they assist PTH to promote osteoclastic bone resorption; they also enhance calcium transport across the cell membrane and thus indirectly promote the process of mineralization.

Parathyroid hormone

Parathyroid hormone is the fine regulator of calcium exchange. It maintains the extracellular calcium concentration between very narrow limits; production and release are stimulated by a fall and suppressed by a rise in plasma ionized calcium.

Target organs are the kidney, bone and (indirectly) the gut. Acting on the *renal tubules,* PTH increases phosphate excretion by restricting its reabsorption, and conserves calcium by increasing its reabsorption. These responses rapidly compensate for any change in plasma ionized calcium. Acting on the *kidney parenchyma,* it controls hydroxylation of the vitamin D metabolite, 25-HCC.

In *bone* PTH promotes osteoclastic resorption and the release of calcium and phosphate into the blood. This is a much slower way of maintaining plasma calcium levels.

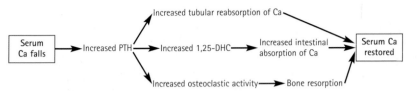

7.6 Calcium homeostasis Algorithm showing the role of PTH in maintaining calcium homeostasis.

Calcitonin

Calcitonin, which is secreted by the C cells of the thyroid, does more or less the opposite of PTH: it suppresses osteoclastic bone resorption and increases renal calcium excretion.

Oestrogen

Oestrogen is thought to stimulate calcium absorption and to protect bone from the unrestrained action of PTH. Its withdrawal leads to osteoporosis; this occurs naturally at the menopause, but it also follows oophorectomy in younger women and a similar effect is seen in other amenorrhoeic states.

Adrenal corticosteroids

Corticosteroids administered in excess cause a pernicious type of osteoporosis due to a combination of increased bone resorption, diminished bone formation, decreased intestinal calcium absorption and increased calcium excretion; collagen synthesis may also be defective.

Local factors

Systemic hormones have a large-scale effect on bone turnover, but many of the cellular activities at the work-front where remodelling takes place are mediated by local factors such as *insulin-like growth factor I (somatomedin C), transforming growth factors, interleukin-1 (IL-1), osteoclast-activating factor (OAF)* and *prostaglandins.*

Bone morphogenetic protein (BMP), which can be extracted from bone matrix, induces chondrogenesis and bone formation. This process – known as bone induction – may be important in fracture healing and bone-graft replacement.

Mechanical stress

The effect of mechanical stress on bone remodelling is embodied in Wolff's Law (page 55). Positive influences on bone formation are produced by gravity, load-bearing, muscle action and vascular pulsation. Weightlessness, prolonged bed-rest, lack of exercise, muscular weakness and limb immobilization are all associated with osteoporosis.

METABOLIC BONE DISORDERS

Most of the common metabolic bone disorders are associated with depletion of bone tissue. They fall into three groups: (1) *osteoporosis,* in which the quantity of bone (bone mass) is abnormally low; (2) *osteomalacia,* in which the osseous connective tissue (osteoid) is present but insufficiently mineralized; and (3) *osteitis fibrosa,* in which PTH over-production leads to bone resorption and replacement by fibrous tissue.

Clinical assessment

Metabolic bone disease usually presents with features of *skeletal failure* (bone pain, fractures and deformity), *hypercalcaemia* (anorexia, abdominal pain, depression, renal stone or metastatic calcification), or an *endocrine disorder.* There may be obvious physical signs, such as the 'moon face' and cushingoid build of hypercortisolism, or an exaggerated thoracic kyphosis due to osteoporotic vertebral compression, and children with rickets may have characteristic deformities. It is important to enquire about previous conditions such as intestinal disease (hints of malabsorption), alcohol abuse, dietary fads and cigarette smoking, and previous medication.

X-ray examination

The commonest x-ray signs are a non-specific loss of radiographic density – *osteopenia* – and *vertebral compression fractures;* less obvious features are *cortical stress fractures* and *cortical erosions.* Children may show features of *rickets* and elderly people should be investigated for signs of *metastatic bone disease* and *myelomatosis.*

Measurement of bone mass

X-ray signs of bone loss are late and unreliable; there are much more accurate ways of measuring bone mineral density (BMD) and bone mass. These are based on the principle that a beam of energy is attenuated as it passes through bone, and the degree of attenuation is related to the mass and mineral content of the bone. BMD is expressed in grams per unit area (g/cm^2) and is recorded in comparison to

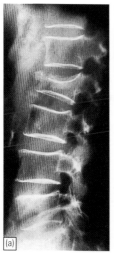

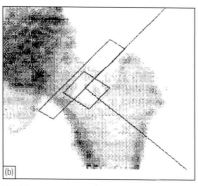

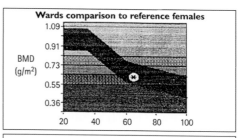

Wards BMD (g/cm²)1	0.619 ± 0.02
Wards % young females	68 ± 3
Wards % age matched	95 ± 3

7.7 Measurement of bone mass (a) X-ray of the lumbar spine shows a compression fracture of L2. The general loss of bone density accentuates the cortical outlines of the vertebral body end-plates. These features are characteristic of diminished bone mass, which can be measured accurately by dual-energy x-ray absorptiometry (b). In this case the value at the femoral neck fell towards the lower limit of normal for the relevant age group.

the sex-specific and age-specific distribution of these values in the general population. The measurements are specific for each location (lumbar spine, femoral neck, distal radius etc.).

The most widely used technique is that of *dual-energy x-ray absorptiometry (DEXA)*. Precision and accuracy are excellent, x-ray exposure is not excessive and measurements can be obtained anywhere in the skeleton.

The main indication for using bone densitometry is to assess the degree and progress of bone loss in patients with clinically diagnosed metabolic bone disease. However, it is also useful as a screening procedure for perimenopausal women with multiple risk factors for osteoporotic fractures.

Biochemical tests

Serum calcium and phosphate concentrations should be measured in the fasting state, and it is the ionized calcium fraction that is important.

Serum alkaline phosphatase concentration is an index of osteoblastic activity; it is raised in osteomalacia and in disorders associated with high bone turnover (hyperparathyroidism, Paget's disease, bone metastases).

Parathyroid hormone activity can be estimated from serum assays of the COOH terminal fragment.

Vitamin D activity is assessed by measuring the serum 25-HCC concentration. Serum 1,25-DHCC levels do not necessarily reflect vitamin uptake but are reduced in advanced renal disease.

Urinary calcium and phosphate excretion can be measured. Significant alterations are found in malabsorption disorders, hyperparathyroidism and other conditions associated with hypercalcaemia.

Urinary hydroxyproline excretion is a measure of bone resorption. It may be increased in high-turnover conditions such as Paget's disease but it is not sensitive enough to reflect lesser increases in bone resorption.

Excretion of pyridinium compounds and telopeptides derived from bone collagen cross-links is a much more sensitive index of bone resorption.

NB. Laboratory reports should always state the normal range for each test, which may be different for infants, children and adults.

OSTEOPOROSIS

In osteoporosis the bone is qualitatively normal but there is less of it than would be expected in a person of that age and sex. The bone cortex is thinner than normal and trabeculae are sparse. Not surprisingly, the bone is also weaker than normal and it fractures relatively easily.

Localized osteoporosis is usually due to disuse (including paralysis) or nearby inflammation.

Generalized osteoporosis may be *physiological (age related,* or *'primary')*, but it is also a feature of many systemic disorders *('secondary')* and its precise elucidation can be difficult.

AGE-RELATED OSTEOPOROSIS

Bone mass decreases slowly but steadily from the age of 40 years. Around the menopause this process is accelerated (see Fig. 7.4). This is due to oestrogen withdrawal and less restrained osteoclastic resorption; the same changes are seen in younger women after oophorectomy. Similar changes occur in men, starting about 15 years later than in women. *Risk factors* for accelerated postmenopausal osteoporosis are a family history of osteoporosis, ectomorphic somatotype, hysterectomy, cigarette smoking and dietary faddism. People of Negroid descent suffer less than Whites or Asiatics.

From about 70 years onwards, additional factors come into play. There is a gradual decrease in the rate of bone formation, a type of involutional change affecting both men and women; in many cases bone loss is further increased because of diminished activity, chronic illness and dietary deficiencies. The risk of osteoporotic fracture increases considerably, and on top of that old people develop an increasing propensity to fall.

Clinical features

Postmenopausal osteoporosis

Women between the ages of 55 and 65 may present with acute back pain due to vertebral compression; with repeated minor fractures, they develop progressive kyphosis. If they fall, they are liable to sustain a fracture of one of the long bones, usually the distal end of the radius (Colles' fracture).

Involutional osteoporosis

Over the age of 70, patients (women and men) are more likely to be seen with a fracture of the femoral neck or the proximal end of the humerus. They may already have a history of previous fractures, or obvious vertebral osteoporosis. It is important, in this age group, to look for features of

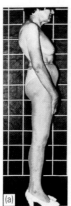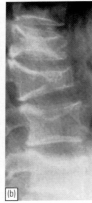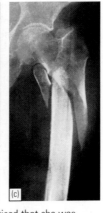

7.8 Osteoporosis (a) This woman noticed that she was becoming more and more round-shouldered; she also had chronic backache and her x-rays (b) show compression of several vertebral bodies. Six years after this x-ray was obtained she fell in her kitchen and sustained the fracture shown in (c).

systemic disease and signs of osteomalacia due to dietary deficiency.

X-rays

X-ray examination may show a typical osteoporotic fracture of one of the long bones or the spine. There is also a general reduction in radiographic bone density and abnormal thinning of the cortices. Bone density can be measured more accurately by DEXA scanning.

Diagnosis

The diagnosis is usually obvious. What is more difficult is to exclude the many specific causes of osteoporosis.

Many elderly patients with 'osteoporotic' fractures also have *osteomalacia*. If there are suspicious features (multiple fractures, Looser zones, pencil-thin cortices, increased alkaline phosphatase), an iliac crest biopsy is justified.

Patients under 45 need full investigation, including biopsy. An important cause in the fifth decade is multiple myeloma.

Prevention

Bone densitometry can be used to identify women who are at more than usual risk of suffering a fracture at the menopause, and prophylactic treatment of this group would seem sensible. However, routine DEXA screening (even in countries where it is available) is still a controversial issue; for practical purposes, it is usually reserved for women with multiple risk factors and particularly those with suspected oestrogen or some other bone-losing disorder, and those who have suffered previous low-energy fractures at the menopause.

Women approaching the menopause should be advised to maintain adequate levels of dietary calcium and vitamin D, to keep up a high level of physical activity and to avoid smoking and excessive consumption of alcohol. If necessary, the recommended daily requirements should be met by taking calcium and vitamin D supplements.

Oestrogen medication (hormone replacement therapy, HRT) is the most effective way of maintaining bone density and reducing the risk of fracture after the menopause; when treatment is stopped, bone loss proceeds at the usual rate. However, there are drawbacks to HRT, notably the risk of recurrent uterine bleeding after the menopause and fears about an increase in the incidence of breast and uterine cancer after long-term treatment. For practical purposes, HRT may be considered for women with low BMD and positive risk factors for osteoporosis; however, it is prudent not to continue with HRT for more than 5 years, and it should not be used at all if risk factors for breast cancer are identified. In women who have not had a hysterectomy, the risk of uterine cancer can be eliminated by administering a combination of oestrogen and progestin.

Bisphosphonates offer a useful alternative to HRT. The newer preparations (especially alendronate) have been shown to prevent bone loss and to reduce the risk of vertebral and hip fractures. Gastrointestinal side-effects are troublesome and suitable precautions should be taken.

Treatment

Initially, treatment is directed at management of the fracture. This will often require internal fixation; the sooner these patients are mobilized and rehabilitated, the better. Patients with muscle weakness and/or poor balance may benefit from gait training and, if necessary, the use of walking aids and rail fittings in the home.

Thereafter, the question of general treatment must be considered. Obvious factors such as concurrent illness, dietary deficiencies, lack of exposure to sunlight and lack of exercise will need attention. If there is any doubt about the adequacy of vitamin D and calcium intake, dietary supplements should be prescribed.

Treatment with bisphosphonates or HRT should also be considered, even in older women; although lost bone will not be restored, at least further loss may be prevented.

 In elderly people, osteoporosis and osteomalacia often go together – both may need treatment.

SECONDARY OSTEOPOROSIS

There are numerous causes of secondary osteoporosis (Table 7.1). *Hyperparathyroidism* is dealt with on page 64. Other common examples are *hypercortisonism, alcohol abuse, malignant disease* and *disuse osteoporosis.*

Hypercortisonism

Prolonged or excessive use of corticosteroids may cause severe osteoporosis, especially if the condition for which the drug is administered is itself associated with bone loss (e.g. rheumatoid arthritis – Fig 7.17). Bone resorption is markedly increased and formation is suppressed.

Treatment presents a problem, because the drug may be essential for the control of some generalized disease. However, corticosteroid dosage should be kept to a minimum; remember that topical and intra-articular preparations are absorbed and may have systemic effects if used repeatedly.

Preventive measures include the use of calcium supplements (at least 1500 mg per day) and vitamin D. In postmenopausal women and elderly men, HRT or bisphosphonates may be effective in reducing bone resorption, though here again prolonged use of HRT should be avoided.

Alcohol abuse

This is a common (and often neglected) cause of osteoporosis at all ages, with the added factor of an increased likelihood of falls and other injuries. Bone changes are due to a combination of decreased calcium absorption, liver failure and a toxic effect on osteoblast function. Alcohol also has a mild glucocorticoid effect.

Multiple myeloma and carcinomatosis

Generalized osteoporosis, anaemia and a high erythrocyte sedimentation rate (ESR) are characteristic features of myelomatosis and metastatic bone disease. Bone loss is due to over-production of local osteoclast-activating factors.

 Osteoporosis in middle-aged men: check for myelomatosis.

Disuse

The worst effects of stress reduction are seen in states of weightlessness; bone resorption,

Table 7.1 Some causes of osteoporosis

Nutritional	Malignant disease
Scurvy	Carcinomatosis
Malnutrition	Multiple myeloma
Malabsorption	Leukaemia
Endocrine disorders	**Non-malignant disease**
Hyperparathyroidism	Rheumatoid arthritis
Gonadal insufficiency	Ankylosing spondylosis
Cushing's disease	Tuberculosis
Thyrotoxicosis	Chronic renal disease
Drug-induced	**Idiopathic**
Corticosteroids	Juvenile osteoporosis
Alcohol	Post-climacteric osteoporosis
Heparin	

unbalanced by formation, leads to hypercalcaemia, hypercalciuria and severe osteoporosis. Lesser degrees of osteoporosis are seen in bedridden patients, and regional osteoporosis is common after immobilization of a limb. The effects can be mitigated by encouraging mobility, exercise and weight-bearing.

RICKETS AND OSTEOMALACIA

Rickets and osteomalacia are different expressions of the same disease: incomplete mineralization of bone due to inadequate absorption and/or utilization of calcium. *Osteomalacia* is the more general term, which describes the most obvious pathological feature – bone 'softening'. *Rickets* refers specifically to children, in whom there is also defective bone growth.

The condition is usually due to lack of vitamin D or its active metabolites, but it can also be caused by hypophosphataemia or severe calcium deficiency.

Pathology

In *rickets* the characteristic changes arise from the inability to calcify the intercellular matrix in the deepest layers of the physis. The cellular part of the physis is thicker than normal but the newly formed bone in the metaphysis is weak and may be indented and cup-shaped. Further away from the physis, the changes are essentially those of osteomalacia.

Osteomalacia is characterized by the appearance of thin trabeculae surrounded by unusually wide uncalcified osteoid seams. In mild cases the bones may look normal but they can be more easily crushed and fractured. In severe cases the long-bone cortices are thinner than normal and may show signs of new or old stress fractures. Vertebral compression fractures are common. In the most advanced cases there may be severe bone deformities.

VITAMIN D DEFICIENCY RICKETS

Vitamin D deficiency rickets, once common in Northern Europe owing to a combination of dietary lack and under-exposure to sunlight, is now seldom seen in its classic form. Infants may present with tetany or convulsions. There is failure to thrive, listlessness and muscular flaccidity.

Early bone changes are deformity of the skull (craniotabes) and thickening of the knees, ankles and wrists from physeal overgrowth. Enlargement of the costochondral junctions ('rickety rosary') and lateral indentation of the chest (Harrison's sulcus) may also appear. Distal tibial bowing has been attributed to sitting or lying cross-legged.

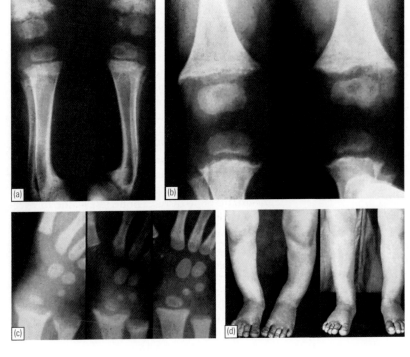

7.9 Rickets (a,b) Typical metaphyseal x-ray changes in florid rickets. (c) Wrist x-rays showing progressive improvement with treatment. (d) Corrective osteotomy may be needed in neglected cases.

Once the child stands, lower limb deformities increase and stunting of growth may be obvious. In severe rickets there may be spinal curvature, coxa vara and bending or fractures of the long bones.

X-rays

In active rickets there is thickening and widening of the physes, distortion of the metaphyses and, sometimes, bowing of the long bones. These changes often leave traces after healing.

Investigations

Serum calcium and phosphate concentrations are diminished and alkaline phosphatase is increased. Urinary calcium excretion is diminished.

Treatment

Untreated patients develop long-bone deformities which may later require corrective osteotomy. The condition responds rapidly to vitamin D administration in the form of calciferol 400–1000 IU per day. After normal growth, residual deformities are usually slight.

HYPOPHOSPHATAEMIC RICKETS

Chronic hypophosphataemia occurs in a number of disorders in which there is impaired renal tubular reabsorption of phosphate. Calcium levels are normal but bone mineralization is defective.

Familial hypophosphataemic rickets (vitamin D-resistant rickets)

This is probably the commonest form of rickets seen today. It is an X-linked genetic disorder with dominant inheritance, starting in infancy or soon after and causing severe bony deformity. The children are below normal height, and deformities such as genu valgum or genu varum are common. There is no myopathy. *X-rays* show changes similar to those of vitamin D-deficiency rickets. Serum calcium levels are normal but phosphate is reduced.

Treatment

Treatment is by large doses of vitamin D (50 000 IU or more) and up to 4 g of inorganic phosphate per day (with careful monitoring to prevent overdosage), continued until growth ceases.

Bony deformities may require bracing or osteotomy. If the child needs to be immobilized, vitamin D must be stopped temporarily to prevent hypercalcaemia from the combined effects of treatment and disuse bone resorption.

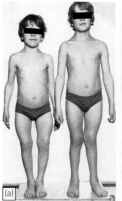
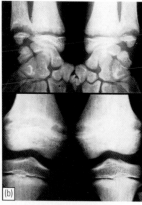

7.10 Familial hypophosphataemic rickets (a) These brothers presented with knee deformities; their x-rays (b) show the typical features of rickets. The physes are increased in depth and the cup-shaped deformities of the metaphyses are particularly well shown in the ulna on each side.

OSTEOMALACIA IN ADULTS

Osteomalacia may result from defects anywhere along the metabolic pathway for vitamin D: nutritional lack, under-exposure to sunlight, intestinal malabsorption or defective conversion to the active metabolites in the liver or kidney.

Clinical features

Symptoms usually appear insidiously and are rather vague. Bone pain, backache and muscle weakness may be present for years before the diagnosis is made. Unexplained pain in the hip or one of the long bones may presage a stress fracture. Often the condition is suspected only when the patient is admitted to hospital with a vertebral compression fracture or an 'insufficiency fracture' of the femur or tibia.

Some of these patients have been living alone, on a poor diet and with little exposure to sunlight. Others are immigrants who have moved from sunny climates to countries with long winters, perhaps retaining customary diets which are lacking in vitamin D. Others again suffer from intestinal malabsorption or disorders of the liver or kidney which affect conversion of vitamin D to the active metabolites. All of these diagnostic possibilities should be explored.

X-rays

Suspicious features are generalized rarefaction of bone and signs of previous fractures of the vertebrae, ribs, pubic rami or long bones. Almost pathognomic is the Looser zone, a thin transverse

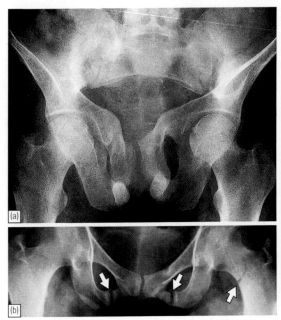

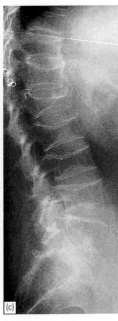

7.11 Osteomalacia Three characteristic features of osteomalacia: (a) indentation of the pelvic walls producing the 'trefoil pelvis'; (b) Looser's zones (stress fractures) in the pubic rami and left femoral neck; (c) biconcave vertebrae.

band of rarefaction due to a poorly healing stress fracture. There may also be signs of secondary hyperparathyroidism.

Investigations

Serum calcium and phosphate concentrations may be diminished, and alkaline phosphatase is raised. More significant are diminished values for 25-HCC and 1,25-DHCC. Biochemical changes are often insignificant and biopsy may be needed for diagnosis; excessive amounts of unmineralized osteoid can be demonstrated.

Having made the diagnosis, it is still necessary to establish the cause. Patients should be investigated for malabsorption syndromes, liver disorders and renal disease.

Treatment

Treatment with vitamin D and calcium supplements is usually effective. Elderly people often need large doses of vitamin D (up to 2000 IU per day). Underlying disorders of the gut, liver or kidney will need treatment as well.

Adult hypophosphataemia

Although rare, this must be remembered as a cause of unexplained bone loss in adults. Patients may also complain of joint pains. The condition responds dramatically to treatment with phosphate, vitamin D and calcium.

HYPERPARATHYROIDISM

Excessive secretion of PTH may be *primary* (usually due to parathyroid adenoma or hyperplasia), *secondary* (due to persistent hypocalcaemia) or *tertiary* (when secondary hyperplasia leads to autonomous over-activity).

Pathology

The cardinal feature of hyperparathyroidism is a rise in serum calcium. Over-production of PTH enhances calcium conservation by stimulating tubular reabsorption and intestinal absorption as well as osteoclastic resorption of bone. The resulting hypercalcaemia so increases glomerular filtration of calcium that there is hypercalciuria despite the augmented tubular reabsorption. Urinary phosphate also is increased, owing to suppressed tubular reabsorption.

The effects of these changes are seen in the *kidneys* (calcinosis, stone formation, recurrent infection and impaired function), the *bones* (osteoporosis and subperiosteal erosions) and in the general manifestations of *hypercalcaemia*, including calcification of soft tissues. In severe cases osteoclastic hyperactivity produces endosteal cavitation and replacement of the marrow spaces by vascular granulations and fibrous tissue *(osteitis fibrosa cystica)*. Haemorrhage and giant-cell reaction within the fibrous stroma may give rise to brownish, tumour-like masses, whose liquefaction leads to fluid-filled cysts *(brown tumours)*.

Clinical features

Primary hyperparathyroidism is quite common; the usual cause is a solitary adenoma in one of the small parathyroid glands.

Patients are middle-aged (40–65 years) and women are affected twice as often as men. Many remain asymptomatic and are diagnosed only because routine biochemistry tests unexpectedly reveal a raised serum calcium level.

Symptoms are due mainly to hypercalcaemia: anorexia, nausea, abdominal pain, depression, fatigue and muscle weakness. Patients may also develop polyuria, kidney stones or nephrocalcinosis due to chronic hypercalciuria. Some complain of joint symptoms, due to chondrocalcinosis. Only a minority (probably less than 10 per cent) present with bone disease – and this is usually generalized osteoporosis rather than the classic features of osteitis fibrosa, bone cysts and pathological fractures.

> A rhyme for hypercalcaemia: 'Moans, stones and porotic bones'.

X-rays

Typical features are osteoporosis (sometimes including vertebral collapse) and areas of cortical erosion. Hyperparathyroid 'brown tumours' should be considered in the differential diagnosis of atypical cyst-like lesions of long bones. However, the classic – and almost pathognomonic – feature, which should always be sought, is subperiosteal cortical resorption of the middle phalanges. Non-specific features of hypercalcaemia are renal calculi, nephrocalcinosis and chondrocalcinosis.

Investigations

Biochemical tests show hypercalcaemia, hypophosphataemia and a raised serum PTH concentration. Serum alkaline phosphatase may be raised.

Treatment

Treatment is usually conservative and includes adequate hydration and decreased calcium intake. If an adenoma is present, it should be removed. The indications for parathyroidectomy are marked and unremitting hypercalcaemia, recurrent renal calculi, progressive nephrocalcinosis and severe osteoporosis.

Postoperatively there is a danger of severe hypocalcaemia due to brisk formation of new bone (the 'hungry bone syndrome'). This must be treated promptly, with one of the fast-acting vitamin D metabolites.

Secondary hyperparathyroidism

Secondary hyperparathyroidism is sometimes seen in rickets and osteomalacia, and accounts for some of the radiological features in these disorders. Treatment is directed at the primary condition.

RENAL OSTEODYSTROPHY

This condition must not be confused with renal tubular phosphate-losing disorders which give rise to hypophosphataemic rickets (page 63).

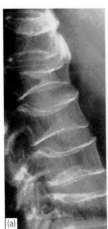
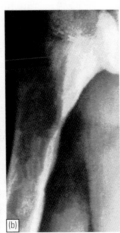
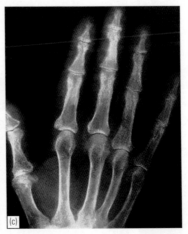

7.12 Hyperparathyroidism (a) Spinal osteoporosis is typical. This patient also complained of pain in the right arm; an x-ray (b) showed cortical erosion of the humerus. Other signs included typical erosions of the phalangeal cortices (c).

Patients with *chronic renal failure* are liable to develop diffuse bone changes due to a combination of rickets or osteomalacia, secondary hyperparathyroidism, osteoporosis and osteosclerosis. Uraemia and phosphate retention are accompanied by a fall in serum calcium which is due partly to the hyperphosphataemia and partly to 1,25-DHCC deficiency. It is now recognized that the bone changes are aggravated by aluminium retention or contamination of dialysis fluids.

Renal abnormalities precede the bone changes by several years. Children are clinically more severely affected than adults: they are stunted, pasty-faced, and have marked rachitic deformities. Myopathy is common.

X-rays

Children show features similar to those of severe rickets. Those with long-standing disease may present with epiphyseal displacement (see Fig. 7.13b). Osteosclerosis is seen mainly in the axial skeleton and is more common in young patients. Signs of secondary hyperparathyroidism can be widespread and severe.

Biochemical features

Characteristic changes are low serum calcium, high serum phosphate and elevated alkaline phosphatase levels. Urinary excretion of calcium and phosphate is diminished. Plasma PTH levels may be raised.

Treatment

Renal failure, if irreversible, may require haemodialysis or renal transplantation.

The osteodystrophy should be treated, in the first instance, with large doses of vitamin D (up to 500 000 IU daily); in resistant cases, small doses of 1,25-DHCC may be effective. Epiphyseolysis may need internal fixation, and residual deformities can be corrected once the disease is under control.

SCURVY

Vitamin C (ascorbic acid) deficiency causes failure of collagen synthesis and osteoid formation. The result is osteoporosis, which in infants is most marked in the juxtaepiphyseal bone. Spontaneous bleeding is common and may cause subperiosteal haematomas.

The infant is irritable and anaemic. The gums may be spongy and bleeding. Subperiosteal haemorrhage causes excruciating pain and tenderness near the large joints. Fractures or epiphyseal separations may occur.

X-rays show generalized bone rarefaction, most marked in the long-bone metaphyses. The normal calcification in growing cartilage produces dense bands in the juxtaepiphyseal metaphyses and around the ossific centres of the epiphyses (the 'ring sign'). The metaphyses may be deformed or fractured. Subperiosteal haematomas show as soft-tissue swellings or periosseous calcification.

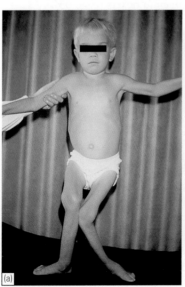
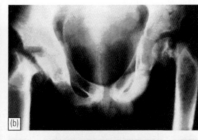
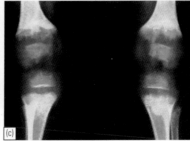

7.13 Renal glomerular osteodystrophy (a) This young boy with chronic renal failure developed severe deformities of (b) the hips and (c) knees. Note the displacement of the upper femoral epiphyses.

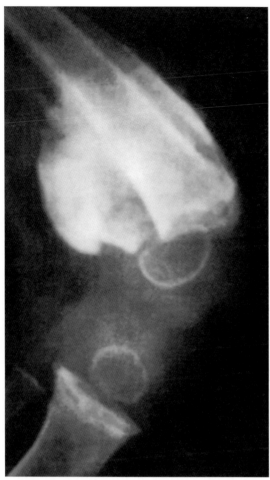

7.14 Scurvy A calcified subperiosteal haematoma may be mistaken for a tumour. Note the typical 'ring sign' in the femoral and tibial epiphyses.

Treatment with large doses of vitamin C produces prompt recovery.

FLUOROSIS

Fluorosis is fairly common in those parts of the world where fluoride appears in the soil and drinking water. Mottling of the teeth is a fairly common manifestation, and in areas where fluoride concentrations in the drinking water are particularly high, widespread skeletal abnormalities are occasionally encountered. Characteristic features in severe cases are sub-periosteal new-bone accretion and osteosclerosis, together with hyperostosis at the bony attachments of ligaments and tendons. Despite the apparent thickening and 'density' of the skeleton, the bones

fracture more easily under bending and twisting loads.

Patients complain of backache, bone pain and joint stiffness. Sometimes the first clinical manifestation is a stress fracture.

The typical x-ray features are osteosclerosis, osteophytosis and ossification of ligamentous and fascial attachments. Changes are most marked in the spine and pelvis, where the bones become densely opaque.

There is no specific treatment for this condition. After exposure ceases, it still takes years for bone fluoride to be excreted.

PAGET'S DISEASE (OSTEITIS DEFORMANS)

Paget's disease is characterized by enlargement and thickening of the bone, but the internal architecture is abnormal and the bone is unusually brittle. The condition has a curious ethnic and geographic distribution, being relatively common in North America, Britain, Germany and Australia (more than 3 per cent of people aged over 40) but rare in Asia, Africa and the Middle East. The cause is unknown.

Pathology

Any bone may be affected; in the worst cases many are involved. Cortices are thickened but irregular, at one stage more porous than usual and at another more sclerotic. This is due to alternating phases of rapid bone resorption and formation. While resorption predominates (the 'vascular' stage), the bone is easily deformed; in the late stage the bone becomes increasingly sclerotic and brittle. The characteristic cellular change is a marked increase in osteoclastic and osteoblastic activity.

Clinical features

Paget's disease affects men and women equally. Only occasionally does it present in patients under the age of 50, but from that age onwards it becomes increasingly common. The disease may remain localized to a single bone for many years, the pelvis and tibia being the commonest sites, and the femur, skull, spine and clavicle the next commonest.

Most people with Paget's disease are asymptomatic, the disorder being diagnosed when an x-ray is taken for some unrelated condition or after the incidental discovery of a raised serum alkaline phosphatase level. When pain occurs it is dull and constant.

Deformities are seen mainly in the lower limbs. The limb looks bent and feels thick, and the skin is unduly warm. If the skull is affected, it enlarges; the patient may complain that old hats no longer fit. The skull base may become flattened (platybasia), giving the appearance of a short neck. In generalized Paget's disease there may also be considerable kyphosis, so the patient becomes shorter and ape-like, with bent legs and arms.

Cranial nerve compression may lead to impaired vision, facial palsy, trigeminal neuralgia or deafness. Vertebral thickening may cause spinal cord or nerve root compression.

X-rays

The appearances are so striking that the diagnosis is seldom in doubt. During the resorptive phase there may be localized areas of osteolysis; later the bone becomes thick and sclerotic, with coarse trabeculation. Occasionally the diagnosis is made only when the patient presents with a pathological fracture.

Investigations

Serum calcium and phosphate levels are usually normal. The most useful test is measurement of the serum alkaline phosphatase level, which correlates with the activity and extent of disease.

Twenty-four-hour urinary excretion of pyridinoline cross-links is a good indicator of disease activity and bone resorption.

Complications

Fractures

Fractures are common, especially in the weight-bearing bones. The fracture line is usually partly transverse and partly oblique, like the line of section of a felled tree. In the femur there is a high rate of non-union; for femoral neck fractures prosthetic replacement and for shaft fractures early internal fixation are recommended.

Nerve compression and spinal stenosis

Occasionally this is the first abnormality to be detected, and may call for definitive surgical treatment.

Bone sarcoma

Osteosarcoma arising in an elderly patient is almost always due to malignant transformation in Paget's disease. The frequency of malignant change is probably around 1 per cent. It should always be suspected if a known site of Paget's disease becomes more painful, swollen or tender. The prognosis is extremely grave.

High-output cardiac failure

Though rare, this is an important general complication. It is due to prolonged, increased bone blood flow.

Hypercalcaemia

Patients who are immobilized for long periods may develop hypercalcaemia.

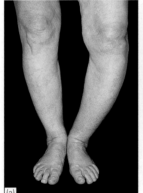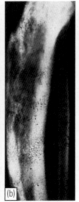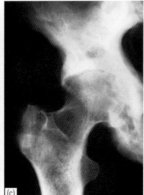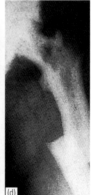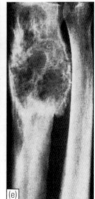

(a) (b) (c) (d) (e)

7.15 Paget's disease (a) Deformity of the tibia due to Paget's disease. (b) X-ray shows that the bone is thickened, coarsened and bent. Complications include (c) erosive arthritis in a nearby joint; (d) fracture; and (e) osteosarcoma of the affected bone.

Treatment

Most patients with Paget's disease never have any symptoms and require no treatment. Indeed, there is no specific therapy, but drugs such as calcitonin and bisphosphonates can control the disease by suppressing bone turnover. Patients should be examined regularly for signs of increased bone activity, such as local tenderness and warmth, or a rise in the alkaline phosphatase level.

The indications for specific treatment are: (1) persistent bone pain; (2) repeated fractures; (3) neurological complications; (4) high-output cardiac failure; (5) hypercalcaemia due to immobilization; and (6) preparation for major bone surgery where there is a risk of excessive haemorrhage.

Calcitonin is the most widely used. It reduces bone resorption by decreasing both the activity and the number of osteoclasts; serum alkaline phosphatase and urinary hydroxyproline levels are lowered. Maintenance injections once or twice weekly may have to be continued indefinitely, but some authorities advocate stopping the drug and resuming treatment if symptoms recur.

Bisphosphonates bind to hydroxyapatite crystals, inhibiting their rate of growth and dissolution. It is claimed that the reduction in bone turnover following their use is associated with the formation of lamellar rather than woven bone and that, even after treatment is stopped, there may be prolonged remission of disease. Etidronate can be given orally (always on an empty stomach) but dosage should be kept low lest impaired bone mineralization results in osteomalacia.

The newer bishosphonates, such as pamidronate and alendronate, are more effective and produce remissions even with short courses of 1 or 2 weeks.

Operative treatment may be needed for a pathological fracture. An osteosarcoma, if detected early, may be resectable, but generally the prognosis is grave.

ENDOCRINE DISORDERS

The endocrine system plays an important part in skeletal growth and maturation, as well as the maintenance of bone turnover. The anterior lobe of the pituitary gland directly affects growth; it also controls the activities of the thyroid, the gonads and the adrenal cortex, each of which has its own influence on bone. Thus endocrine abnormalities may cause problems at several levels: (a) local effects due to glandular enlargement (e.g. pressure on cranial nerves from a pituitary adenoma); (b) over-secretion or under-secretion of hormone by the primarily affected gland; and (c) over-activity or under-activity of other glands which are controlled by the primary dysfunctional gland.

For the sake of clarity, the descriptions which follow have been somewhat simplified.

PITUITARY DYSFUNCTION

The *posterior lobe* of the pituitary gland has no influence on the musculoskeletal system. The *anterior lobe* is responsible for the secretion of pituitary growth hormone, as well as thyrotropic, gonadotropic and adrenocorticotropic hormones.

Hypopituitarism

Anterior pituitary hyposecretion may be caused by *intrinsic disorders* (such as infarction, haemorrhage and intrapituitary tumours) or by *extrinsic lesions* (such as a craniopharyngioma) which press on the anterior lobe of the pituitary. Space-occupying lesions are likely to have other intracranial pressure effects.

Children

In childhood and adolescence, two distinct clinical disorders are encountered. In the *Lorain syndrome* the predominant effect is on growth: the child fails to grow but the body proportions are normal. In *Fröhlich's syndrome* delayed skeletal maturation is associated with adiposity and hypogonadism. Weakness of the physes combined with disproportionate adiposity may result in slipping of the proximal femoral or proximal tibial epiphyses.

Adults

Panhypopituitarism causes a variety of symptoms and signs, including those of cortisol and sex-hormone deficiency. The only important skeletal effect is premature osteoporosis.

Treatment

Treatment will depend on the cause and the degree of dwarfism. If a tumour is identified (e.g. a craniopharyngioma), it can be removed or ablated.

Growth-hormone deficiency has been successfully treated by the administration of biosynthetic growth hormone (somatotropin). The response should be checked by serial plots on the growth chart.

Hyperpituitarism

Over-secretion of pituitary growth hormone is usually due to an acidophil adenoma. The effects vary according to the age of onset.

Gigantism

Growth-hormone over-secretion in childhood and adolescence causes excessive growth of the entire

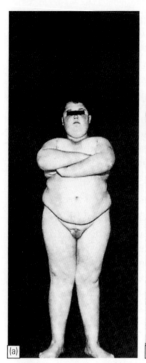
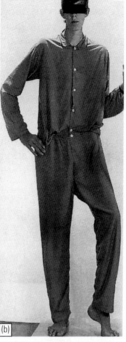

7.16 Endocrine disorders (a) *Hypopituitarism:* a boy of 12 with the unmistakable build of Frölich's syndrome.
(b) *Hyperpituitarism:* this 16-year-old giant suffered from a pituitary adenoma.

skeleton. The condition may be suspected quite early, and it is important to track the child's development by regular clinical and x-ray examination. In addition to being excessively tall, patients may develop deformity of the hip due to epiphyseal displacement.

Treatment is directed at early removal of the pituitary tumour.

Acromegaly

Over-secretion of pituitary growth hormone in adulthood causes enlargement of the bones and soft tissues, but without the very marked elongation that is seen in gigantism. The bones are thickened, rather than lengthened; there is also hypertrophy of articular cartilage, which leads to enlargement of the joints. Bones such as the mandible, the clavicles, ribs, sternum and scapulae, which develop secondary growth centres in late adolescence or early adulthood, may go on growing longer than usual. Thickening of the skull, prominence of the orbital margins, overgrowth of the jaw and enlargement of the nose, lips and tongue produce the characteristic facies of acromegaly. The chest is broad and barrel-shaped and the hands and feet are large. Thickening of the bone ends may cause

secondary osteoarthritis. About 10 per cent of acromegalics develop diabetes, and cardiovascular disease is more common than usual.

Treatment

The indications for operation are the presence of a tumour in childhood and cranial nerve pressure symptoms at any age. Trans-sphenoidal surgery has a high rate of success, provided the diagnosis is made reasonably early and the tumour is not too large.

ADRENOCORTICAL DYSFUNCTION

The adrenal cortex secretes both mineralocorticoids (aldosterone) and glucocorticoids (cortisol). The latter has profound effects on bone and mineral metabolism, causing suppression of osteoblast activity, reduced calcium absorption, increased calcium excretion and enhanced PTH activity. Bone resorption is increased and formation is suppressed.

Hypercortisonism (Cushing's syndrome)

Glucocorticoid excess may be caused by increased pituitary secretion of adrenocorticotrophic hormone (ACTH) – the original Cushing's disease – by independent over-secretion by the adrenal cortex (usually due to a steroid-secreting tumour) or by prolonged or excessive treatment with glucocorticoids (probably the commonest cause). Whatever the cause, the clinical picture is much the same and is generally referred to as *Cushing's syndrome.*

Clinical features

Patients have a characteristic appearance: the face is rounded and looks somewhat puffy ('moon face') and the trunk is obese, often with abdominal striae. However, the legs are quite thin and there may be proximal wasting and weakness.

X-rays

Hypercortisonism is one of the causes of generalized osteoporosis; compression fractures of the vertebrae are common. CT may show an adrenal tumour.

Complications

Wounds and fractures heal slowly, bones provide little purchase for internal fixation, and postoperative infection is more common than usual. A common complication of high-dosage corticosteroid therapy is avascular necrosis (see Chapter 6).

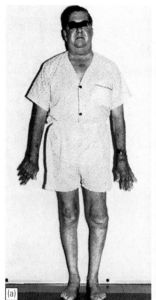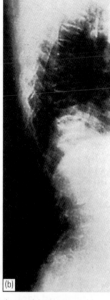

7.17 Cushing's syndrome (a) A patient with rheumatoid arthritis on long-term corticosteroid treatment. (b) On x-ray, the bones look washed-out and there are compression fractures at multiple levels.

Management

Systemic corticosteroids should be used only when essential and in low dosage. If treatment is prolonged, calcium supplements (at least 1500 mg per day) and vitamin D should be given.

THYROID DYSFUNCTION

Hypothyroidism

Congenital hypothyroidism (cretinism) may be caused by developmental abnormalities of the thyroid, but it also occurs in endemic form in areas of iodine deficiency. Unless the condition is treated immediately (and diagnosis at birth is not easy!), the child becomes severely dwarfed and mentally retarded. X-rays may show irregular epiphyseal ossification. Treatment with thyroid hormone is essential.

Hyperthyroidism

Hyperthyroidism in adults may give rise to osteoporosis. Treatment of the primary disorder results in improved bone mass.

CHAPTER 8

GENETIC DISORDERS, DYSPLASIAS AND MALFORMATIONS

Abnormal development of cartilage and bone may give rise to a variety of physical abnormalities which are loosely described as skeletal dysplasias and malformations. Hundreds of such disorders have been described, and more are being added every year as advances in genetic analysis uncover previously unrecognized defects. Conditions affecting the skeletal system can be divided into three broad categories: single gene disorders, chromosome disorders and embryonal damage.

CHROMOSOMES AND GENES

The life-imparting material in the nucleus of every cell is *deoxyribonucleic acid (DNA)*. Each of the 46 *chromosomes* in the cell nucleus consists of a single molecule of DNA; unravelled, it would be several centimetres long, a double-stranded chain along which thousands of segments are defined and demarcated as *genes*. These are the basic units of inherited biological information, each gene coding for the synthesis of a specific protein. Working as a set (or *genome*), they tell the cells how to develop, differentiate and function in specialized ways.

Of the 46 chromosomes in each cell, 44 (the *autosomes*) are disposed in 22 homologous pairs; one strand of each pair, carrying the same type of genetic information, is derived from each parent. The remaining two are the *sex chromosomes*:

females have two X chromosomes (one from each parent); males have one X chromosome (from the mother) and one Y chromosome (from the father).

Each gene occurs at a specific point, or locus, on the chromosome. Since the chromosomes are paired, there are two forms, or *alleles*, of each gene (one maternal, one paternal) at each locus; if the two alleles coding for a particular trait are identical, it is said to be a *homozygous* trait; if they are not identical, it is a *heterozygous* trait.

The full genetic make-up of an individual is called the *genotype*. The finished person – a product of inherited traits and environmental forces – is the *phenotype*.

An important part of the unique human genotype is the *major histocompatibility complex (MHC)*, also known as the *HLA system* (after human leucocyte antigen). This is a cluster of genes on chromosome 6 that is responsible for immunological specificity.

Single gene disorders

Gene mutation may occur by insertion, deletion, substitution or fusion of amino acids or nucleotides in the DNA chain. This can have profound consequences for cartilage growth, collagen structure, matrix patterning and marrow cell metabolism. The abnormality is then passed on to future generations according to simple mendelian rules (see below). There are literally thousands of single gene disorders, accounting for more than 5 per cent of child deaths, yet it is rare to see any one of them in an orthopaedic practice.

Chromosome disorders

Changes in chromosomal structure usually have serious consequences, the affected fetuses being either stillborn or developing with severe physical and mental abnormalities. Unlike genetic disorders, these conditions are not transmitted in future generations.

Embryonal damage

Many fetal abnormalities result from injury to the developing embryo. Most are of unknown aetiology but some are due to specific teratogenic agents which damage the embryo or the placenta during the first few months of gestation. Suspected or known teratogens include viral infections (e.g. rubella), certain drugs (e.g. thalidomide) and ionizing radiation. The resulting defects are usually asymmetrical and localized, ranging from mild anatomical faults to severe malformations such as non-development of an entire limb.

Patterns of inheritance

If it is certain that both parents of a child with a genetic disorder are normal, the defect must have been caused by a *mutant gene*. From then, the genetic abnormality will be transmitted to future offspring according to well-defined patterns of inheritance, which may be either *autosomal* or *X-linked,* and *dominant* or *recessive*.

Autosomal dominant transmission means that the abnormality is inherited even if only one allele of a pair is abnormal, i.e. only one parent need have been affected and the condition is *heterozygous.* In that case, half the children of either sex are likely to develop the disease, though it may appear in varying degrees of severity *(variable expressivity).*

Autosomal recessive transmission means that both alleles of a pair have to be abnormal for the child to be affected, i.e. the condition is *homozygous.* Each parent contributes a faulty gene, though if both are heterozygous, they themselves will be clinically normal. Theoretically, one in four of their children will then be homozygous sufferers, two out of four will be *heterozygous carriers* of the faulty gene and one will be completely normal. It is easy to see why the rare recessive disorders are seen mainly in the children of consanguineous marriages or in closed communities where many people are related to each other.

X-linked disorders are caused by a faulty gene in the X chromosome. Characteristically, therefore, they never pass directly from father to son because the father's X chromosome inevitably goes to the daughter and the Y chromosome to the son. The best known example is haemophilia: an affected man will have normal children but all his daughters will be carriers and half of his sons will be bleeders.

Genetic markers

Many common disorders show an unusually close association with certain blood groups, tissue types or other serum proteins that occur with higher than expected frequency in the patients and their relatives. These are referred to as genetic markers. A good example is ankylosing spondylitis: more than 90 per cent of patients and 60 per cent of their first-degree relatives are positive for HLA-B27.

DIAGNOSIS

Prenatal diagnosis

Many genetic disorders can be diagnosed before birth, thus giving the parents the choice of elective abortion. *High-resolution ultrasound imaging* is harmless and is now done almost routinely. On the other hand, tests that involve *amniocentesis* or *chorionic villus sampling* carry a risk of injury to the fetus and are therefore used only when there is an increased likelihood of some abnormality, e.g. if the mother is over 35 years old or if there is a history of previous chromosomal or genetic abnormalities.

Diagnosis in childhood

Physical abnormalities may be obvious *at birth,* for example disproportionately short limbs, suggesting achondroplasia. *During infancy,* the reasons for presentation are failure to grow normally, disproportionate shortness of the limbs, delay in walking or repeated fractures.

Older children are more obviously abnormal. Features which attract attention are retarded growth, deformities of the spine and/or limbs, unusual facial characteristics and a history of repeated fractures. *Remember, though, that multiple fractures in different stages of healing are also suggestive of non-accidental injury* (the 'battered baby' syndrome).

The *family history* is important and may reveal a characteristic pattern of inheritance. Remember, however, that even an apparently normal parent may be very mildly affected, a fact which will not come out if one relies entirely on the 'history', without the benefit of direct observation.

Special investigations may be indicated to identify specific enzyme or metabolic abnormalities.

Presentation in adults

Dysmorphic individuals who reach adulthood may lead active lives, marry and have children of their own. Nevertheless, they often seek medical advice for problems such as abnormally short stature, local bone deformities, spinal stenosis, repeated fractures, secondary osteoarthritis or joint instability. As in children, family history and special investigations for enzyme or metabolic abnormalities are important.

Note. When dealing with these patients, terms such as 'dwarf' and 'dwarfism' should be avoided, as they are often perceived to have pejorative associations.

PRINCIPLES OF MANAGEMENT

Management should address not only the problems which the patient will encounter as he or she grows up, but also the needs and concerns of the entire family. This involves treatment of the genetic defect or its immediate effects, prevention and correction of developmental deformities, and counselling.

Specific treatment

The ideal form of treatment would be modification or replacement of the faulty gene. For the present, however, treatment is directed mainly at identifying the defining protein or enzyme abnormality resulting from the genetic defect and then, where possible, administering the essential ingredient that will restore physiological function or counteract the pathological effects of the abnormality. One example is the treatment of Gaucher's disease by administering the missing enzyme, alglucerase.

Correction of deformities

Bony deformities, if they interfere with function, should be corrected and joint replacement may be needed in later life. Severe spinal anomalies may be amenable to corrective surgery, but such operations should be performed only in specialized units. Limb lengthening is occasionally performed for people with abnormally short stature.

Counselling

This should include a full explanation of the problem and expert advice about the risks for future children.

 Growth disorders affecting the spine may cause odontoid hypoplasia and atlantoaxial instability; this calls for special care during anaesthesia.

CLASSIFICATION

There is no completely satisfactory classification of developmental disorders. The same genetic abnormality may be expressed in different ways, while a variety of gene defects may cause almost

Table 8.1 A practical grouping of generalized developmental disorders

---

1. **Genetic disorders of cartilage and bone growth (chondro-osteodystrophies)**
   Dysplasias with predominantly physeal and metaphyseal changes
   Hereditary multiple exostosis
   Achondroplasia
   Hypochondroplasia
   Metaphyseal chondrodysplasia
   Dyschondroplasia (enchondromatosis, Ollier's disease)

   Dysplasias with predominantly epiphyseal changes
   Multiple epiphyseal dysplasia
   Spondyloepiphyseal dysplasia

   Dysplasias with predominantly diaphyseal changes
   Osteopetrosis (marble bones, Albers–Schönberg disease)
   Diaphyseal dysplasia (Engelmann's disease, Camurati's disease)
   Candle bones, spotted bones and striped bones

2. **Collagen disorders**
   Osteogenesis imperfecta (brittle bones)
   Mild
   Lethal
   Severe
   Moderate

   Generalized joint laxity

   Ehlers–Danlos syndrome

   Larsen's syndrome

3. **Enzyme defects and metabolic disorders**
   Mucopolysaccharidoses
   Hurler's syndrome (MPS I)
   Hunter's syndrome (MPS II)
   Morquio–Brailsford syndrome (MPS IV)

   Gaucher's disease

   Homocystinuria

   Alkaptonuria

4. **Chromosome disorders**
   Down's syndrome

identical clinical syndromes. The grouping presented in Table 8.1 is no more than a convenient way of cataloguing the least rare of the clinical syndromes. Only a few representative conditions are described in this chapter.

DISORDERS OF CARTILAGE AND BONE GROWTH

HEREDITARY MULTIPLE EXOSTOSIS (DIAPHYSEAL ACLASIS)

This, the most common of all skeletal dysplasias, is a congenital disorder in which multiple exostoses appear at the metaphyses as the child grows. It is inherited by autosomal dominant transmission and appears to represent a failure of growth-plate modelling.

Each exostosis is covered by a cartilage cap and is, effectively, an osteochondroma; it grows only while the child grows and any enlargement after that may herald malignant change to a chondrosarcoma. The failure of modelling results in deformities of the long bones.

Clinical features

The condition is usually discovered in childhood; hard lumps appear at the ends of the long bones and along the apophyseal borders of the scapula and pelvis. The child may be slightly short, with bowing of the forearms and valgus knees.

Occasionally one of the lumps becomes tender or causes trouble due to pressure on a tendon.

X-rays show the pathognomonic exostoses as well as broadening and lumpiness of the metaphyses.

Management

If an exostosis is troublesome (and certainly if it starts to 'grow' after the parent bone has stopped), it should be removed.

ACHONDROPLASIA

This is the classic example of chondrodysplasia, and the commonest form of short-limbed diminution of stature. It is inherited as an autosomal dominant trait, but because most of the affected individuals do not have children, new cases usually appear sporadically due to gene mutation.

Clinical features

Severe, disproportionate shortening of the limb bones may be diagnosed by x-ray before birth. The abnormality is certainly obvious in childhood: growth is severely stunted, the limbs (particularly the proximal segments) are disproportionately short, and the skull is quite large with prominent forehead and saddle-shaped nose. The fingers appear stubby and somewhat splayed (trident hands). The trunk seems too long by comparison

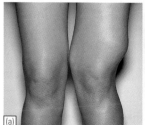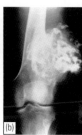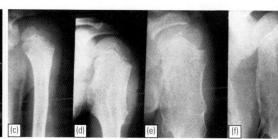

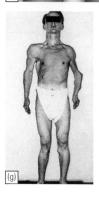

8.1 Hereditary multiple exostosis (a) The patient (or a parent) notices a hard 'bump' close to a joint; the x-ray (b) shows it to be an exostosis – actually an osteochondroma. This turns out to be one of several such lesions and serial x-rays (c–f) reveal more extensive defects in bone growth. (g) Adult with multiple exostoses and typical deformities of the arms and legs.

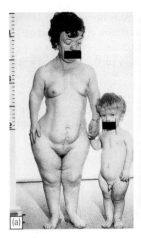
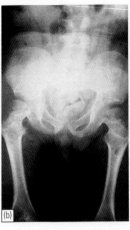
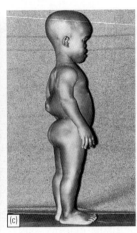

8.2 Achondroplasia
(a) Mother and child with the typical features of achondroplasia. (b) X-ray showing the short femora and flat pelvis. (c) Some children develop a prominent thoracolumbar gibbus.

with the limbs, and the posture when standing is typical: the back is excessively lordotic, the buttocks prominent, the hips flexed, the legs bowed and the elbows bent. In infancy there is often a thoracolumbar gibbus, which disappears after a few years.

These features are more striking in adults, whose height is usually around 122 cm (48 inches). In addition, shortening of the vertebral pedicles may lead to lumbar spinal stenosis.

X-rays show the short bones, anteroposterior narrowing of the pelvis and, sometimes, changes in the spine.

Diagnosis

Achondroplasia should not be confused with other types of short-limbed dysplasia. In some (e.g. Morquio's disease), the shortening affects distal segments more than proximal and there may be widespread associated abnormalities. Others (e.g. the epiphyseal dysplasias) are distinguished by the fact that the head and face are quite normal whereas the epiphyses show characteristic changes on x-ray examination.

Management

During childhood, operative treatment may be needed for lower limb deformities (usually genu varum). Occasionally the thoracolumbar kyphosis fails to correct itself; if there is significant deformity (angulation of more than 40 degrees) by the age of 5 years, there is a risk of cord compression and operative correction may be needed.

During adulthood, spinal stenosis may require decompression. Intervertebral disc prolapse superimposed on a narrow spinal canal should be treated as an emergency.

Advances in methods of external fixation have made lower limb lengthening a feasible option. However, there are drawbacks: complications, including non-union, infection and nerve palsy, may be disastrous – and the cosmetic effect of long legs and short arms may be less pleasing than anticipated.

MULTIPLE EPIPHYSEAL DYSPLASIA (MED)

This is a familial disorder (autosomal dominant) in which the long-bone epiphyses develop abnormally.

Clinical features

Children may present with stunted growth or, occasionally, with joint pain and progressive deformity. The face, skull and spine are normal. In adult life, residual bone defects may lead to joint incongruity and secondary osteoarthritis.

X-ray changes are apparent from early childhood. Epiphyseal ossification is irregular or abnormal in outline. In the growing child the epiphyses are misshapen, and in the hips this may be mistaken for bilateral Perthes' disease. At maturity, the femoral heads and femoral condyles are flattened; secondary osteoarthritis may ensue and, if many joints are involved, the patient can be severely crippled.

Spondyloepiphyseal dysplasia (SED)

This condition represents a heterogeneous group of disorders in which MED is associated with vertebral changes.

Management

Children may complain of slight pain and limp, but little can (or need) be done about this. At

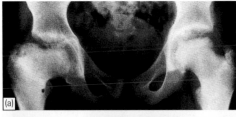

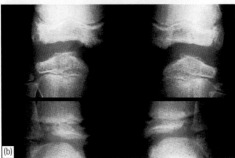

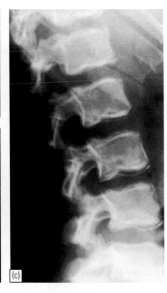

8.3 Multiple epiphyseal dysplasia (a,b) X-rays show epiphyseal distortion and flattening at multiple sites, in this case the hips, knees and ankles. (c) The ring epiphyses of the vertebral bodies also may be affected; in spondyloepiphyseal dysplasia this is the dominant feature.

maturity, bony deformities sometimes require corrective osteotomy. In later life, secondary osteoarthritis may need reconstructive surgery.

Patients with SED may also need treatment for back pain.

COLLAGEN DISORDERS

Heritable defects of collagen synthesis give rise to a number of disorders involving either the soft connective tissues or bone, or both. In many cases the specific collagen defect has now been identified.

OSTEOGENESIS IMPERFECTA

Osteogenesis imperfecta (OI) is one of the commonest of the heritable bone disorders, with an estimated incidence of 1 in 20 000. It is due to defective synthesis of type I collagen, with generalized involvement of the bones, teeth, ligaments, sclerae and skin. It is a heterogeneous condition and there are at least four subgroups showing variations in phenotype and pattern of inheritance. What they have in common are (1) osteopenia, (2) proneness to fracture and (3) laxity of ligaments. About two-thirds of patients have (4) blue sclerae, and about half have (5) 'crumbling teeth', or dentinogenesis imperfecta.

Clinical features

Four clinical types of OI have been identified: mild, lethal, severe and moderately severe.

OI type I (mild)

This, the commonest variety, is a comparatively mild autosomal dominant disorder. Fractures occur throughout life but severe deformity is uncommon. Characteristically the sclerae are blue and the joints are hypermobile.

X-rays show osteopenia and thinning of the cortices. Old fractures are usually evident and there may be some bowing of the long bones.

OI type II (lethal)

This severe, recessive disorder may be diagnosed before birth by x-ray or ultrasound imaging. Some infants are still-born, and those who survive have multiple fractures and deformities of the long bones.

OI type III (severe, deforming)

This is the classic, though not the commonest, form of OI. It is sometimes diagnosed at birth and by the age of 6 years the child has had numerous fractures and has usually developed severe deformities. It is not as severe as type II, but few of the children survive into adulthood; those who do are markedly deformed and disabled.

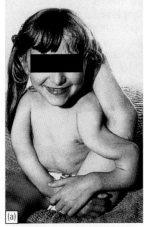

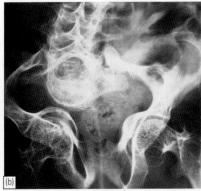

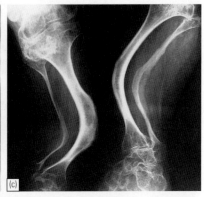

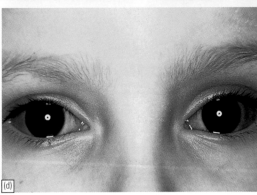

8.4 Osteogenesis imperfecta (a) This young girl had severe deformities of all her limbs, the result of multiple mini-fractures of the long bones over time. This is the classic (type III) form of osteogenesis imperfecta (OI). (b,c) X-ray features in a slightly older patient with the same condition. (d) Blue sclerae usually occur in the milder, type I OI.

OI type IV (moderately severe)

This autosomal dominant disorder is similar to type I but the sclerae are only a pale blue and they become normal in colour during adult life.

Management

The most severe forms of OI defy treatment, and none is indicated apart from sympathetic nursing care. For other types of OI, treatment is aimed at: (1) gentle nursing of infants, to prevent fractures as far as possible; (2) prompt splinting when fractures do occur, to prevent unnecessary deformity; (3) mobilization, to prevent further osteoporosis; and (4) correction of deformities, if necessary by multiple osteotomies, bone realignment and intramedullary fixation.

GENERALIZED JOINT LAXITY

About 5 per cent of people have hypermobile joints. This trait runs in families and is inherited as a mendelian dominant. The condition is not in itself disabling, but it may predispose to congenital

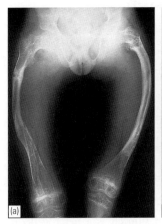

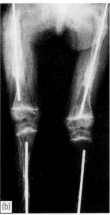

8.5 Osteogenesis imperfecta (a) Moderately severe (type IV) disease. These deformities can be corrected by multiple osteotomies and 'rodding' (b).

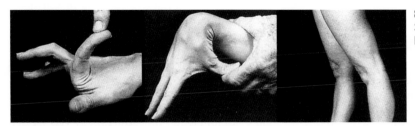

8.6 Generalized joint laxity Simple tests for joint hypermobility.

dislocation of the hip in the newborn or recurrent dislocation of the patella or shoulder in later life. Transient joint pains are common and there is an increased risk of ankle sprains.

MARFAN'S SYNDROME

This is a generalized autosomal dominant disorder affecting the bones, ligaments, eyes and cardiovascular structures. It is thought to be due to a cross-linkage defect in collagen and elastin.

Clinical features

Patients are tall, with disproportionately long legs and arms; typically, arm span exceeds height. The digits are unusually long, giving rise to the term 'arachnodactyly' or 'spider fingers'. Spinal abnormalities include spondylolisthesis and scoliosis. There is an increased incidence of slipped upper femoral epiphysis. Generalized joint laxity is usual and patients may develop flat-feet or dislocation of the patella or shoulder. Associated abnormalities include a high arched palate, hernias,

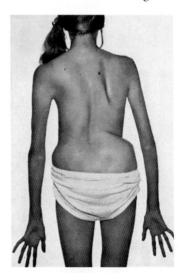

8.7 Marfan's syndrome The combination of disproportionately long arms, 'spider fingers' and scoliosis is characteristic.

lens dislocation, retinal detachment, aortic aneurysm and mitral or aortic incompetence.

Management

Patients occasionally need treatment for progressive scoliosis or flat-feet. The heart should be carefully checked before operation.

EHLERS–DANLOS SYNDROME

Ehlers–Danlos syndrome (EDS) designates a heterogeneous group of connective tissue disorders characterized by joint hypermobility, skin laxity and (in some cases) blood vessel fragility. The syndrome comprises at least ten distinct types; almost all cases are associated with autosomal dominant inheritance.

Classic EDS (types I and II)

These account for about 80 per cent of cases. Babies show marked hypotonia. Hypermobility persists and older patients are often capable of bizarre feats of contortion. The skin is soft, hyperelastic and easily damaged. Deformities to look for are sloping shoulders and ribs and thoracolumbar scoliosis.

Type III EDS

In this condition there is marked joint laxity but almost normal skin. Joint dislocation (usually shoulder or patella) is common.

Type IV EDS

These patients usually have neither joint hypermobility nor skin laxity; the effects are seen in blood vessels and internal organs and include arterial rupture, intracranial bleeding, bowel rupture and even uterine rupture. Tissue fragility makes repair of visceral ruptures very difficult.

Other types of EDS

A number of groups show combinations of the above features. They include odd recessive and X-linked disorders.

Management

Complications (e.g. recurrent dislocation or scoliosis) may need treatment. However, if joint laxity is marked, soft-tissue reconstruction usually fails to cure the tendency to dislocation. Blood vessel fragility may cause severe bleeding at operation, and wound healing is often poor.

Joint instability may lead to osteoarthritis, which will require treatment in later life.

NEUROFIBROMATOSIS

Neurofibromatosis is one of the commonest single-gene disorders affecting the skeleton. Two types are recognized: *type 1 (neurofibromatosis, NF-1)* – also known as von Recklinghausen's disease – has an incidence of about 1 in 3500 live births. The abnormality is located in the gene which codes for neurofibromin, on chromosome 17. It is transmitted as autosomal dominant, with almost 100 per cent penetrance, but more than 50 per cent of cases are due to new mutations. The most characteristic lesions are neurofibromata (Schwann cell tumours) and patches of skin pigmentation (*café au lait* spots), but other features are remarkably protean and musculoskeletal abnormalities are seen in almost half of those affected. *Type 2 (NF-2)* is very rare and is seldom associated with skeletal defects.

Clinical features of NF-1

Almost all patients have the typical widespread patches of skin pigmentation and multiple cutaneous neurofibromata which usually appear before puberty. Less common is a single, large plexiform neurofibroma, or an area of soft-tissue overgrowth in one of the limbs.

The orthopaedic surgeon is most likely to encounter the condition in a child or adolescent who presents with *scoliosis;* the most suggestive deformity is a very short, sharp curve. *Local tumours* in the spine can cause symptoms resembling those of disc prolapse, and x-rays may show scalloping of the posterior aspects of the vertebral bodies, erosion of the pedicles or intervertebral foraminal enlargement.

Congenital tibial dysplasia and *pseudarthrosis* are rare conditions, but almost 50 per cent of patients with these lesions have some evidence of neurofibromatosis.

Malignant change occurs in 2–5 per cent of affected individuals and is the most common complication in elderly patients.

Treatment

A local tumour causing nerve compression should be removed. Treatment may be needed also for associated conditions such as scoliosis or tibial pseudarthrosis.

METABOLIC DISORDERS

Many single-gene disorders are expressed as under-secretion of an enzyme that controls a specific stage in the metabolic chain; the undegraded substrate accumulates and may be stored, with harmful effects, in various tissues. All these inborn errors of metabolism are inherited as recessive traits. Two examples involving the musculoskeletal system are the mucopolysaccharidoses and Gaucher's disease.

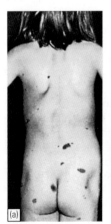
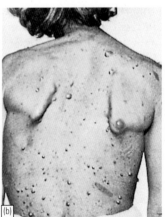
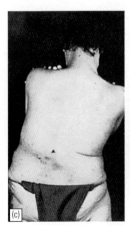
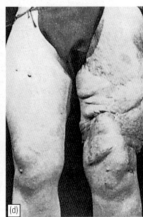

8.8 Neurofibromatosis (a) Café-au-lait spots; (b) multiple neurofibromata and slight scoliosis; (c,d) a patient with scoliosis and soft-tissue overgrowth ('elephantiasis').

MUCOPOLYSACCHARIDOSES

The mucopolysaccharidoses are a group of metabolic disorders in which, because of lack of certain essential degradative enzymes, there is incomplete breakdown and excessive storage of glycosaminoglycans (GAGs). Partially degraded GAGs accumulate in the liver, spleen, bones and other tissues and spill over into the blood and urine, where they can be detected by suitable biochemical tests. These inborn errors of metabolism are inherited as recessive traits.

Clinical features

Depending on the specific enzyme deficiency and the type of GAG storage, at least ten clinical syndromes have been defined. As a group, they have certain recognisable features: marked shortness of stature with vertebral deformity, coarse facies, hepatosplenomegaly and (in some cases) mental retardation. X-rays show bone dysplasia affecting the vertebral bodies, epiphyses and metaphyses; typically, the bones have a spatulate appearance. The diagnosis can be confirmed by testing for abnormal GAG excretion or demonstrating the enzyme deficiency in blood cells or cultured skin fibroblasts.

Management

Specific treatment for these disorders is not yet possible, but enzyme replacement is being developed. Deformities may need correction by osteotomy, though this should be delayed until growth has ceased.

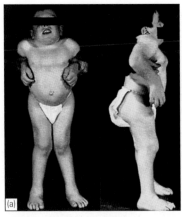
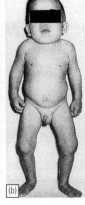

8.9 Mucopolysaccharidoses (a) A young boy showing the characteristic features of Morquio–Brailsford syndrome. (b) A child with Hunter's syndrome.

GAUCHER'S DISEASE

The genetic disorder described by Gaucher more than 100 years ago is caused by lack of a specific enzyme which is responsible for the breakdown and excretion of cell membrane products from defunct cells. This is a classic example of a lipid storage disease with secondary effects in bone.

When cells die, a glucocerebroside is released from the cell membrane; before it can be excreted, the glycoside bond holding the glucose molecule has to be split by a specific enzyme – glucosylceramide β-glucosidase. If this enzyme is lacking, the glucocerebroside cannot be excreted and instead is stored in the lysosomal bodies of macrophages of the reticuloendothelial system, notably in the marrow, spleen and liver. Accumulation of these abnormal macrophages leads to enlargement of the spleen and liver, and secondary changes in the marrow and bone.

Most patients suffer from a chronic form of the disorder, with changes predominantly in the marrow, bone and spleen, and varying degrees of pancytopenia *(Type I)*. A rare form of the disease affecting the central nervous system *(Type II)* appears in infancy and usually causes death within a year. *Type III* is a subacute disorder characterized by the appearance of hepatosplenomegaly in childhood and skeletal and neurological abnormalities during adolescence.

Like other storage disorders, Gaucher's disease is transmitted as an autosomal recessive trait.

Clinical features

Children usually present with pain, and sometimes loss of movement, in one of the larger joints. The spleen may be enlarged (or it may already have been removed!). Older patients may develop back pain due to vertebral osteopenia and compression fractures; femoral neck fractures also are not uncommon. A suggestive finding (when positive) is elevation of the serum acid phosphatase level.

A common complication is *osteonecrosis,* usually of the femoral head. The patient (often a child or adolescent) may present with an acute 'bone crisis': unrelenting pain, local tenderness and restriction of movement accompanied by pyrexia, leucocytosis and an elevated erythrocyte sedimentation rate (ESR). The clinical features resemble those of osteomyelitis or septic arthritis; diagnosis is further confused by the fact that Gaucher's disease predisposes to true bone infection.

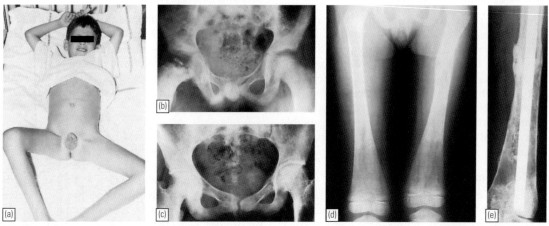

8.10 Gaucher's disease (a) A distressed young boy during an acute Gaucher crisis. The right hip is intensely painful and abduction is restricted. The x-ray (b) shows avascular necrosis of the right femoral head. (c) X-ray of an older patient with a sclerotic left femoral head, the result of previous ischaemic necrosis. (d) Bilateral failure of femoral tubularization (the Erlenmeyer flask appearance). (e) Pathological fractures sometimes occur and can be treated by internal fixation. The sclerotic patches in the interior part of the bone are typical of old medullary infarcts.

Imaging

X-rays may show the distinctive feature of an expanded distal half of femur (the so-called Erlenmeyer flask appearance). Typical signs of osteonecrosis sometimes appear in the femoral head, femoral condyles, talus or humeral head. A *radioisotope bone scan* may help to distinguish a crisis episode from infection: the former is usually 'cold', the latter 'hot'. *MRI* is the most reliable way of defining marrow involvement.

Treatment

Bone pain may need symptomatic treatment. For the acute crisis, analgesic medication and bed-rest followed by a period of non-weight-bearing is recommended. Specific therapy is now available (albeit costly) in the form of the replacement enzyme alglucerase. This has been shown to reverse the blood changes and reduce the size of the liver and spleen. The bone complications also are diminished.

Osteonecrosis of the femoral head may require operative treatment (see Chapter 6).

CHROMOSOME DISORDERS

DOWN'S SYNDROME (TRISOMY 21)

This condition results from having an extra copy of chromosome 21. It is much more common than any of the skeletal dysplasias, with an overall incidence of 1 per 800 live births – and 1 in 250 if the mother is over 37 years of age. Affected infants can be recognized at birth: the head is foreshortened and the eyes slant upwards, with prominent epicanthic folds; the nose is flattened, the lips are parted and the tongue protrudes. There may be abnormal palmar creases, clinodactyly and spreading of the first and second toes. The babies are unusually floppy (hypotonic) and skeletal development is delayed. Children are short and, because of their characteristic facial appearance, they tend to resemble each other. They show varying degrees of mental retardation. Joint laxity may lead to sprains or subluxation (e.g. of the patella).

Associated anomalies, particularly cardiac defects, are common, and there is diminished resistance to infection. Life expectancy is about 35 years.

There is no specific treatment, but surgery can offer considerable cosmetic improvement. Attentive care will allow many of these individuals to pursue a pleasant and productive life.

LOCALIZED MALFORMATIONS

Localized malformations of the vertebrae or limbs are common. The majority cause no disability and may be discovered incidentally during investigation of some other disorder. Some have a genetic background and similar malformations are seen in association with generalized skeletal dysplasia. Most are sporadic and probably non-genetic – i.e. caused by injury to the developing embryo, especially during the first 3 months of pregnancy. In some cases there is a known teratogenic agent, for example maternal infection or drug administration. Usually, however, the exact cause is unknown.

VERTEBRAL ANOMALIES

The commonest vertebral anomaly is spina bifida (see page 102). Others appear as complete *agenesis, hemivertebrae* or *fused vertebrae;* they may lead to severe deformity (kyphoscoliosis) and paralysis. Operative treatment may be needed for cord compression.

In *Sprengel's deformity* there is elevation of the scapula, with or without vertebral anomalies. Treatment is seldom necessary.

LIMB ANOMALIES

These include extra bones, absent bones, hypoplastic bones and fusions. Occasionally a whole limb or part of a limb fails to develop.

These conditions all require specialized reconstructive surgery, often during the first few years of life.

CONGENITAL PSEUDARTHROSIS

A curious anomaly is congenital pseudarthrosis, usually of the tibia. The baby is born with a fractured lower third of tibia, or with a bent fibula which later breaks. The fracture is resistant to conventional methods of treatment, but specialized techniques, including bone-grafting, may be successful.

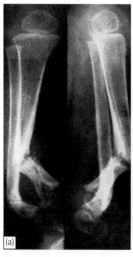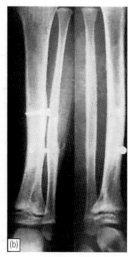

8.11 Congenital pseudarthrosis The tibia is the most common site (a); in this case bone-grafting was successful (b).

CHAPTER 9

TUMOURS

A simple classification of the more common tumours and tumour-like lesions of bone is set out in Table 9.1. It should be remembered, however, that the commonest malignant tumours in bone are metastatic deposits, which are not, strictly speaking, 'bone tumours' (i.e. of mesenchymal origin).

DIAGNOSIS

Most tumours cause *pain, swelling* and local *tenderness;* occasionally a lesion is discovered accidentally during x-ray examination, or as the result of a *pathological fracture.*

It is not always easy to tell whether a bone tumour is benign or malignant, but rapid growth, warmth, tenderness and an ill-defined edge suggest malignancy. If treatment is to be rational, we must know the precise diagnosis and also the extent of the lesion, its relationship to perivascular spaces, and the likelihood of distant spread. Therefore, in all cases of suspected malignancy (and sometimes even with unusual benign lesions), investigations should include high-quality radiography, CT or MRI, bone scanning and a carefully planned biopsy before definitive treatment begins.

Imaging

Plain x-rays are the most useful of all imaging techniques. There may be an obvious abnormality in the bone – a discrete lump, bone destruction, cortical thickening, or something that looks like a 'cyst' in the bone. The site of the lesion, whether solitary or multiple and whether well defined or ill-defined are all helpful clues to the diagnosis.

Remember that 'cystic' lesions are not necessarily hollow cavities: any radiolucent material (e.g. a

Table 9.1 A classification of the less rare primary bone tumours

Cell type	Benign	Malignant
Bone	Osteoid osteoma	Osteosarcoma
Cartilage	Chondroma	Chondrosarcoma
	Osteochondroma	
Fibrous tissue	Fibroma	Fibrosarcoma
Marrow	Haemangioma	Angiosarcoma
Uncertain	Giant-cell tumour	Malignant giant-cell tumour

Ask

Where is the lesion?

Is it solitary or multiple?

Does it look like a cyst?

Is the centre calcified?

Are the margins well defined?

Or poorly defined?

Is there cortical destruction?

Or periosteal reaction?

fibroma or a chondroma) may look like a cyst. If the boundary of the 'cyst' is sharply defined, it is probably benign; if it is hazy and diffuse, it suggests an invasive tumour. Stippled calcification inside a vacant area is characteristic of cartilage tumours.

Look carefully at the bone surfaces and beyond: periosteal new-bone formation and extension of the tumour into the soft tissues are suggestive of malignant change.

> **Periosteal hypertrophy: exclude infection, stress fracture and soft-tissue bruising as well as tumour.**

CT and *MRI* are useful for assessing the true extent of the tumour and its relationship to surrounding structures.

Radionuclide scanning with ^{99m}Tc-HDP shows non-specific reactive changes in bone; this can be helpful in revealing the site of a small tumour (e.g. an osteoid osteoma) or the presence of skip lesions or silent secondary deposits.

Biopsy

With few exceptions, biopsy is essential for both diagnosis and planning of treatment. If sufficient expertise is available, the biopsy can be done with a *large-bore needle;* however, *open biopsy* is more reliable. The site is selected so that it can be included in any subsequent ablative operation. As little as possible of the tumour is exposed and a block of tissue is removed – ideally in the boundary zone, so as to include normal tissue, pseudocapsule and abnormal tissue. A *frozen section* should be examined – not so much to make a definitive diagnosis but to ensure that representative tissue has been obtained. If necessary, several samples can be taken. If bone is removed, the raw area is covered with bone wax or methylmethacrylate cement. If a tourniquet is used, it should be released and full haemostasis achieved before closing the wound. Drains should be avoided, so as to minimize the risk of tumour contamination.

Tumour biopsy should never be regarded as a 'minor' procedure. Complications include haemorrhage, wound breakdown, infection and pathological fracture. The person doing the biopsy should have a clear idea of what may be done next and where operative incisions or skin flaps will be placed. Errors and complications are far less likely if the biopsy is performed in a specialist centre.

For tumours that are almost certainly benign, an *excisional biopsy* is permissible (the entire lesion is removed); with cysts, representative tissue can be obtained by careful curettage.

When dealing with tumours that could be malignant, there is a strong temptation to perform the biopsy as soon as possible; as this may alter the CT and MRI appearances, it is important to delay the operation until all the imaging studies have been completed.

Differential diagnosis

Conditions notorious for mimicking bone tumours are infection and stress fractures.

Chronic osteomyelitis typically causes pain and swelling, and x-rays may show an area of bone destruction in the metaphysis and periosteal new-bone formation. If systemic features have been suppressed by antibiotics, these changes may be mistaken for those of a destructive tumour. Tissue should be submitted for both bacteriological and histological examination.

Stress fractures are another source of misdiagnosis. The patient is often a young adult with localized pain near a large joint; x-rays show a dubious area of cortical 'destruction' and overlying periosteal new bone; if a biopsy is performed, the healing callus may show histological features resembling those of osteosarcoma. Proper consultation between surgeon, radiologist and pathologist should prevent any error.

PRINCIPLES OF TREATMENT

Benign lesions that are asymptomatic

If the diagnosis is beyond doubt, one can temporise: treatment may never be needed. Otherwise a biopsy is advisable, either an excisional biopsy or curettage.

Benign lesions that become symptomatic or start to enlarge

Painful lesions and tumours that continue to enlarge after the end of normal bone growth always require biopsy and confirmation of the diagnosis. Unless they are unusually aggressive, they can generally be removed by complete local excision.

Suspected malignant tumours

If there is any suspicion that the lesion could be a primary malignant tumour, the patient is admitted for detailed assessment in order (a) to confirm the diagnosis, (b) to establish the grade of malignancy and (c) to define precisely how far the tumour has spread. The various treatment options can then be discussed; they include local excision, wide excision with limb sparing, amputation, and different types of adjuvant therapy. The patient must be fully informed about the pros and cons of each.

Tumours are graded according to cytological characteristics which indicate how aggressive they are, i.e. the likelihood of recurrence and spread after surgical removal. *Benign lesions,* by definition, occupy the lowest grade and are usually amenable to local (marginal) excision with little risk of recurrence. *Sarcomas* are divided into *low grade* and *high grade;* the former are only moderately aggressive (the estimated risk of metastasis is less than 25 per cent) and take a long time to metastasize (e.g. secondary chondrosarcoma or parosteal osteosarcoma), whereas the latter are usually very aggressive and metastasize early (e.g. osteosarcoma or fibrosarcoma).

Assuming that there are no metastases, the local extent of the tumour is the most important factor in deciding how much tissue has to be removed. This is best shown by CT and MRI.

Intracompartmental lesions – i.e. those that are confined to an enclosed tissue space such as a single bone or a muscle group within its fascial envelope – are more amenable to complete excision than *extracompartmental lesions* – i.e. those that extend into interfascial or extrafascial planes with no natural barrier to proximal or distal spread.

In general terms, low-grade lesions which are still intracompartmental can be treated by wide excision without exposing the tumour. High-grade sarcomas confined to bone may need more radical excision, with or without bone-graft or prosthetic replacement; and high-grade lesions with extracompartmental spread need either radical excision and prosthetic replacement or amputation. In addition, the patient may need chemotherapy to reduce the risk of metastasis.

Limb-sparing surgery seems preferable to amputation, provided there are no skip lesions and the limb is still functional. However, it should only be undertaken where expert facilities are available, and even then the complication rate is considerable (e.g. wound breakdown, infection and prosthetic failure). If there is any doubt about the extent or aggressiveness of the tumour, *amputation* is the better option.

Multi-agent chemotherapy is the preferred method of adjuvant treatment for malignant bone tumours. Drugs currently in use are methotrexate, doxorubicin (adriamycin), cyclophosphamide, vincristine and cisplatin. Treatment is started 8–12 weeks preoperatively and the effect is assessed by examining the resected tumour. If there is little or no necrosis, a different drug is selected for postoperative treatment; otherwise maintenance chemotherapy is continued for another 6–12 months.

Radiotherapy is suitable for highly sensitive tumours (such as Ewing's sarcoma); it is then combined with adjuvant chemotherapy.

BENIGN BONE LESIONS

NON-OSSIFYING FIBROMA (FIBROUS CORTICAL DEFECT)

This, the commonest benign lesion of bone, is a developmental defect in which a nest of fibrous tissue appears within the bone and persists for some years before ossifying. It is asymptomatic and is almost always encountered in children as an incidental finding on x-ray. The usual sites are the metaphyses of long bones; occasionally there are multiple lesions.

X-ray

The appearance is unmistakable. There is a more or less oval radiolucent area in or adjacent to the cortex. Although it looks cystic on x-ray, it is a solid lesion consisting of unremarkable fibrous tissue. As the bone grows, the defect becomes less obvious and it eventually heals spontaneously. However, it sometimes enlarges and there may be a pathological fracture.

Treatment

Except for a pathological fracture, treatment is unnecessary.

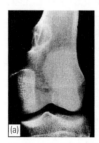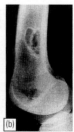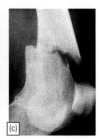

9.1 Non-ossifying fibroma (a) The x-ray always shows a cortical defect, although in some projection planes this looks deceptively like a medullary 'cyst' (b). The bone may fracture through the weakened area (c).

FIBROUS DYSPLASIA

Fibrous dysplasia is a developmental disorder in which areas of trabecular bone are replaced by fibrous tissue, osteoid and woven bone. At operation the lesional tissue has a coarse, gritty feel, due to the specks of immature bone. The condition may affect one bone *(monostotic)*, one limb *(monomelic)* or many bones *(polyostotic)*. Malignant transformation to fibrosarcoma occurs in 5–10 per cent of patients with polyostotic lesions, but only rarely in monostotic lesions.

Clinical features

Small, single lesions are asymptomatic. Large, monostotic lesions may cause pain and bone deformity, or may be discovered only when the patient develops a pathological fracture.

X-rays

Cyst-like areas in the metaphysis or shaft have a hazy (so-called ground-glass) appearance. The weight-bearing bones may be bent, and one of the classic features is the 'shepherd's crook' deformity of the proximal femur.

Pathology

The histological picture is of cellular fibrous tissue with patches of woven bone and scattered giant cells.

Treatment

Small lesions need no treatment. Those that are large and painful or threatening to fracture (or have fractured) can be curetted and grafted, but there is a strong tendency for the abnormality to recur. Deformities may need correction by suitably designed osteotomies.

OSTEOID OSTEOMA

This is a benign tumour consisting of osteoid and newly formed bone. It is small (usually less than 1 cm in size), round or oval in shape, and encased in dense bone. It is usually seen in patients aged under 30, and more than half the cases occur in the femur or tibia.

The leading symptom is pain, which is sometimes severe and is usually relieved by aspirin but not by rest.

X-ray

The important feature is a tiny radiolucent area, the so-called 'nidus'. In the diaphysis, the nidus is surrounded by dense bone and the cortex is thickened. Lesions in the metaphysis show less cortical thickening. It is sometimes difficult to distinguish an osteoid osteoma from a small Brodie's abscess without biopsy.

Treatment

The only effective treatment is complete removal of the nidus. The lesion is carefully localized by x-ray and/or CT and then excised in a small block of bone; the specimen should be x-rayed immediately to confirm that it does contain the little tumour.

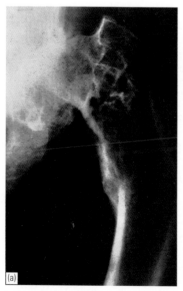
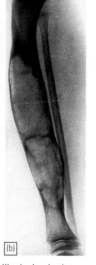

9.2 Fibrous dysplasia (a) The large cyst-like lesion in the proximal femur has resulted in a so-called shepherd's crook deformity. (b) X-ray showing the typical ground-glass appearance of fibrous dysplasia in the tibia.

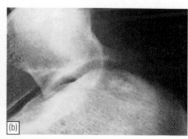
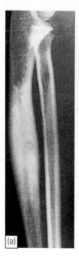

9.3 Osteoid osteoma The x-ray appearance depends on the site of the lesion. (a) Cortical tumours cause marked reactive bone thickening around a small lucent nidus. (b) Lesions in cancellous bone cause far less periosteal reaction and are easily mistaken for a Brodie's abscess.

CHONDROMA (ENCHONDROMA)

Islands of cartilage may persist in the metaphyses of bones formed by endochondral ossification; sometimes they grow and take on the characteristics of a benign tumour. The lesional tissue is indistinguishable from normal hyaline cartilage, but parts of the tumour may show areas of degeneration and calcification.

Clinical features

Chondromas are usually asymptomatic and are discovered incidentally on x-ray or after a pathological fracture. They are seen at any age (but mostly in young people) and in any bone preformed in cartilage. Lesions may be solitary or multiple and part of a generalized dysplasia.

X-ray

The tumour appears as a central, sometimes expanded, radiolucent area near the bone end. What distinguishes it from other cyst-like lesions is the appearance of tiny flecks of calcification within the lucent area.

Treatment

If the tumour is painful or appears to be enlarging, or if it presents as a pathological fracture, it should be removed as thoroughly as possible by curettage; the defect is filled with bone-graft.

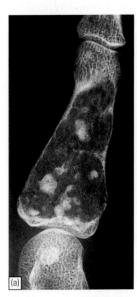
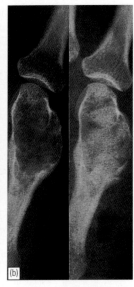

(a)   (b)

9.4 Chondroma The hand is a common site. Though the lesion in (a) looks like a cyst, it is in fact a solid but radiolucent tumour with central patches of calcification – a typical feature of chondroma. The lesion in (b) was treated by curettage and bone-grafting.

Prognosis

There is a small but significant risk of *malignant change;* suspicious features in adult patients are (1) the onset of pain, (2) enlargement of the lesion and (3) cortical erosion. If these features are present, and especially in older patients, the tumour should be treated as a low-grade malignancy.

OSTEOCHONDROMA (CARTILAGE-CAPPED EXOSTOSIS)

Pathology

This, one of the commonest 'tumours' of bone, is a developmental lesion which starts as a small overgrowth of cartilage at the edge of the physeal plate and develops by endochondral ossification into a bony protuberance still covered by the cap of cartilage. Any bone that develops in cartilage may be involved; the commonest sites are the fast-growing ends of long bones and the crest of the ilium. Multiple lesions may develop as part of a heritable disorder – hereditary multiple exostosis – in which there is abnormal bone growth resulting in characteristic deformities (see page 75).

There is a small risk of malignant transformation. This is seen most often with pelvic exostoses – not because they are inherently different but because considerable enlargement may, for long periods, pass unnoticed. The exact incidence is difficult to assess because troublesome lesions are usually removed before they show histological features of malignancy; estimates range from 1 per cent for solitary lesions to 6 per cent for multiple.

Clinical features

The patient is usually a teenager or young adult when the lump is first discovered. The exostosis may go on enlarging up to the end of the normal growth period for that bone; *any further enlargement after that is suggestive of malignant change.*

X-ray

What is seen on x-ray is a well-defined bony protuberance (exostosis) emerging from the metaphysis. It looks smaller than it feels because the cartilage cap does not show on x-ray; however, large lesions undergo cartilage degeneration and calcification and then the x-ray shows the bony exostosis surrounded by blotches of calcified material.

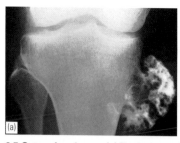
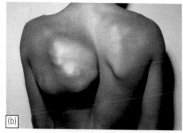
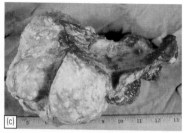

9.5 Osteochondroma (a) The lesion typically forms as a cartilage-capped exostosis near the end of one of the long bones. The 'cap' does not show on x-ray unless it is calcified, as in this case. (b,c) This 20-year-old man had known about the lump on his left scapula for many years. He stopped growing at the age of 18, but the tumour continued to enlarge. The scapula was removed and further sections from the depth of the lesion showed features of malignant change.

Treatment

If the tumour causes symptoms, it should be excised; if, in an adult, it has recently become bigger or painful, operation is urgent, for these features suggest malignancy, even if the histology looks 'benign'.

CHONDROBLASTOMA

This rare tumour of immature cartilage cells is one of the very few lesions to appear primarily in the epiphysis, usually of the proximal humerus, femur or tibia. The presenting symptom is aching and tenderness adjacent to the joint. The characteristic *x-ray* appearance is of a well-demarcated radiolucent area in the epiphysis.

Treatment

In children, the risk of damage to the physis makes it risky to remove the lesion. In adults this is not a problem; however, there is a high risk of recurrence after incomplete removal, and if this happens repeatedly, there may be serious damage to the nearby joint.

CHONDROMYXOID FIBROMA

Like other benign cartilaginous lesions, this is seen mainly in adolescents and young adults. It may occur in any bone but is more common in those of the lower limb.

Patients seldom complain, and the lesion is usually discovered by accident or after a pathological fracture.

On *x-ray* examination this looks like an ovoid cyst situated eccentrically in the metaphysis. However, it is a solid tumour of mixed cartilage, fibrous and myxomatous tissues.

Where feasible, the lesion should be excised, but often one can do no more than a thorough curettage, followed by autogenous bone-grafting.

SIMPLE BONE CYST

This is a true solitary or unicameral bone cyst. It appears during childhood, typically in the metaphysis of one of the long bones and most commonly in the proximal humerus or femur. It is not a tumour, tends to heal spontaneously and is seldom seen in adults. The condition is usually discovered after a pathological fracture or as an incidental finding on x-ray.

X-ray

The appearance on x-ray is of a large bubble inside the bone. It may occupy the entire metaphysis but does not extend beyond the physeal plate.

Treatment

Asymptomatic lesions in older children can be left alone, but the patient should be cautioned to avoid injury which might cause a fracture. 'Active' cysts (those in young children, usually abutting against the physeal plate and obviously enlarging in sequential x-rays) should be treated, in the first instance, by aspiration of fluid and injection of 80–160 mg of methylprednisolone. This has been found to stop further enlargement and promote healing of the cyst; however, there is doubt as to whether it is the prednisolone or the act of injection that does the trick. If the cyst goes on enlarging, or if there is a pathological fracture, the cavity should be curetted and then packed with bone chips.

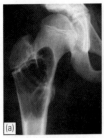 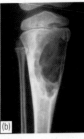 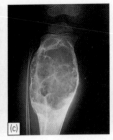 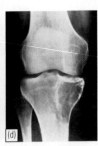

9.6 Cyst-like lesions (a) *Simple bone cyst*: Fills the medullary cavity but does not expand the bone. (b) *Chondromyxoid fibroma*: Looks cystic but is actually a radiolucent benign tumour; always in the metaphysis; hard boundary tailing off towards the diaphysis. (c) *Aneurysmal bone cyst*: Expansile cystic tumour, always on the metaphyseal side of the physis. (d) *Giant-cell tumour*: Hardly ever appears before epiphysis has fused; the pathognomonic feature is that it extends right up to the subarticular bone plate; sometimes malignant.

ANEURYSMAL BONE CYST

This is a cystic, tumour-like lesion which occurs chiefly in the spine and the metaphyses of long bones, usually affecting young adults. It may expand the bone and cause marked thinning of the cortex. When the cyst is opened, it is found to contain clotted blood, and during curettage there may be considerable bleeding from the fleshy lining membrane. Histologically the membrane consists of fibrous tissue with vascular spaces, deposits of haemosiderin and multinucleated giant cells. There is no risk of malignant transformation.

X-ray

In a growing tubular bone the cyst is always situated in the metaphysis and may resemble a simple cyst. In adults it can be mistaken for a giant-cell tumour but, unlike the latter, its boundary stops well short of the articular margin.

Treatment

The cyst should be thoroughly curetted and then packed with chipped bone grafts. Sometimes the grafts are resorbed and the cyst recurs, necessitating a second or third operation.

GIANT-CELL TUMOUR

Pathology

Giant-cell tumour is a lesion of uncertain origin that appears after the end of bone growth, most commonly in the distal femur, proximal tibia, proximal humerus and distal radius. The tumour has a reddish, fleshy appearance; it comes away in pieces quite easily when curetted but is difficult to remove completely from the surrounding bone. Aggressive lesions have a poorly defined 'floor' and appear to extend into the surrounding bone. Histologically the striking feature is an abundance of multinucleated giant cells scattered on a background of stromal cells, with little or no visible intercellular tissue.

About one-third of these tumours remain truly benign; one-third become locally invasive and one-third metastasize.

Clinical features

The patient is usually a young adult who complains of pain at the end of a long bone; sometimes there is slight swelling. Pathological fracture occurs in 10–15 per cent of cases.

Imaging

Although this is a solid tumour, it appears on x-ray as a 'cystic' (i.e. radiolucent) area situated eccentrically at the end of a long bone. *Unlike any of the other 'cystic' lesions, it always extends right up to the subchondral bone plate.* The endosteal margin is usually clear-cut, but in invasive lesions it is ill-defined.

Considering the tumour's potential for aggressive behaviour, detailed staging procedures are essential. CT scans and MRI will reveal the extent of the tumour, both within the bone and beyond. It is important to establish whether the articular surface has been broached; arthroscopy may be helpful. Biopsy is essential.

Treatment

Well-confined, slow-growing lesions with benign histology can safely be treated by thorough curettage and 'stripping' of the cavity with burrs and gouges, followed by swabbing with hydrogen peroxide or by the application of liquid nitrogen; the cavity is then packed with bone chips. More aggressive tumours, and recurrent lesions, should be treated by excision, followed, if necessary, by bone-grafting or prosthetic replacement.

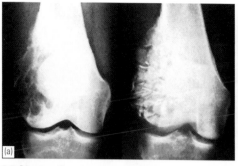 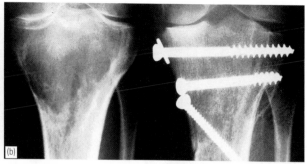

9.7 Giant-cell tumour – treatment (a) Local removal and packing with bone-grafts. (b) Block resection and replacement with a large corticocancellous allograft.

PRIMARY MALIGNANT BONE TUMOURS

OSTEOSARCOMA

Pathology

In its classic form, osteosarcoma is a highly malignant tumour arising within the bone and spreading rapidly outwards to the periosteum and surrounding soft tissues. The histological appearances show considerable variation. Some areas may consist of characteristic spindle cells in an osteoid matrix; others may contain cartilage cells or fibroblastic tissue with little or no osteoid.

Clinical features

Osteosarcoma occurs predominantly in children and adolescents. It may affect any bone but most commonly the long-bone metaphyses, especially around the knee and at the proximal end of the humerus. Pain is usually the first symptom; it is constant, worse at night, and gradually increases in severity. Sometimes the patient presents with a lump. On examination there may be some swelling and local tenderness. In late cases there is a palpable mass and the overlying tissues may look inflamed. The erythrocyte sedimentation rate (ESR) is usually raised and there may be an increase in serum alkaline phosphatase.

Imaging

On *x-ray*, some tumours are entirely osteolytic, others show alternating areas of lysis and increased bone density. The tumour margins are poorly defined. Often the cortex is breached and the tumour extends into the adjacent tissues; when this happens, streaks of new bone appear, radiating outwards from the cortex – the so-called 'sunburst' effect. Where the tumour emerges from the cortex, reactive new bone forms in the angle between periosteum and cortex (Codman's triangle). While both the sunburst appearance and Codman's triangle are typical of osteosarcoma, they can also be seen in other rapidly growing tumours.

Other imaging studies are essential for staging purposes. *Radioisotope* scans may reveal skip lesions, but a negative scan does not exclude them. *CT* and *MRI* reliably show the extent of the tumour. Chest x-rays are done routinely, but *pulmonary CT* is a much more sensitive detector of lung metastases. *About 10 per cent of patients have pulmonary metastases by the time they are first seen.*

Diagnosis

In most cases the diagnosis can be made on the x-ray appearances. However, atypical lesions can be mistaken for more benign conditions, and non-neoplastic conditions such as chronic bone infection, large gouty tophi and stress fractures sometimes masquerade as malignant lesions.

A biopsy should always be performed before commencing treatment; it must be planned to allow for complete removal of the track when the tumour is excised.

Treatment

The principles of treatment are outlined on page 85. Multi-agent chemotherapy is given for 8–12 weeks and then, provided the tumour is resectable and there are no skip lesions, a wide resection is carried out. It is important to eradicate the primary lesion completely; the mortality rate after local recurrence is far worse than following effective ablation at the first encounter. Depending on the site of the tumour, preparations would have been made to replace that segment of bone with either a large bone-graft or a custom-made implant; in some cases an amputation may be more appropriate.

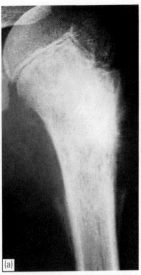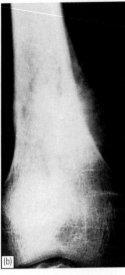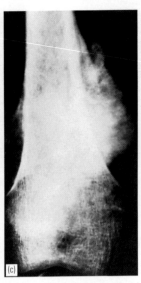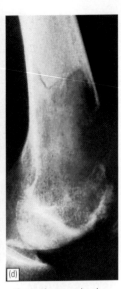

9.8 Osteosarcoma (a,b) Characteristic appearance with sun-ray spicules and Codman's triangle where the periosteum begins to be lifted away from the shaft; (c) same patient as (b) after radiotherapy; (d) a predominantly osteolytic tumour.

The pathological specimen is examined to assess the response to preoperative chemotherapy. If tumour necrosis is marked, chemotherapy is continued for another 6–12 months; if the response is poor, a different chemotherapeutic agent is substituted.

Pulmonary metastases, especially if they are small and peripherally situated, may be completely resected with a wedge of lung tissue.

Outcome

Long-term survival after wide resection and chemotherapy is higher than 60 per cent. Tumour-replacement implants usually function well. There is a fairly high complication rate (mainly wound breakdown and infection), but in patients who survive, the risk of aseptic loosening at 10 years is around 10 per cent for hip prostheses and 30 per cent for prostheses around the knee.

CHONDROSARCOMA

Pathology

Chondrosarcoma occurs either as a *primary* tumour or as a *secondary* change in a pre-existing benign chondroma or osteochondroma. Cartilage-capped exostoses of the pelvis and scapula seem to be more susceptible than others to malignant change, but perhaps this is simply because at these sites the tumour can grow without being detected and removed at an early stage.

A *low-grade chondrosarcoma* may show histological features no different from those of an aggressive benign cartilaginous lesion.

High-grade tumours are more cellular, and there may be abnormal features such as cellular plumpness, hyperchromasia and mitoses.

Clinical features

Chondrosarcomas have their highest incidence in the fourth and fifth decades, and men are affected more often than women. The tumours are slow growing and are usually present for many months before being discovered. Patients may complain of a dull ache or a gradually enlarging lump. Medullary lesions may present as a pathological fracture.

Imaging

Primary chondrosarcoma can occur in any bone that develops in cartilage but is usually seen in the metaphysis of one of the tubular bones. *X-ray examination* shows a radiolucent area with central flecks of calcification. Some lesions look like benign chondromas; others are associated with unmistakable features of bone destruction.

Secondary chondrosarcoma usually arises in the cartilage cap of an osteochondroma that has been present since childhood. Large osteochondromas with widespread calcification in the cartilage cap should be viewed with suspicion, and any osteochondroma that increases in size after the end of normal bone growth should be regarded as

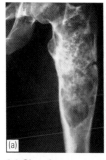
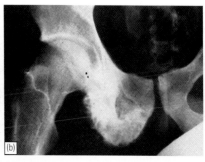
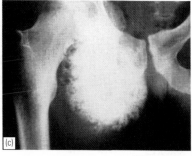

9.9 Chondrosarcoma (a) Primary chondrosarcoma appears in the x-rays as a large lucent area encroaching upon or expanding the cortex. A characteristic feature is patchy calcification in the centre of the lesion, well demonstrated in this case. Note that the lateral cortex has fractured. (b,c) Secondary chondrosarcoma usually rises in the cartilage cap of an osteochondroma. In this case the tumour started in the right inferior pubic ramus and went on enlarging after the end of the normal growth period. Although the first biopsy looked benign, continued tumour growth was highly suspicious and a second biopsy showed features of malignancy.

definitely malignant; in that case *CT and MRI should be performed before biopsy.*

Treatment

Chondrosarcomas are usually slow growing and metastasize late. They present the ideal case for wide excision and prosthetic replacement, provided it is certain that the lesion can be completely removed without exposing the tumour and without causing an unacceptable loss of function. Otherwise amputation may be a safer option. The tumour does not respond to either radiotherapy or chemotherapy.

EWING'S SARCOMA

Pathology

Ewing's sarcoma is believed to arise from endothelial cells in the bone marrow. It occurs most commonly between the ages of 10 and 20 years, usually in a tubular bone, and especially in the tibia, fibula or clavicle. Macroscopically the tumour is lobulated and often fairly large. Microscopically, sheets of small dark polyhedral cells with no regular arrangement and no ground substance are seen.

Clinical features

The patient presents with pain – often throbbing in character – and swelling. Generalized illness and pyrexia, together with a warm, tender swelling and a raised ESR, may suggest a (mistaken) diagnosis of osteomyelitis.

Imaging

X-ray usually shows an area of bone destruction which, unlike that in osteosarcoma, is predominantly in the mid-diaphysis. New-bone formation may extend along the shaft and sometimes it appears as fusiform layers of bone around the lesion – the so-called *'onion-peel'* effect. *CT* and *MRI* will reveal any large extraosseous component, and *radioisotope scans* may disclose multiple lesions elsewhere in the skeleton.

Diagnosis

The condition which should be excluded as rapidly as possible is bone infection. On biopsy, the essential step is to recognize this as a malignant round-cell tumour, distinct from osteosarcoma. Other round-cell tumours that may resemble Ewing's are *reticulum-cell sarcoma and metastatic neuroblastoma.*

Treatment

The prognosis is always poor and surgery alone does little to improve it. Radiotherapy has a dramatic effect on the tumour but overall survival is not much enhanced. Chemotherapy is much more effective, offering a 5-year survival rate of about 50 per cent. The best results are achieved by a combination of all three methods.

MULTIPLE MYELOMA

Pathology

Multiple myeloma is a malignant B-cell lymphoproliferative disorder of the marrow, with plasma cells predominating. The effects on bone are due to marrow-cell proliferation and increased osteoclastic activity, resulting in *osteoporosis* and the appearance of discrete *lytic lesions* throughout the skeleton *(myelomatosis)*. A particularly large colony of plasma cells may form what appears to be a solitary tumour *(plasmacytoma)* in one of the bones, but sooner or later most of these cases turn out to be examples of the same widespread disease.

At operation the affected bone is soft and crumbly. The typical microscopic picture is of sheets of plasmacytes with a large eccentric nucleus containing a spoke-like arrangement of chromatin.

Clinical features

The patient, typically aged 45–65, presents with weakness, backache, bone pain or a pathological fracture. Hypercalcaemia may cause symptoms such as thirst, polyuria and abdominal pain.

Associated features of the marrow-cell disorder are *plasma protein abnormalities, increased blood viscosity* and *anaemia*. Bone resorption leads to *hypercalcaemia* in about one-third of cases. Late secondary features are due to *renal dysfunction* and *spinal cord* or *root compression* caused by vertebral collapse.

The prognosis in established cases is poor, with a median survival of 2 or 3 years.

X-ray

X-rays often show nothing more than generalized osteoporosis; but remember that *myeloma is one of the commonest causes of osteoporosis and vertebral compression fracture in men over the age of 45 years.* The 'classic' lesions are multiple punched-out defects in the skull, pelvis and proximal femur, a crushed vertebra, or a solitary lytic tumour in a large-bone metaphysis.

Investigations

Mild anaemia is common, and an almost constant feature is a high ESR. Blood chemistry may show a raised creatinine level and hypercalcaemia. More than half the patients have Bence-Jones protein in their urine, and serum protein electrophoresis shows a characteristic abnormal band. A sternal

marrow puncture may show plasmacytosis, with typical 'myeloma' cells.

Diagnosis

If the only x-ray change is osteoporosis, the differential diagnosis must include all the *other causes of bone loss.* If there are lytic lesions, the features can be similar to those of *metastatic bone disease.*

Paraproteinaemia is a feature of other (benign) *gammopathies;* it is wise to seek the help of a haematologist before reaching a clinical diagnosis.

Treatment

The immediate need is for pain control and, if necessary, treatment of pathological fractures. General supportive measures include correction of fluid balance and treatment for hypercalcaemia.

Limb fractures are best managed by internal fixation and packing of cavities with methylmethacrylate cement (which also helps to staunch the profuse bleeding that sometimes occurs). Perioperative antibiotic prophylaxis is important as there is a higher than usual risk of infection and wound breakdown.

Spinal fractures carry the risk of cord compression and need immediate stabilization, either by effective bracing or by internal fixation. Unrelieved cord pressure may need decompression.

Specific therapy is with alkylating cytotoxic agents (e.g. melphalan). Corticosteroids are also used – especially if bone pain is marked – but this probably does not alter the course of the disease. Solitary plasmacytomas can be treated by radiotherapy.

METASTATIC BONE DISEASE

In patients over 50 years, bone metastases are seen more frequently than all primary malignant bone tumours together. The commonest source is carcinoma of the breast; next in frequency are carcinomas of the prostate, kidney, lung, thyroid, bladder and gastrointestinal tract. In about 10 per cent of cases no primary tumour is found.

The commonest sites for bone metastases are the vertebrae, pelvis, the proximal half of the femur and the humerus.

Metastases are usually osteolytic, and pathological fractures are common. Bone resorption is due either to the direct action of tumour cells or to tumour-derived factors that stimulate osteoclastic activity. Osteoblastic lesions are uncommon; they usually occur in prostatic carcinoma.

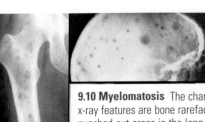

9.10 Myelomatosis The characteristic x-ray features are bone rarefaction and punched-out areas in the long bones and skull.

Clinical features

The patient is usually aged 50–70 years; with any destructive bone lesion in this age group, the differential diagnosis must include metastasis.

Pain is the commonest – and often the only – clinical feature. The sudden appearance of backache or thigh pain in an elderly person (especially someone known to have been treated for carcinoma in the past) is always suspicious. If x-rays do not show anything, a radionuclide scan might.

Some deposits remain clinically silent and are discovered incidentally on x-ray, or after a pathological fracture. Sudden collapse of a vertebral body or a fracture of the mid-shaft of a long bone in an elderly person is an ominous sign; if there is no history and no clinical clue pointing to a primary carcinoma, a biopsy of the fracture area is essential.

Symptoms of hypercalcaemia may occur (and are often missed) in patients with skeletal metastases. These include anorexia, nausea, thirst, polyuria, abdominal pain, general weakness and depression.

Imaging

On x-ray examination, skeletal deposits usually appear as rarefied areas in the medulla or patches of bone destruction in the cortex. Vertebral collapse is also common. Osteoblastic deposits are seen in late cases of prostatic carcinoma. *Radioscintigraphy,* using ^{99m}Tc-HDP, is the most sensitive method of detecting 'silent' metastatic deposits in bone; areas of increased activity are selected for x-ray examination.

Special investigations

The ESR may be increased and the haemoglobin concentration is usually low. The serum alkaline phosphatase concentration is often increased, and in prostatic carcinoma the acid phosphatase also is elevated.

Treatment

By the time a patient has developed secondary deposits, the prognosis for survival is almost hopeless. Occasionally, radical treatment (by combined surgery and radiotherapy) of a solitary secondary deposit and of its parent primary may be rewarding and even apparently curative. This applies particularly to hypernephroma and thyroid tumours; but in the great majority of cases, and certainly in those with multiple secondaries, treatment is entirely symptomatic. For that reason, elaborate witch-hunts to discover the source of an occult primary tumour are avoided, though it may be worthwhile investigating for tumours that are amenable to hormonal manipulation.

Despite the ultimately hopeless prognosis, patients deserve to be made comfortable, to enjoy (as far as possible) their remaining months or years, and to die in a peaceful and dignified way. The active treatment of skeletal metastases contributes to this in no small measure. In addition, patients need sympathetic counselling and practical assistance with their material affairs.

Control of pain and metastatic activity

Most patients require *analgesics,* but the more powerful narcotics should be reserved for the terminally ill.

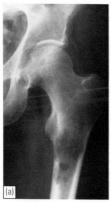
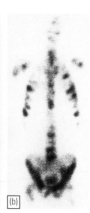
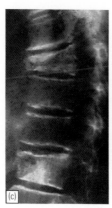
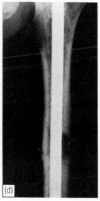

9.11 Metastatic tumours (a,b) This patient presented with pain in the right upper thigh. X-ray showed what appeared to be a single metastasis in the upper third of the femur. However, the radioisotope scan revealed many deposits in other parts of the skeleton. (c) Patients over 60 with vertebral compression fractures may simply be very osteoporotic, but they should always be investigated for metastatic bone disease and myelomatosis. (d) Prophylactic nailing for a femoral metastasis which might otherwise have resulted in a pathological fracture.

Unless specifically contraindicated, *radiotherapy* is used both to control pain and to reduce metastatic growth. This is often combined with other forms of treatment (e.g. internal fixation).

Secondary deposits from breast or prostate can often be controlled by *hormone therapy:* stilboestrol for prostatic secondaries and androgenic drugs or oestrogens for breast carcinoma. Disseminated secondaries from breast carcinoma are sometimes treated by oophorectomy combined with adrenalectomy or by hypophyseal ablation.

Hypercalcaemia may have serious consequences, including renal acidosis, nephrocalcinosis, unconsciousness and coma. It should be treated by ensuring adequate hydration, reducing the calcium intake and, if necessary, administering bisphosphonates.

Treatment of fractures

Surgical timidity may condemn the patient to a painful, lingering death, so shaft fractures should almost always be treated by internal fixation and (if necessary) packing with methylmethacrylate cement. Pain is immediately relieved, nursing is made easier, and the patient can get up and about or attend for other types of treatment without unnecessary discomfort. The fractures usually unite satisfactorily.

In most cases, intramedullary nailing is the most effective method; fractures near joints (e.g. the distal femur or proximal tibia) may need fixation with plates or blade-plates. Fractures of the femoral neck rarely, if ever, unite and are best treated by prosthetic replacement.

Postoperative irradiation is essential to prevent further extension of the metastatic lesion.

Prophylactic fixation

Large deposits that threaten to result in fracture should be treated by internal fixation while the bone is still intact. A preoperative radionuclide scan will show whether other lesions are present in that bone, thus calling for more extensive fixation and postoperative radiotherapy.

Spinal stabilization

Vertebral fractures usually require some form of support. If the spine is stable, a well-fitting brace may be sufficient. However, spinal instability may cause severe pain, making it almost impossible for the patient to sit or stand – with or without a brace. For these patients, operative stabilization is indicated – usually a posterior spinal fusion – followed by radiotherapy.

Preoperative assessment should include CT or MRI, and sometimes myelography, to establish whether the cord is threatened; if it is, spinal decompression should be carried out at the same time.

If there are overt symptoms and signs of cord compression, treatment is urgent. If the patient is expected to live for some time, surgical decompression and fusion are indicated. However, if the patient is in a terminal stage, it may be more humane to give radiotherapy, alone or together with corticosteroids and narcotics, to control oedema and pain.

CHAPTER 10

NEUROMUSCULAR DISORDERS

Of the vast range of neurological disorders, those which most commonly give rise to orthopaedic problems are:

- Cerebral palsy and stroke (upper motor neuron, spastic disorders)
- Compressive lesions of the spinal cord
- Neural tube defects (spina bifida)
- Anterior poliomyelitis
- Degenerative motor neuron disorders
- Nerve root disorders
- Peripheral neuropathies.

This chapter also deals with two types of 'muscle disorder':

- Arthrogryposis
- Muscular dystrophy.

CLINICAL ASSESSMENT

Cerebral palsy and spina bifida present during infancy; poliomyelitis usually occurs in childhood; spinal cord lesions and peripheral neuropathies are more common in adults. However, the residual effects of neurological disease, such as muscle weakness and deformity, may need attention throughout life.

Clinical assessment comprises a complete neurological examination (see Chapter 1) as well as examination of the neck and back. Attention should also be paid to natural posture, gait, sense of balance, involuntary movements and autonomic functions.

Gait and posture

Typical patterns of walking can often be recognized.

A *spastic gait* is stiff and jerky, often with the feet in equinus, the knees somewhat flexed and the hips adducted ('scissoring').

A *drop-foot gait* is due to peripheral neuropathy or injury of the nerves supplying the dorsiflexors of the ankle. During the swing phase the foot falls into equinus ('drops'), and if it were not lifted higher than usual the toes would drag along the ground.

A *high-stepping gait* signifies either bilateral foot-drop or a problem with proprioception and balance.

A *waddling gait,* in which the trunk is thrown from side to side with each step, may be due to dislocation of the hips or to weakness of the abductor muscles.

Ataxia produces a more obvious and irregular loss of balance, which is compensated for by a broad-based gait, or sometimes uncontrollable staggering.

Deformity

When all muscle groups are equally weak *(balanced paralysis),* the joint simply assumes the position imposed on it by gravity. It is unstable and the limb feels floppy or flail. Deformity occurs when one group of muscles is too weak to balance the pull of antagonists *(unbalanced paralysis).* At first the deformity can be corrected passively but with time it becomes fixed. In children, paralysis may affect bone growth.

Muscle weakness

This may be due to *upper motor neuron lesions* (spastic paresis), *lower motor neuron lesions* (flaccid paresis) or *muscle disorders*. Muscle power is usually graded on the Medical Research Council Scale, as follows: 0 = total paralysis; 1 = barely detectable contraction; 2 = not enough power to act against gravity; 3 = strong enough to act against gravity; 4 = still stronger but less than normal; 5 = normal power.

Sensory changes

Numbness and paraesthesia may be the main complaints. It is important to establish their exact distribution as this will help to localize the lesion (Fig. 10.1).

Autonomic functions

The sympathetic and parasympathetic systems are concerned with functions such as involuntary muscle contraction, sphincter control, peripheral blood flow and sweating.

Table 10.1 Nerve root supply and actions of main muscle groups

Sternomastoids	Spinal accessory C2, 3, 4
Trapezius	Spinal accessory C3, 4
Diaphragm	C3, 4, 5
Deltoid	C5, 6
Supraspinatus and infraspinatus	C5, 6
Serratus anterior	C5, 6, 7
Pectoralis major	C5, 6, 7, 8
Elbow flexion	C5, 6
extension	C7
Supination	C5, 6
Pronation	C6
Wrist extension	C6, (7)
flexion	C7, (8)
Finger extension	C7
flexion	C7, 8, T1
abduction and adduction	C8, T1
Hip flexion	L1, 2, 3
extension	L5, S1
adduction	L2, 3, 4
abduction	L4, 5, S1
Knee extension	L(2), 3, 4
flexion	L5, S1
Ankle dorsiflexion	L4, 5
plantarflexion	S1, 2
inversion	L4, 5
eversion	L5, S1
Toe extension	L5
flexion	S1
abduction	S1, 2

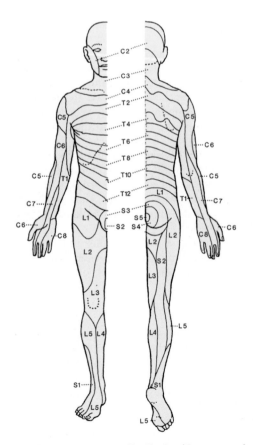

10.1 Sensory nerve root distribution (dermatomes)

Cauda equina syndrome

Neurological lesions of the conus medullaris or cauda equina may result in urinary and faecal retention and impairment of penile erection. These are important signs in patients with spinal injuries and lumbar intervertebral disc prolapse; if the neurological compression is not relieved within hours, the effects may be irreversible.

Horner's syndrome

Sympathetic blockade in the vicinity of C7 and T1 may result in a characteristic combination of ipsilateral ptosis (drooping eyelid), miosis (contraction of the pupil), facial hyperaemia (flushing) and anhidrosis (loss of sweating). This is an important clue in the diagnosis of cervicothoracic tumours, cord compression, mediastinal tumours, apical tumours of the lung and pre-ganglionic damage to the nerve roots in a brachial plexus injury.

IMAGING

Plain x-rays of the skull or spine are routine for all disorders of the central nervous system. Specialized imaging of the brain and spinal cord may be necessary to reveal degenerative or space-occupying lesions. Narrowing of the spinal canal is best demonstrated by *CT.* Destructive lesions of the spine may require both *CT and MRI* to show the extent of cord involvement.

SPECIAL INVESTIGATIONS

Electrodiagnosis

Electromyography and nerve conduction studies are helpful in establishing (1) whether weakness is due to nerve or muscle disorder, and (2) whether (and where) a peripheral nerve is compressed or damaged.

Muscle biopsy

A biopsy may yield valuable diagnostic information, but only if there are facilities for light microscopy, electron microscopy and histochemical processing.

CEREBRAL PALSY

The term 'cerebral palsy' includes a group of disorders which result from non-progressive brain damage during early development. The incidence is about 2 per 1000 live births. Known *causal factors* are prematurity, perinatal anoxia, kernicterus and postnatal brain infections or injury. The main consequence is the development of neuromuscular inco-ordination, dystonia (abnormal posturing and movement), weakness and spasticity; in addition there may be convulsions, perceptual problems, speech disorder and mental retardation.

Early diagnosis

A history of perinatal difficulties may suggest the diagnosis, but at birth the disease is rarely recognized. Early symptoms include difficulty in sucking and swallowing, with dribbling at the mouth; the mother may notice that the baby feels stiff or wriggles awkwardly. Gradually it becomes apparent that the developmental milestones are delayed: the normal child usually holds its head up at 3 months, sits up at 6 months and begins walking at about 1 year. Neonatal reflexes also may be delayed.

 Unusual baby: check developmental milestones.

Late diagnosis

The clinical picture emerges slowly and varies considerably from case to case. Some patients have severe athetosis; others are ataxic; but by far the majority have a spastic paresis. As the name implies, there is both spasticity and weakness, although the presence of the former may make it difficult to assess the latter. Tendon reflexes are brisk and plantar responses extensor. Sensation is normal.

The children are often emotionally unstable and sometimes suffer from fits. Intelligence may be impaired.

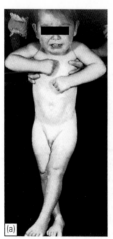 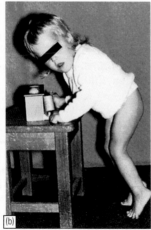 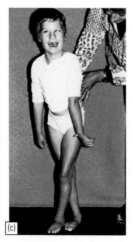 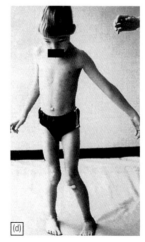

10.2 Cerebral palsy (a) Adductor spasm (scissors stance); (b) flexion deformity of hips and knees with equinus of the feet; (c) general posture and characteristic facial expression; (d) ataxic type of palsy.

Types of motor dysfunction

Spastic paresis is the commonest variety, accounting for more than 60 per cent of all cases. It may appear as *hemiplegia* (affecting one side of the body), *diplegia* (affecting mainly the lower limbs), *total-body* involvement, in which all four limbs and the head and neck are affected (often associated with a low IQ), or *isolated asymmetrical* paresis.

Athetosis manifests as continuous, involuntary writhing movements. Tongue and speech muscles may also be involved.

Ataxia appears as muscular inco-ordination during voluntary movements. Balance is poor and the child walks with a characteristic wide-based gait.

Characteristic deformities

The combination of muscle imbalance and spasticity gives rise to characteristic deformities and postures, which are exaggerated when the child attempts to stand or walk:

■ flexion of the elbows and wrists, with fingers clasped,
■ tight adduction of the hips (scissors posture),
■ knees slightly flexed and unable to be straightened,
■ ankles and feet in equinus.

Treatment

Treatment is best carried out in a special centre where the child can enjoy the benefits of combined physiotherapy, occupational therapy, speech therapy and remedial education. If the facilities are available, further assessment may be carried out in a gait laboratory.

Medication may be needed to control fits and reduce hyperactivity. *Physical therapy* is started during the first year of life, before abnormal motor patterns have become established, and may be continued into adolescence. *Splintage* is often necessary to counteract spastic deformities or to hold position after corrective surgery. In recent years intramuscular *botulinum A toxin* has been used to reduce muscle tone in the hope that this will prevent the development of soft-tissue contractures. Even a temporary reduction in spasticity may help in deciding what type of operation (if any) would be useful.

Corrective surgery

The indications for surgery are: (1) a spastic posture which cannot be controlled by conservative measures; (2) a fixed deformity that interferes with function; (3) secondary complications such as bony deformities, dislocation of the hip and joint instability.

Patients with *hemiplegia* respond well to both conservative and operative treatment, and all of them should eventually be able to walk unaided. Those with *diplegia* are more difficult to manage, but most of them will eventually be able to walk. Patients with *total-body involvement* have a poor prognosis for walking, yet even in this group surgery may be needed to improve spinal stability. Low intelligence is no bar to surgery.

Timing is important. As long as the spastic deformity is controlled by lesser measures, there is no urgency about operations; indeed, one approach is to put off all operations until the condition stabilizes after the age of 6 or 7 years and then do all the necessary corrective operations at one or two sittings. However, if it becomes difficult to maintain position, it may be better to operate before function deteriorates, and certainly before fixed deformity supervenes. The physiotherapist's advice is often the most valuable.

Surgical options are limited. (1) Tight muscles can be released or their tendons lengthened, but this will also diminish muscle power. Nerve transection may have a similar effect. (2) Weak muscles can be augmented by tendon transfers, but there is a risk that the combined effect of enhancing power on one side of a joint and taking away the spastic antagonist may result in severe over-correction! (3) Fixed deformities can be corrected by osteotomy, by fusing the joint or by arthroplasty. Always consider what effect this will have on the position of other joints and on overall function.

A general rule should be to tackle soft-tissue problems first and bony problems later.

Regional survey

For a regional survey of corrective operations, the reader is referred to *Apley's System of Orthopaedics and Fractures,* 8th edition (published by Arnold, London, 2001).

STROKE

Cerebral damage following a stroke may cause persistent spastic paresis in the adult; disturbance of proprioception and stereognosis may coexist. In the early recuperative stage, physiotherapy and splintage are important in preventing fixed contractures; all affected joints should be put through a full range of movement every day, and deformities should be corrected and splinted until controlled muscle power returns. Proprioception

Table 10.2 Treatment of the principal deformities of the limbs

	Deformity	**Splintage**	**Surgery**
Foot	Equinus	Spring-loaded dorsiflexion	Lengthen tendo Achilles
	Equinovarus	Bracing in eversion and dorsiflexion	Lengthen tendo Achilles and transfer lateral half of tibialis anterior to cuboid
Knee	Flexion	Long caliper	Hamstring release
Hip	Adduction	–	Obturator neurectomy
			Adductor muscle release
Shoulder	Adduction	–	Subscapularis release
Elbow	Flexion	–	Release elbow flexors
Wrist	Flexion	Wrist splint	Lengthen or release wrist flexors; may need fusion or carpectomy
Fingers	Flexion	–	Lengthen or release flexors

and co-ordination can be improved by occupational therapy. Once maximal motor recovery has been achieved – usually by 9 months – residual deformity or joint instability may need surgical correction or permanent splinting.

LESIONS OF THE SPINAL CORD

With lesions of the spinal cord, patients complain of muscle weakness, numbness or loss of balance; bladder and bowel control may be impaired and men may complain of impotence. Examination reveals a spastic upper motor neuron (UMN) paresis, with exaggerated reflexes and a Babinski response. There may be a fairly precise boundary of sensory change, suggesting the level of cord involvement. Extradural compression may also involve nerve roots and cause lower motor neuron (LMN) signs.

Patterns of cord dysfunction

The pattern of motor and sensory impairment suggests the level of cord involvement.

- *Cervical cord* – LMN weakness and sensory loss in arms; UMN signs in the lower limbs.
- *Thoracic cord* – UMN paresis in lower limbs; variable sensory impairment.
- *Lumbar cord* – combination of UMN and LMN signs in lower limbs.
- *Cauda equina* – LMN signs and sensory loss in lower limbs, plus urinary retention with overflow.

Diagnosis

The more common causes of spinal cord dysfunction are listed in Table 10.3. Traumatic and compressive lesions are the ones most likely to be

Table 10.3 Causes of spinal cord dysfunction

Acute injury
Vertebral fractures
Fracture–dislocation

Infection
Epidural abscess
Poliomyelitis

Intervertebral disc prolapse
Sequestrated disc
Disc prolapse in spinal stenosis

Vertebral canal stenosis
Congenital stenosis
Acquired stenosis

Spinal cord tumours
Neurofibroma
Meningioma

Intrinsic cord lesions
Tabes dorsalis
Syringomyelia
Other degenerative disorders

Miscellaneous
Spina bifida
Vascular lesions
Multiple lesions
Multiple sclerosis
Haemorrhagic disorders

seen by orthopaedic surgeons. Plain x-rays will show structural abnormalities of the spine; cord compression can be visualized by myelography, alone or combined with CT. Intrinsic lesions of the cord require further investigation by blood tests, cerebrospinal fluid (CSF) examination and MRI.

Management

Acute compressive lesions require urgent diagnosis and treatment if permanent damage is to be prevented. Bladder dysfunction is ominous: whereas motor and sensory signs may improve after decompression, *loss of bladder control, if present for more than 24 hours, may be irreversible*.

With chronic lesions, one can afford to temporise. Once the diagnosis is certain, appropriate treatment can be applied.

SPINA BIFIDA

Spina bifida is a congenital disorder in which the two halves of the posterior vertebral arch (or several arches) have failed to fuse. This is often associated with maldevelopment of the neural tube and the overlying skin; the combination of faults is called *dysraphism*. It usually occurs in the lumbar or lumbosacral region. If neural elements are involved, there may be paralysis and loss of sensation and sphincter control.

Spina bifida occulta

In the mildest forms of dysraphism there is a midline defect between the laminae and nothing more; hence the term *occulta* (meaning secret). However, there may be tell-tale defects in the overlying skin: a dimple, a pit or a tuft of hair.

Spina bifida cystica

In severe forms of dysraphism the vertebral laminae are missing and the contents of the vertebral canal prolapse through the defect – either as a CSF-filled meningeal sac (or *meningocele*) or as a sac containing part of the spinal cord and nerve roots, a *myelomeningocele* (the commonest lesion). The cord may be in its primitive state, the unfolded neural plate forming part of the roof of the sac; this is an *'open' myelomeningocele* or *rachischisis*. In a *'closed' myelomeningocele* the neural tube is fully formed and covered by membrane and skin.

Hydrocephalus

Distal tethering of the cord may cause herniation of the cerebellum and brainstem through the foramen magnum, resulting in obstruction to CSF circulation and hydrocephalus. The ventricles dilate and the skull enlarges by separation of the cranial sutures. Persistently raised intracranial pressure may cause cerebral atrophy and mental retardation.

Neurological dysfunction

Myelomeningocele is always associated with neurological deficit below the level of the lesion. This may also occur – though less frequently and much less severely – in spina bifida occulta.

Incidence and screening

Isolated laminar defects are seen in more than 5 per cent of lumbar spine x-rays. By comparison, cystic spina bifida is rare, at 2–3 per 1000 live births, but if one child is affected the risk for the next child is ten times greater.

Neural tube defects are associated with high levels of α-fetoprotein in the amniotic fluid and serum. This offers an effective method of antenatal screening during the 15th to 18th weeks of pregnancy.

Clinical features

Spina bifida occulta

Isolated laminar defects are often seen in normal people and usually they can be ignored. However, a posterior midline dimple, a tuft of hair or a pigmented naevus is more serious; patients may present at any age with neurological symptoms and signs.

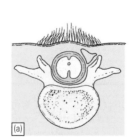 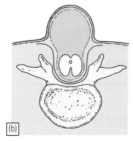 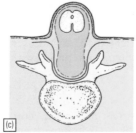 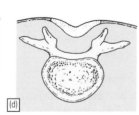

10.3 Dysraphism (a) Spina bifida occulta. (b) Meningocele. (c) Myelomeningocele. (d) Open myelomeningocele.

Spina bifida cystica

The saccular lesion over the lumbosacral spine is obvious at birth. It may be covered only with membrane, or with membrane and skin. In open myelomeningoceles the neural elements form the roof of the cyst. Hydrocephalus is common.

The baby's posture may suggest the type of paralysis and sometimes indicates its neurological level. There is generally a flaccid weakness of muscle groups in the lower limbs; sensibility is impaired and there may be urinary and bowel incontinence. The precise neurological deficit varies according to the level of the lesion.

Deformities such as hip dislocation, genu recurvatum and talipes may be present at birth, or they may develop later owing to muscle imbalance.

Management

Folic acid, taken daily before conception and continuing through the first 12 weeks of pregnancy, reduces the risk of neural tube defects in the fetus.

Selection of patients for operative closure of the spinal lesion is ethically controversial. Most centres avoid urgent operation if the neurological level is high (above L1), if spinal deformities are severe or if there is marked hydrocephalus. In the remainder (about half) the skin lesion is closed within 48 hours in order to prevent drying and ulceration.

Subsequent management may involve neurosurgery (for hydrocephalus), urological surgery (for bladder incontinence) and orthopaedic surgery (for muscle imbalance and joint deformity). Surgical treatment must, however, always be backed up by prolonged and skilled physiotherapy, occupational therapy and splintage, preferably carried out in a specialized centre.

Except in the mildest cases, the late functional outcome cannot be predicted with any confidence until the child's neuromuscular condition is assessed at the age of 3 or 4 years. Most patients with myelomeningocele will never be functionally independent. More important than walking is the development of upper limb function and intellectual skills and the ability to cope with the basic activities of daily living. These objectives can be achieved from a wheelchair just as well as from unsteady legs.

Joint deformities should be corrected – initially by gentle physiotherapy (beware of causing iatrogenic fractures!) and later by splintage with lightweight orthoses. Surgical correction may be needed if these measures fail. Prolonged immobilization carries the risk of pathological fracture and should therefore be avoided.

Children with lesions below L4 will have quadriceps control and active knee extension; they should therefore be encouraged to walk. Children with high lumbar lesions may start off walking with the aid of lower limb braces, but they will eventually opt for a wheelchair.

Urinary problems develop in 90 per cent of cases; they range from poor control to bladder paralysis, urinary retention and hydronephrosis. Simple measures such as manual expression may be needed from an early age. In males, urinary retention with overflow can be managed by fitting a penile appliance; in females, bladder neck resection or urinary diversion may be necessary.

POLIOMYELITIS

Poliomyelitis is a viral infection of the anterior horn cells of the spinal cord which may lead to permanent paralysis of isolated groups of muscles.

Following a trivial and often unrecognized minor illness (a sore throat or diarrhoea), the patient develops meningitis. Two or 3 days afterwards paralysis may follow, and the muscles are both weak and painful. If the patient does not succumb from respiratory paralysis, pain and

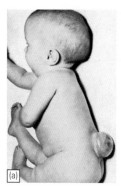
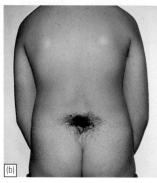
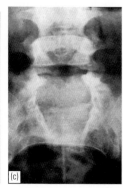

10.4 Spina bifida (a) Baby with spina bifida cystica (a myelomeningocele). (b) Tuft of hair over the lumbosacral junction. X-ray in this case showed a sacral defect (c).

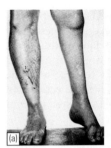
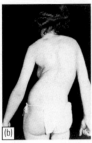
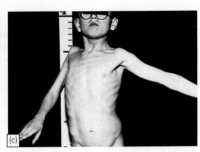

10.5 Poliomyelitis
(a) Shortening and wasting of the left leg, with equinus of the ankle. (b) This long curve is typical of a paralytic scoliosis. (c) Paralysis of the right deltoid and supraspinatus makes it impossible for this boy to abduct his right arm.

pyrexia subside – the convalescent stage has been reached.

Some anterior horn cells will have been destroyed by the virus; others, merely damaged by oedema, survive, and the muscles they supply can regain their lost power. Such recovery may continue for about 2 years, but after that any residual weakness is permanent. The clinical features of this stage will be described.

Clinical features

The patient is fit (except for residual paralysis), although if the trunk muscles were involved, he or she may have respiratory difficulty or may develop scoliosis. An affected limb often looks bluish, wasted and deformed; there are frequently extensive chilblains and the skin feels cold. Paralysis may be obvious, but lesser degrees of weakness are discovered only by systematic examination. Sensation is unaffected. When a badly paralysed limb is picked up it has a floppy feel which, in the presence of normal sensation, is characteristic. If the disease occurred in childhood, there may also be shortening of the limb.

Principles of treatment

In some countries immunization has been so successful that poliomyelitis has become a rare disease. However, the victims of earlier epidemics continue to pose challenging problems.

During the acute stage bed-rest and sedation are all that can be offered. When paralysis occurs, supportive treatment becomes increasingly important. Painful limb muscles need warmth and gentle physiotherapy.

During the long period of recovery physiotherapy is stepped up and every effort is made to regain maximum power; because of the associated trophic changes, hydrotherapy also is useful. Between exercise periods, splintage may be needed to prevent fixed deformities.

During the stage of residual paralysis orthopaedic treatment comes into its own. Four types of problem in particular may need attention.

1. *Isolated muscle weakness without deformity.* Quadriceps paralysis may make walking impossible; it is best managed with a splint or caliper which holds the knee straight. Elsewhere, isolated weakness (e.g. of thumb opposition) may be treated by tendon transfer.

2. *Residual deformity.* Unbalanced paralysis which is passively correctable can at first usually be counteracted by splintage. However, an appropriate tendon transfer may solve the problem permanently. Fixed deformity cannot be corrected by either splintage or tendon transfer alone; it is necessary to restore alignment operatively, and to stabilize the joint (if necessary, by arthrodesis). This is especially applicable to fixed deformities of the ankle and foot, but the same principle applies in treating paralytic scoliosis. Occasionally fixed deformity is an advantage: e.g. an equinus foot may help to compensate mechanically for quadriceps weakness and, if so, it should not be corrected.

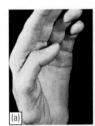
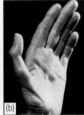
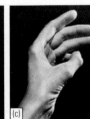
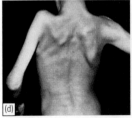
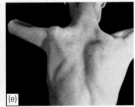

10.6 Poliomyelitis – treatment (a–c) Superficialis tendon transfer for opponens paralysis. In (b) the tendon can be seen in action at the start of thumb opposition (c). (d,e) Arthrodesis of the left shoulder to restore abduction after paralysis of the deltoid.

3. *Flail joint.* Balanced paralysis, because it causes no deformity, may need no treatment. However, if the joint is unstable it must be stabilized, either by permanent splintage or by arthrodesis.

4. *Shortening.* Leg length inequality of up to 3 cm can be compensated for by building up the shoe. Anything more is unsightly, and operative lengthening of the femur or tibia (or shortening of the opposite limb) might be preferable.

MOTOR NEURON DISORDERS

Rare degenerative disorders of the motor neurons and/or anterior horn cells of the cord cause progressive and sometimes fatal paralysis.

Motor neuron disease affects both UMNs and anterior horn cells, causing widespread symptoms and signs. Patients may present in middle age with muscle weakness (e.g. clumsy hands or unexplained foot-drop) and wasting in the presence of exaggerated reflexes. Sensation and bladder control are normal. The disease is progressive and incurable. Patients usually end up in a wheelchair and have increasing difficulty with speech and eating. Most of them die within 5 years from a combination of respiratory weakness and aspiration pneumonia. Supportive treatment includes nursing, occupational therapy and the use of various mechanical and electronic aids to assist in essential activities.

Spinal muscular atrophy is the term applied to a rare group of heritable disorders in which there is widespread anterior horn cell degeneration leading to progressive LMN weakness. In the worst cases the infant is weak and floppy at birth and death usually occurs within a year. In less severe forms, adolescents or young adults present with limb weakness, proximal muscle wasting and 'paralytic' scoliosis. Patients may live to 30–40 years of age but are usually confined to a wheelchair. Spinal braces are used to improve sitting ability; if this cannot prevent the spine from collapsing, operative instrumentation and fusion is advisable.

CHRONIC PERIPHERAL NEUROPATHIES

Disorders of the peripheral nerves may affect motor, sensory or autonomic functions; may be localized to a short segment or may involve the full length of the nerve fibres, including their cell bodies in the anterior horn (motor neurons), posterior root ganglia (sensory neurons) and autonomic ganglia. In some cases spinal cord tracts are involved as well.

There are essentially three types of peripheral nerve pathology: (1) acute interruption of axonal continuity; (2) axonal degeneration; and (3) demyelination – loss of the lipoprotein coating which 'insulates' all motor axons and the larger sensory axons serving touch, pain and proprioception. In all three, conduction is disturbed or completely blocked, with consequent loss of motor and/or sensory function. *Axonal degeneration* is the most damaging, and recovery, if it occurs at all, is slow and often incomplete. *Demyelination* is less harmful, may be localized to a short segment of nerve, and is usually followed by spontaneous recovery over a period of a few weeks. Most of the chronic neuropathies show a mixture of degeneration and demyelination.

Localized nerve injuries and *nerve entrapments* are dealt with in Chapter 11.

Classification

The peripheral neuropathies are divided into:

- *mononeuropathy* – involvement of a single nerve,
- *multiple mononeuropathy* – involvement of several isolated nerves (e.g. leprosy),
- *polyneuropathy* – widespread symmetrical dysfunction (e.g. diabetic neuropathy, alcoholic neuropathy or vitamin deficiency); in more than 50 per cent of cases no specific cause is found.

Disorders may be predominantly sensory, predominantly motor, or mixed. Chronic motor loss with no sensory component is usually due to anterior horn cell disease rather than polyneuropathy.

Clinical features

Patients usually complain of 'pins and needles' (paraesthesiae) or numbness. They may also notice weakness or loss of balance in walking. Occasionally (in the predominantly motor neuropathies) the main complaint is of progressive deformity, for example claw-hand or cavus foot.

The onset may be rapid (over a few days) or very gradual (over weeks or months). Sometimes there is a history of injury, infection, a known disease such as diabetes or malignancy, alcohol abuse or nutritional deficiency.

Examination may reveal weakness in a particular muscle group and/or loss of peripheral sensation. In the polyneuropathies the limbs are involved symmetrically, usually legs before arms and distal before proximal parts. In mononeuropathy, sensory loss follows the 'map' of the affected nerve. In polyneuropathy there is a symmetrical 'glove' or 'stocking' distribution.

Trophic skin changes may be present. Deep sensation is also affected and some patients develop ataxia. If pain sensibility and proprioception are depressed, there may be joint instability or breakdown of the articular surfaces (neuropathic joint disease or 'Charcot joints').

Clinical examination alone may establish the diagnosis. Further help is provided by electromyography (which may suggest the type of abnormality) and nerve conduction studies (which may show exactly where the lesion is). It is then still necessary to establish the cause (e.g. diabetes or alcoholism) though frequently none can be identified.

NEURALGIC AMYOTROPHY (ACUTE BRACHIAL NEURITIS)

This unusual cause of severe cervicobrachial pain and weakness is believed to be due to a viral infection of the cervical nerve roots; there is often a history of a recent viral infection and sometimes a small epidemic occurs among inmates of an institution.

The onset of pain around the scapula or in the shoulder and arm is often so sudden that the patient can recall the exact moment when it began. It may continue for days or weeks. Other symptoms are paraesthesiae in the arm or hand and weakness of the muscles of the shoulder, forearm or hand.

Muscle wasting may be obvious after a few days, and winging of the scapula (due to serratus

anterior weakness) is common. Shoulder movement is limited by pain but this limitation is invariably transient. Sensory loss in one or more of the cervical dermatomes is not uncommon.

The feature that distinguishes neuralgic amyotrophy from an acute cervical disc herniation is the involvement of multiple nerve root levels.

There is no specific treatment; pain is controlled with analgesics. The prognosis is usually good, but full neurological recovery may take months or years.

 Sudden upper limb pain plus neurological symptoms: ?neuralgic amyotrophy.

LEPROSY

Although uncommon in Europe and North America, this is still a frequent cause of peripheral neuropathy in Africa and Asia.

Mycobacterium leprae, an acid-fast organism, causes a diffuse inflammatory disorder of the skin, mucous membranes and peripheral nerves. Depending on the host response, several forms of disease may evolve. The most severe neurological lesions are seen in *tuberculoid leprosy.* Anaesthetic skin patches develop over the extensor surfaces of the limbs; loss of motor function leads to weakness and deformities of the hands and feet. Thickened nerves may be felt as cords under the skin or where they cross the bones (e.g. the ulnar nerve behind the medial epicondyle of the elbow). Trophic ulcers are common and may predispose to osteomyelitis.

Lepromatous leprosy is associated with a symmetrical polyneuropathy, which occurs late in the disease.

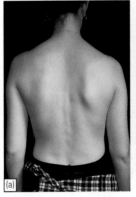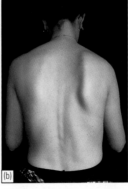

10.7 Neuralgic amyotrophy A common feature of neuralgic amyotrophy is winging of the scapula due to serratus anterior weakness. Even at rest (a) the right scapula is prominent in this young woman. When she thrusts her arms forwards against the wall (b) the abnormality is more pronounced.

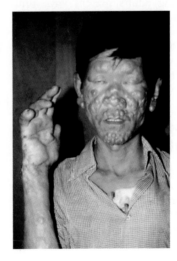

10.8 Leprosy – ulnar nerve paralysis Ulnar nerve paralysis is relatively common in long-standing leprosy. This patient has the typical ulnar claw-hand deformity.

Treatment

Combined chemotherapy (mainly rifampicin and dapsone) is continued for 6 months to 2 years, depending on the response. Muscle weakness – particularly the intrinsic muscle paralysis due to ulnar nerve involvement – may require multiple tendon transfers.

DIABETIC NEUROPATHY

Diabetes, especially if poorly controlled, is one of the commonest causes of peripheral neuropathy. Hyperglycaemia interferes with Schwann cell function, leading to demyelination and axonal degeneration. Microvascular occlusion may also play a part. Patients complain of numbness and paraesthesiae in the foot and hands. The onset is insidious and the condition often goes undiagnosed until complications arise – neuropathic ulcers of the feet, regional osteoporosis and fractures of the foot bones, or Charcot joints in the ankles and feet. There may be muscular weakness and loss of reflexes. A late feature is loss of balance.

Treatment

Management of the diabetic foot is discussed on page 250. Treatment consists essentially of skin care, management of fractures, and splintage or arthrodesis of grossly unstable or deformed joints. The underlying disorder should, of course, be controlled.

HEREDITARY NEUROPATHIES

These rare disorders present in childhood and adolescence, usually with muscle weakness and deformity.

Hereditary motor and sensory neuropathy (HMSN)

This is a group of conditions which includes *peroneal muscular atrophy* and *Charcot–Marie–Tooth disease,* the least rare of the inherited neuropathies, which are usually passed on as autosomal dominant disorders. HMSN type I is seen in young children, who have difficulty walking and develop claw-toes and pes cavus or cavovarus. There may be severe wasting of the legs and (later) the upper limbs. Spinal deformity is common. This is a demyelinating disorder and nerve conduction velocity is markedly slowed. The diagnosis can be confirmed by finding demyelination on sural nerve biopsy. Type II HMSN occurs in adolescents and young adults and is much less disabling than type I; it affects only the lower limbs, causing mild pes

cavus and wasting of the peronei. Nerve conduction velocity is only slightly reduced, indicating primary axonal degeneration.

If foot deformities are progressive or disabling, operative correction may bring a marked improvement.

Friedreich's ataxia

This autosomal recessive disorder is characterized by spinocerebellar dysfunction, but there may also be degeneration of the posterior root ganglia and peripheral nerves. Patients present at around the age of 6 years with gait ataxia, lower limb weakness and deformities similar to those of severe Charcot–Marie–Tooth disease. The muscle weakness, which may also involve the upper limbs and the trunk, is progressive; by the age of 20 years the patient has usually taken to a wheelchair and is likely to die of cardiomyopathy before the age of 45. Despite the poor prognosis, surgical correction of deformities is worthwhile.

ARTHROGRYPOSIS MULTIPLEX CONGENITA

This unwieldy term is applied to a group of rare congenital disorders characterized by multiple (often symmetrical) joint contractures. *Neurogenic* and *myogenic* varieties are described. In addition to the contractures there is stiffness of several joints, shapeless, cylindrical limbs and absence of skin creases. The deformities are associated with unbalanced muscle weakness, which follows a neurosegmental distribution. Deformities and contractures develop in utero and remain largely unchanged throughout life.

The most easily recognisable form of arthrogryposis is that affecting all four limbs. Typically, the shoulders are internally rotated and adducted, the elbows stiff in either flexion or extension, the wrists in flexion and ulnar deviation, the hips flexed and adducted, the knees usually hyperextended and the feet in equinovarus. When only a few joints are involved, the diagnosis can be more difficult. However, a characteristic 'localized' feature is bilateral rigid and intractable club-foot deformity.

Management

Treatment begins soon after birth and initially consists of gentle manipulation and muscle-stretching exercises, later combined with splintage to prevent (or slow down) recurrence of joint contractures. If progress is slow, tendon release, tendon transfers and osteotomies may become necessary. Arthrogrypotic club-foot usually

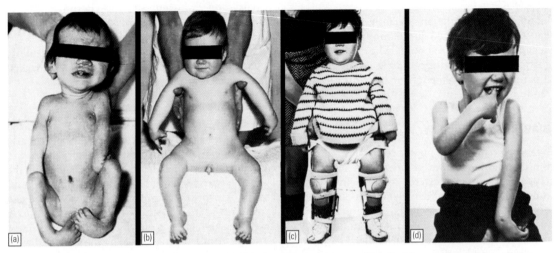

10.9 Arthrogryposis multiplex congenita (a,b) Severe deformities are present at birth. In this case all four limbs are affected. (c,d) Operative treatment is often worthwhile. In this young boy the lower limbs were tackled first and the feet and knees are held in splints. In the upper limbs, the minimum aim is to enable a hand to reach the mouth.

demands operative correction. Dislocation of the hip, likewise, often defies conservative treatment, and open reduction is needed. Whatever the form of treatment, parents should be warned that recurrent deformity is common. Remember that the aims of treatment are to provide these children with the ability to walk and upper limb function adequate to the needs of their most important daily activities, rather than the restoration of full movement.

MUSCULAR DYSTROPHY

The muscular dystrophies are extremely rare and only one of them will be considered. *Pseudohypertrophic muscular dystrophy (Duchenne dystrophy)* is a progressive disorder of sex-linked recessive inheritance. It is usually unsuspected until the child, always a boy, starts to walk. He has difficulty standing and falls frequently. Calf muscles may look bulky (pseudohypertrophy) but

this is due to fat and belies the weakness, which is progressive and generalized. By 10 years of age the child is unable to walk and he rarely survives into adult life. Manipulation, splintage or even tendon operations may help to prevent and correct deformities and to keep the child mobile.

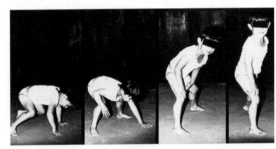

10.10 Muscular dystrophy This boy, with a Duchenne type of dystrophy, has to climb up his legs in order to achieve the upright position.

CHAPTER 11

PERIPHERAL NERVE INJURIES

Peripheral nerves are bundles of *axons* conducting efferent (motor) impulses from cells in the anterior horn of the spinal cord to the muscles, and afferent (sensory) impulses from peripheral receptors, via cells in the posterior root ganglia, to the cord. They also convey sudomotor and vasomotor fibres from ganglion cells in the sympathetic chain. Some nerves are predominantly motor, some predominantly sensory; the larger trunks are mixed, with motor and sensory axons running in separate bundles.

A single motor neuron supplies ten to several thousand muscle fibres, the ratio depending on the degree of dexterity demanded of the particular muscle (the smaller the ratio, the finer the movement). Similarly, the peripheral branches of each sensory neuron may serve anything from a single muscle spindle to a comparatively large patch of skin; here again, the fewer the end receptors served by a single axon, the greater the degree of discrimination.

The signal, or action potential, carried by motor neurons is transmitted to the muscle fibres by the release of a chemical transmitter, acetylcholine, at the terminal bouton of the nerve. Sensory signals are similarly conveyed to the dorsal root ganglia and from there up the ipsilateral column of the spinal cord, through the brainstem and thalamus, to the opposite (sensory) cortex. Proprioceptive impulses from the muscle spindles and joints bypass this route and are carried to the anterior horn cells as part of a local reflex arc. The economy of this system ensures that 'survival' mechanisms such as balance and sense of position in space are activated with great speed.

In the peripheral nerves, all motor axons and the large sensory axons serving touch, pain and proprioception are coated with *myelin,* a multilayered lipoprotein membrane derived from the accompanying *Schwann cells.* Every few millimetres the myelin sheath is interrupted, leaving short segments of bare axon called the *nodes of Ranvier.* Nerve impulses leap from node to node with the speed of electricity, much faster than would be the case if these axons were not insulated by the myelin sheaths. Depletion of the myelin sheath causes slowing – and eventually complete blocking – of axonal conduction.

Most axons – in particular the small-diameter fibres carrying crude sensation and the efferent sympathetic fibres – are unmyelinated but wrapped in Schwann cell cytoplasm. Damage to these axons causes unpleasant or bizarre sensations and various sudomotor and vasomotor effects.

Outside the Schwann cell membrane the axon is covered by a connective tissue stocking, the *endoneurium.* The axons that make up a nerve are separated into bundles (fascicles) by fairly dense membranous tissue, the *perineurium.* In a transected nerve, these fascicles are seen pouting from the cut surface, their perineurial sheaths well defined and strong enough to be grasped by fine instruments. The groups of fascicles that make up a nerve trunk are enclosed in an even thicker connective tissue coat, the *epineurium.*

The nerve is richly supplied by *blood vessels* that

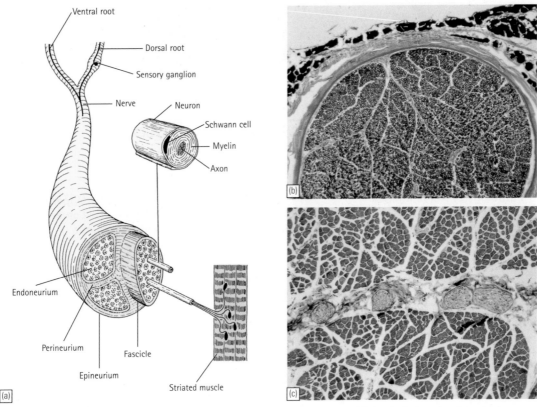

11.1 Nerve structure (a) Diagram of the structural elements of a peripheral nerve. (b) Histological section through a large nerve. The epineurium and perineurial septa are well defined; axons appear as tiny black dots. (c) High-power view, showing blood vessels in the perineurium.

run longitudinally in the epineurium before penetrating the various layers to become the *endoneurial capillaries.* These fine vessels may be damaged by stretching or rough handling.

PATHOLOGY OF NERVE INJURIES

Nerves can be injured by ischaemia, compression, traction, laceration or burning. Damage varies in severity from transient and quickly recoverable loss of function to complete interruption and degeneration.

Transient ischaemia

Acute nerve compression causes numbness and tingling within 15 minutes, loss of pain sensibility after 30 minutes and muscle weakness after 45 minutes. Relief of compression is followed by intense paraesthesiae lasting up to 5 minutes (the familiar 'pins and needles' after a limb 'goes to

sleep'); feeling is restored within 30 seconds and full muscle power after about 10 minutes. These changes are due to transient endoneurial anoxia and they leave no trace of nerve damage.

Neurapraxia

Herbert Seddon, in 1943, coined the term 'neurapraxia' to describe a reversible block to nerve conduction in which there is loss of sensation and muscle power, followed by spontaneous recovery after a few days or weeks. The nerve is intact but mechanical pressure has caused demyelination of axons in a limited segment.

Axonotmesis

This is a more severe form of injury in which there is interruption of the axons in a segment of nerve. It is seen typically after closed fractures and dislocations. There is loss of conduction but the nerve is in continuity and the neural tubes are intact. Distal to the lesion, and for a few millimetres proximal to it, axons disintegrate and are resorbed by phagocytes. This *Wallerian degeneration* (named after the physiologist Augustus Waller) takes only a few days and is accompanied by proliferation of Schwann cells and fibroblasts lining the endoneurial tubes. The denervated motor end-plates and sensory receptors gradually atrophy, and if they are not re-innervated within 2 years they will never recover.

Axonal regeneration starts within hours of nerve damage. The proximal stumps sprout numerous unmyelinated tendrils, many of which find their way into the cell-clogged endoneurial tubes. These new axonal processes grow at a speed of 1–2 mm per day, the larger fibres slowly acquiring a new myelin coat. Eventually they join to the denervated end-organs, which enlarge and start functioning again.

Neurotmesis

In Seddon's original classification, neurotmesis meant division of the nerve trunk, such as may occur in an open wound. It is now recognized that severe injury can be inflicted without actually dividing the nerve; in such cases there may be degrees of damage between that of axonotmesis, which is potentially recoverable,

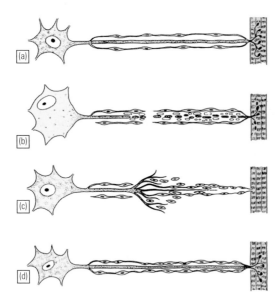

11.2 Nerve injury and regeneration (a) Normal axon and target organ (striated muscle). (b) Following nerve injury, the distal part of the axon disintegrates and the myelin sheath breaks up. (c) New axonal tendrils grow into the mass of proliferating Schwann cells. One of the tendrils will find its way into the old endoneurial tube and (d) the axon will slowly regenerate.

and complete neurotmesis which will never recover without surgical intervention. As in axonotmesis there is rapid Wallerian degeneration, but here the endoneurial tubes are destroyed over a variable segment and scarring thwarts any hope of regenerating axons entering the distal segment and regaining their target organs. Instead, regenerating fibres mingle with proliferating Schwann cells and fibroblasts in a jumbled knot, or 'neuroma', at the site of injury. Even after surgical repair many new axons fail to reach the distal segment, and those that do may not find suitable Schwann tubes, or may not reach the correct end-organs in time, or may remain incompletely myelinated. Function may be adequate but is never normal.

CLINICAL FEATURES

Acute nerve injuries are easily missed, especially if associated with fractures or dislocations, the symptoms of which may overshadow those of the nerve lesion. *Always test for nerve injuries following any significant trauma. And test again after manipulation or operation, in case the nerve has been damaged during treatment!*

Ask the patient if there is numbness, tingling or muscle weakness in the target area. Then examine the injured limb systematically for signs of abnormal posture (e.g. a wrist-drop in radial nerve palsy), weakness in specific muscle groups and changes in sensibility. The pattern of change is usually sufficiently characteristic to provide an anatomical diagnosis (see Table 10.1 and Fig. 10.1 on page 98).

If a nerve injury is present, it is crucial also to look for an accompanying vascular injury.

Diagnosis

Having established the presence of a *nerve injury* and, in most cases, the likely anatomical *level* of the injury, it is still necessary to diagnose the *type* of injury and the *degree* of damage. Nerve loss in low-energy injuries is likely to be due to neurapraxia, and in high-energy injuries and open wounds to axonotmesis or neurotmesis. In doubtful cases, one may have to wait a few weeks to see if signs of recovery appear, which would exclude complete nerve division. Muscles supplied by the nerve should be tested repeatedly: assuming that nerve regeneration occurs at the rate of 1 mm per day, one can estimate the expected time of recovery in muscles closest to the site of injury. With open wounds, however, early exploration is the best policy.

Diagnosis
Are there neurological symptoms?
Are there neurological signs?
What is the level of the lesion?
What type of lesion is it?
Are there signs of nerve recovery?

Tinel's sign

A classic sign of progressive nerve recovery is peripheral tingling provoked by percussing the nerve at the site of injury (because of sensitivity of the regenerating axons). After a delay of a few weeks, the sensitive spot should begin to advance down the limb at a rate of 1 mm per day. Failure of Tinel's sign to advance suggests a severe degree of nerve injury and the need for operative exploration.

Electrodiagnostic tests

Nerve conduction tests and electromyography may help to establish the level and severity of the injury, as well as the progress of nerve recovery.

PRINCIPLES OF TREATMENT

Open injuries

Nerve injuries associated with an open wound (even a small stab wound) should be explored and, if necessary, repaired as part of the patient's primary treatment. If the nerve is cleanly divided, end-to-end suture may be possible. A ragged cut will need paring of the stumps with a sharp blade. If this leaves too large a gap, or if the nerve stumps have retracted so that they cannot be brought together without tension, some slack can be gained by mobilizing the nerve, but if it is still difficult to bring the ends together without tension, nerve-grafts (from the sural nerve) can be used to span the interval. The nerve stumps should be anatomically oriented and fine (10/0) sutures inserted in the epineurium. This is specialized surgery, which must be performed under magnification.

Postoperatively, physiotherapy is applied to retain joint movement. However, if there is the least doubt about tension on the nerve, the limb should be splinted in a position which keeps the nerve relaxed for about 2 weeks before starting physiotherapy.

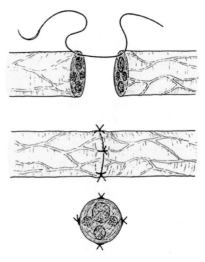

11.3 Nerve repair The stumps are correctly oriented and attached by fine sutures through the epineurium.

Closed injuries

With closed nerve lesions it is more difficult to decide what to do, especially during the first few weeks after injury. In most cases the nerve sheath is intact (neurapraxia or axonotmesis), so one can afford to wait at least until the muscle whose nerve supply arises just below the injury should have recovered (see page 111, 'Diagnosis'). If at that time there is still no sign of recovery, the nerve should be explored.

Delayed repair

Late repair – i.e. weeks or months after the injury – may be indicated because (1) a closed injury was left alone but showed no sign of recovery at the expected time, (2) the diagnosis was missed and the patient presented late, or (3) primary repair has failed. The options must be weighed carefully: if the patient has adapted to the functional loss, if it is a high lesion and re-innervation is unlikely within the critical 2-year period, or if there is a pure motor loss which can be treated by tendon transfer, it may be best to leave well alone. Excessive scarring and intractable joint stiffness may, likewise, make nerve repair questionable; yet in the hand it is still worthwhile simply to regain protective sensation.

The lesion is exposed, working from normal tissue above and below towards the scarred area. If the nerve is in continuity, only slightly thickened and soft, or if there is conduction across the lesion, resection is not advised; if the nerve is scarred and there is no conduction on electrical stimulation, the scar should be resected, paring back the stumps until healthy fascicles are exposed. Nerve suture or grafting is then performed as described above.

Care of paralysed parts

While recovery is awaited, the skin must be protected from friction damage and burns. The joints should be moved through their full range twice daily to prevent stiffness and minimize the work required of muscles when they recover. 'Dynamic' splints may be helpful.

Tendon transfers

Motor recovery may not occur if the regenerating axons fail to reach the muscle within 18–24 months of injury. In such circumstances, tendon transfers should be considered. The following principles must be observed: (1) the donor muscle should be expendable and have adequate power; (2) the recipient site must be mobile and stable; (3) the transferred tendon should be routed subcutaneously in a straight line of pull.

NERVE INJURIES AFFECTING THE UPPER LIMB

BRACHIAL PLEXUS INJURIES

The brachial plexus is formed by the confluence of nerve roots from C5 to T1. The network is most vulnerable to injury where the nerves run from the cervical spine, between the muscles of the neck and beneath the clavicle en route to the arm – either a stab wound or severe traction caused by a fall on the side of the neck or the shoulder. *Supraclavicular lesions* typically occur in motorcycle accidents. *Infraclavicular lesions* are usually associated with fractures or dislocations of the shoulder. Fractures of the clavicle rarely damage the plexus, and then only if caused by a direct blow.

The injury may affect any level of the plexus. *Pre-ganglionic lesions* (i.e. disruption of nerve roots proximal to the dorsal root ganglion) cannot recover and are surgically irreparable. *Post-ganglionic lesions* can be repaired and are capable of recovery. Lesions in continuity have a better prognosis than complete ruptures.

Clinical features

Clinical examination should establish (a) the level of the lesion, (b) whether it is pre-ganglionic or post-ganglionic, and (c) the type of damage.

The level of the lesion

Upper plexus injuries (C5 and 6) cause paralysis of the shoulder abductors and external rotators and the forearm supinators; typically the arm hangs close to the body and internally rotated. Sensation is lost along the outer aspect of the arm and forearm. *Pure lower plexus injuries* are rare; the intrinsic hand muscles are paralysed, resulting in

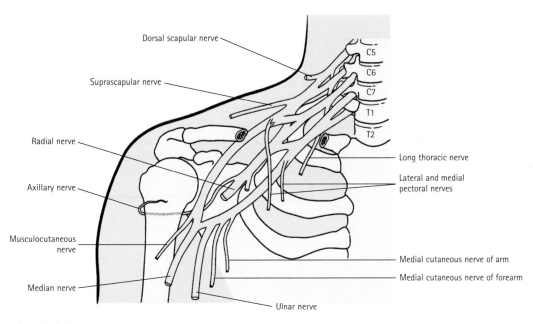

11.4 Brachial plexus Diagram of the brachial plexus and its relationship to the clavicle.

clawing, and sensation is lost along the inner (ulnar) aspect of the arm. *Total plexus lesions* result in paralysis and numbness of the entire limb.

Pre-ganglionic or post-ganglionic

It is important to establish whether the lesion is proximal or distal to the dorsal root ganglion: the former is irreparable; the latter can be repaired and may recover. Features suggesting pre-ganglionic root avulsion are (1) burning pain in an anaesthetic hand, (2) paralysis of scapular muscles or diaphragm, (3) Horner's syndrome (see page 98), (4) severe vascular injury, (5) associated fractures of the cervical spine and (6) spinal cord dysfunction.

The *histamine test* is helpful. Intradermal injection of histamine normally causes a reflex triple response in the surrounding skin (central capillary dilatation, a wheal and a surrounding flare). If the flare reaction persists in an anaesthetic area of skin, the lesion must be proximal to the posterior root ganglion – i.e. it is probably a root avulsion. With a post-ganglionic lesion, the test will be negative because nerve continuity between the skin and the dorsal root ganglion is interrupted.

CT myelography or MRI may show pseudomeningoceles produced by root avulsion.

The type of damage

In post-ganglionic lesions it helps to know how severely the nerve has been damaged. With low-velocity injuries, a period of observation is justified; neurapraxia and axonotmesis should show signs of recovery by 6 or 8 weeks. If neurotmesis seems likely, early operative exploration is called for.

Management

The patient is likely to be admitted to a general unit where fractures and other injuries will be given priority. Emergency surgery is required for brachial plexus lesions associated with penetrating wounds, vascular injury or severe (high-energy) soft-tissue damage, whether open or closed; clean-cut nerves should be repaired or grafted. This is best performed by a team specializing in this kind of work.

All other closed injuries are left until detailed examination and special investigations have been completed. Patients with root avulsion or severe, mutilating injuries of the limb will be unsuitable for nerve surgery, at least until the prognosis for limb function becomes clear.

Progress of the neurological features is carefully monitored. As long as recovery proceeds at the expected rate, watchful observation is in order. If recovery falters, or if special investigations suggest

neurotmesis, the patient should be referred to a special centre for surgical exploration of the brachial plexus and nerve repair, grafting or a nerve transfer procedure. The sooner this decision is made, the better: during the early days, operative exposure is easier and the response to repair more reliable. Repairs performed after 6 months are unlikely to succeed.

Prognosis

Pure upper plexus lesions have the best prognosis. Hand function is spared and muscles innervated from the upper roots often recover after plexus repair or nerve transfer. With avulsion of C7, C8 and T1, even if shoulder and elbow movements are restored, the loss of hand function causes severe disability.

Late reconstruction

If the patient is not seen until very late after injury, or if plexus reconstruction has failed, tendon transfers may restore a moderate level of function.

OBSTETRICAL BRACHIAL PLEXUS INJURIES

Obstetrical palsy is caused by excessive traction on the brachial plexus during childbirth. Two patterns are seen: (1) *upper root injury (Erb's palsy)*, typically in overweight babies with shoulder dystocia at delivery; or (2) *complete plexus injury (Klumpke's palsy)*, usually after breech delivery of smaller babies.

Clinical features

The diagnosis is usually obvious at birth: after a difficult delivery the baby has a floppy or flail arm. Further examination a day or two later will define the type of brachial plexus injury.

Erb's palsy

Injury of C5, C6 and (sometimes) C7 causes paralysis of the abductors and external rotators of the shoulder and the forearm supinators. The arm is held to the side, internally rotated and pronated.

Klumpke's palsy

A complete plexus lesion is much less common, but more severe. The arm is flail and pale; all finger muscles are paralysed, and there may also be vasomotor impairment and an ipsilateral Horner's syndrome (see page 98).

 Prolonged labour and/or shoulder dystocia: examine for brachial plexus injury.

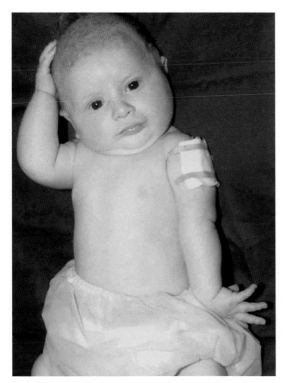

11.5 Erb's palsy Paralysis of the abductors and external rotators of the shoulder, as well as the forearm supinators, results in the typical posture demonstrated in this baby with Erb's palsy of the left arm.

Treatment

If there is no biceps recovery by 3 months, operative intervention should be considered. Unless the roots are avulsed, it may be possible to excise the scar and bridge the gap with free sural nerve-grafts; if the roots are avulsed, nerve transfer may give a worthwhile result. This is advanced surgery which should be undertaken only in specialized centres.

The shoulder is prone to fixed internal rotation and adduction deformity. If diligent physiotherapy does not prevent this, a subscapularis release will be needed, sometimes supplemented by a tendon transfer. In older children, the deformity can be treated by rotation osteotomy of the humerus.

LONG THORACIC NERVE

The nerve to serratus anterior may be damaged in shoulder or neck injuries, or by carrying heavy loads on the shoulder.

The classic sign of serratus anterior palsy is winging of the scapula. This is displayed by asking the patient to push forwards forcefully against a wall.

Except after direct injury or division, the nerve usually recovers spontaneously, though this may take a year or longer.

X-rays should be taken to exclude fractures of the shoulder or clavicle.

Management

Over the next few weeks, one of the following may happen.

Paralysis may recover completely

Upper root lesions often recover spontaneously. A reliable indicator is return of biceps activity by the third month.

Paralysis may improve and then remain static

A total lesion may partially resolve, leaving the infant with either an upper or a complete root syndrome which is unlikely to change.

Paralysis may remain unaltered

This is more likely with complete lesions, especially in the presence of Horner's syndrome.

While waiting for recovery, physiotherapy is applied to keep the joints mobile.

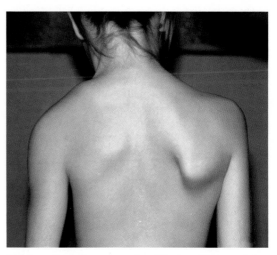

11.6 Long thoracic nerve palsy Winging of the scapula is demonstrated by the patient pushing forwards against the wall. If the serratus anterior is paralysed, the scapula cannot be held firmly against the rib-cage.

SPINAL ACCESSORY NERVE

The spinal accessory nerve supplies the sternomastoid muscle and then runs obliquely across the posterior triangle of the neck to innervate the upper half of the trapezius. Because of its superficial course, it is easily injured in stab wounds and operations in the posterior triangle of the neck.

Following an open wound or operation, the patient complains of pain in the shoulder and weakness on abduction of the arm. There is mild winging of the scapula on active abduction against resistance. In late cases there may be wasting of the trapezius and drooping of the shoulder.

Stab injuries and operative injuries should be explored immediately and the nerve repaired. If the exact cause of injury is uncertain, it is prudent to wait for 6 weeks for signs of recovery. If this does not occur, the nerve should be repaired or grafted.

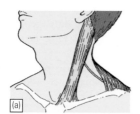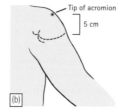

11.7 Dangerous landmarks (a) The accessory nerve runs across the middle of the posterior triangle of the neck and is easily damaged during lymph node biopsy in this area. (b) The axillary nerve runs from behind the shoulder around the outer aspect of the arm about 5 cm below the tip of the acromion process. Incisions across the top of the shoulder must stop short of this level if injury to the axillary nerve is to be avoided.

AXILLARY NERVE

The axillary nerve (C5) is sometimes injured during shoulder dislocation or fractures of the humeral neck. The patient cannot abduct the shoulder (even when pain subsides) owing to deltoid weakness. There may be a small patch of numbness over the deltoid (C5 dermatome).

The nerve usually recovers spontaneously, but if there is no sign of recovery by 8 weeks and electro-diagnostic tests suggest denervation, the nerve should be explored and grafted. A good result can be expected if surgery is performed within 12 weeks of injury. However, if the operation fails, shoulder arthrodesis or tendon transfer should be considered.

RADIAL NERVE

The radial nerve may be injured at the elbow, in the upper arm or in the axilla.

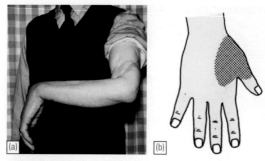

11.8 Radial nerve palsy (a) This man developed a complete drop-wrist palsy following a severe open fracture of the humerus and division of the radial nerve. (b) The typical area of sensory loss.

Low lesions are usually due to fractures or dislocations at the elbow, or an open wound or surgical accident. The patient cannot extend the metacarpophalangeal joints.

High lesions occur with fractures of the humerus or after prolonged tourniquet pressure. They are also seen in patients who fall asleep with the arm dangling over the back of a chair (Saturday night palsy). There is an obvious wrist-drop due to weakness of the wrist extensors and a small patch of sensory loss on the back of the hand at the base of the thumb.

Very high lesions are usually due to pressure in the axilla ('crutch palsy'). The triceps muscle is wasted and paralysed. Spontaneous recovery is the rule.

Open wounds should be explored and the nerve repaired or grafted as soon as possible.

The lesion associated with a fractured humerus is usually an axonotmesis, and function eventually returns. One can therefore afford to wait. However, if there is no sign of recovery by 8–12 weeks, the nerve should be explored and repaired or grafted.

If it is certain that there was no nerve injury on admission and the signs appear only after manipulation or operative treatment, the chances of an iatrogenic injury are high and the nerve should be explored and repaired.

In all cases, while recovery is awaited, the wrist should be splinted in extension and the meta-carpophalangeal and finger joints kept moving.

In radial nerve lesions that do not recover, the disability can be largely overcome by suitable tendon transfers.

ULNAR NERVE

Injuries of the ulnar nerve are usually either near the wrist or near the elbow, although open wounds may damage it at any level.

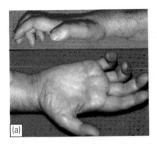
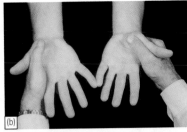
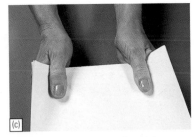

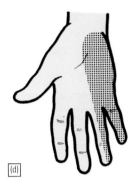

11.9 Ulnar nerve palsy (a) Clawing of the ring and little fingers and wasting of the intrinsic muscles. (b) A good test for interosseous muscle weakness. Ask the patient to spread his fingers (abduct) as strongly as possible and then force his hands together with the little fingers apposed; the weaker side will collapse (the left hand in this case).
(c) *Froment's sign:* the patient is asked to grip a card firmly between thumbs and index fingers; normally this is done using the thumb adductors while the interphalangeal joint is held extended. In the right hand, because the adductor pollicis is weak, the patient grips the card only by acutely flexing the interphalangeal joint of the thumb (flexor pollicis longus is supplied by the median nerve). (d) Typical area of sensory loss.

Low lesions may be caused by pressure (e.g. from a deep ganglion) or a laceration at the wrist. There is hypothenar wasting and the hand is clawed due to paralysis of the intrinsic muscles. Finger abduction is weak, and the loss of thumb adduction makes pinch difficult. Sensation is lost over the ulnar one and a half fingers.

High lesions occur with elbow fractures; they are also seen (much later) if malunion produces marked cubitus valgus with tension on the nerve where it skirts the medial epicondyle. Remember that ulnar nerve symptoms can also be caused by nerve entrapment in the cubital tunnel, especially in patients lying for long periods with the elbows flexed and pressing on the bed. Curiously, the visible deformity is not marked, because the ulnar half of flexor digitorum profundus is paralysed and the fingers are therefore less 'clawed'. Otherwise motor and sensory loss are the same as in low lesions.

Exploration and suture of a divided ulnar nerve are more easily achieved than with most other nerves; large gaps can be bridged because one can gain length by transposing the nerve to the front of the elbow. If recovery does not occur, hand function is significantly impaired because of the loss of power in metacarpophalangeal flexion, finger abduction, pinch and grip. Tendon transfers are possible, but usually restore only a modest level of function.

MEDIAN NERVE

The median nerve is commonly injured near the wrist or high up in the forearm.

Low lesions may be caused by cuts in front of the wrist or by carpal dislocations. The thenar eminence is wasted and thumb abduction and opposition are weak. Sensation is lost over the radial three and a half digits, and trophic changes may be seen.

High lesions are generally due to forearm fractures or elbow dislocation, but stabs and gunshot wounds may damage the nerve at any level. The signs are the same as those of low lesions but, in

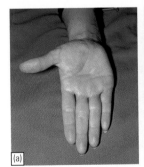
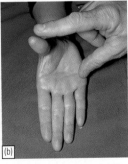

11.10 Median nerve – testing for abductor power (a) The hand must remain flat, palm upwards. (b) The patient is told to point the thumb towards the ceiling against the examiner's resistance.

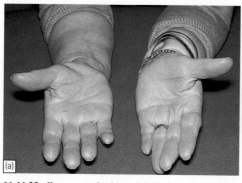
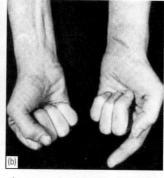
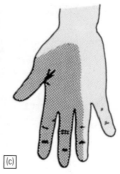

11.11 Median nerve lesions (a) Wasting of the thenar eminence on the right side. (b) In high median nerve lesions, the long flexors to the thumb and index fingers are also paralysed and the patient shows the 'pointing index sign'. (c) Typical area of sensory loss.

addition, the long flexors to the thumb, index and middle fingers are paralysed (Fig 11.11b).

If the nerve is divided, suture should always be attempted; if this cannot be done without producing tension, nerve-grafts can be placed in the gap. If no recovery occurs, disability is severe – mainly because of sensory loss. Tendon transfer can restore thumb opposition, but useful function depends on having sensation as well.

NERVE INJURIES AFFECTING THE LOWER LIMB

FEMORAL NERVE

The femoral nerve may be injured by a gunshot wound, by traction during an operation or by bleeding into the thigh. There is weakness of knee extension (quadriceps) and numbness of the anterior thigh and medial aspect of the leg. The knee jerk is depressed.

This is a disabling lesion and early treatment is essential. A thigh haematoma may need to be evacuated. A clean cut of the nerve may be treated successfully by careful suturing or grafting.

SCIATIC NERVE

Division of the main sciatic nerve is rare except in gunshot wounds or operative (iatrogenic) accidents. Traction and compression are more common and occur with local trauma.

The patient complains of foot-drop, numbness and paraesthesia in the leg and foot; if there has been direct injury to the nerve, the limb may also be painful. Muscles below the knee are paralysed and sensation is absent in most of the leg. If only the deep (peroneal) component of the nerve is affected, paralysis is incomplete and the signs are

easily mistaken for those of a common peroneal nerve injury. Late features are wasting of the calf and trophic ulcers.

If the nerve injury follows hip dislocation or fracture, this must be attended to urgently. Open wounds should be explored and the nerve repaired. While recovery is awaited, a drop-foot splint should be fitted.

The chances of recovery are generally poor and, at best, it will be long delayed and incomplete. Partial lesions can sometimes be managed by tendon transfers. However, if there is no recovery whatever, amputation may be preferable to a flail, deformed, insensitive limb.

Iatrogenic lesions

Sciatic nerve palsy is one of the recognized complications of hip replacement. Usually it is a partial lesion, which is sometimes misdiagnosed as a common peroneal compression injury. There is little to guide one as to whether the sciatic injury is due to direct trauma or to traction on the nerve. If direct injury is suspected, the nerve should be explored. Otherwise it is best to wait for spontaneous recovery, which may take several weeks. In all cases the foot should be splinted to prevent a permanent equinus deformity.

PERONEAL NERVES

The *common peroneal nerve* may be damaged in lateral ligament injuries when the knee is forced into varus, or by pressure from a splint or a plaster cast, or from lying with the leg externally rotated. The patient develops a drop-foot in which both dorsiflexion and eversion are weak. Sensation is lost over the front and outer half of the leg and the dorsum of the foot.

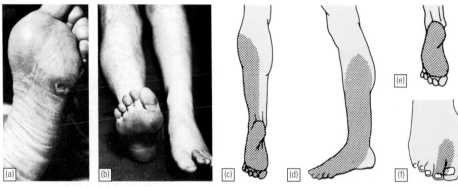

11.12 Sciatic and peroneal nerve lesions (a) One of the late complications is trophic ulceration due to loss of sensibility in the foot. (b) Loss of dorsiflexion causes foot-drop. Characteristic areas of sensory loss are shown: (c) complete sciatic nerve injury, (d) common peroneal nerve injury, (e) posterior tibial nerve injury, and (f) anterior tibial (deep peroneal) nerve injury.

 Following hip surgery, symptoms and signs of 'peroneal nerve injury' are usually, in fact, due to partial sciatic nerve injury.

If only the *superficial branch* is involved, the peroneal muscles are paralysed and eversion is lost, but dorsiflexion is intact. There is loss of sensation over the outer side of the leg and foot.

The *deep branch* may be threatened in an anterior compartment syndrome (see page 378). The patient complains of pain, abnormal sensation and weakness of dorsiflexion; on testing, there may be an area of sensory loss around the first web space on the dorsum of the foot.

Treatment depends on the local circumstances. A threatened compartment syndrome must be treated as an emergency and may need immediate decompression. If there is an open wound, the nerve should be explored and sutured.

While recovery is awaited, a splint is worn to control the foot-drop; the skin must be protected against ulceration. If recovery does not occur, disability can be improved by tendon transfers or foot stabilization.

NERVE ENTRAPMENT SYNDROMES

Wherever peripheral nerves traverse fibro-osseous tunnels, they are at risk of entrapment or compression, especially if the soft tissues increase in bulk, as they may in pregnancy, myxoedema or rheumatoid arthritis, or if there is a local obstruction (e.g. a ganglion or osteophytic spur). The most common sites are the *carpal tunnel* at the wrist (median nerve) and the *cubital tunnel* at the elbow (ulnar nerve). Less common sites are the fascial septa elsewhere in the *forearm,* the *tarsal tunnel* below the ankle (posterior tibial nerve) and the lateral part of the *inguinal ligament* (lateral cutaneous nerve of the thigh). A special case is the *thoracic outlet,* where the subclavian vessels and trunks of the brachial plexus cross the first rib between the scalenus anterior and medius muscles. In these cases there may be vascular as well as neurological signs in the upper limb.

Patients with long-standing, mild, possibly unrecognized, polyneuropathies (for example due to diabetes or alcohol abuse) are particularly prone to symptoms of localized nerve compression. A general neurological assessment is therefore advisable in all patients with features of local nerve compression.

Clinical features

The patient complains of unpleasant tingling or pain or numbness. Symptoms are usually intermittent and related to specific postures which compromise the nerve. Thus, in the *carpal tunnel syndrome,* they occur when the wrist is held still in flexion or hyperextension (often at night when the patient is asleep), and relief is obtained by changing posture or shaking the hand 'to get the circulation going'. In *ulnar neuropathy,* symptoms may be brought on by leaning on the elbow or holding the elbow in flexion for long periods, for example when lying down and reading a book or newspaper, when driving, or when talking on the telephone.

Areas of altered sensation, motor weakness and muscle wasting are so characteristic that the diagnosis and the site of compressive trauma are immediately suggested. The clinical features of altered peripheral nerve function are described in the preceding pages.

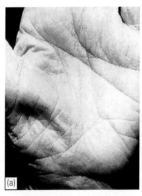
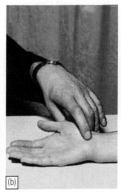
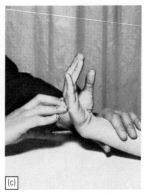
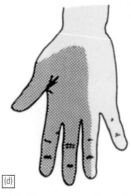

(a) (b) (c) (d)

11.13 Carpal tunnel syndrome (a) Wasting of the thenar eminence is not usually as obvious as this. However, even if muscle bulk looks normal, testing for abductor power will usually show that it is weaker than that in the normal hand (see Figure 11.10). (b) Tinel's sign may be present and (c) holding the wrist in flexion for a few minutes may induce the patient's symptoms (Phalen's test). (d) Area of diminished sensibility.

The likely site of compression should be carefully examined for any local cause – for example in ulnar nerve entrapment a long-standing valgus deformity of the elbow, or in the carpal tunnel syndrome an old Colles' fracture.

The diagnosis may be confirmed by measuring nerve conduction velocity, which is likely to be impaired in the affected segment of the nerve. It is well to remember, though, that this test is not infallible and it should not be used as substitute for careful clinical assessment.

Treatment

In early cases, simple measures such as advising the patient to avoid compromising postures of the affected limb, or preventing flexion of the wrist or elbow with a light-weight splint, may help. If an inflammatory disorder is suspected, corticosteroid injection into the entrapment area can reduce local tissue swelling. The condition is often self-limiting, so there is no hurry about operative treatment. If symptoms persist, or if there is muscle weakness and wasting, operative decompression is indicated. Once axonal degeneration occurs, tunnel decompression may fail to give complete relief.

Median nerve decompression is achieved by dividing the transverse carpal ligament at the wrist. The operation is usually very successful in relieving symptoms. Patients who go on complaining should be investigated for cervical spondylosis.

Ulnar nerve decompression can usually be achieved by simply splitting the aponeurosis covering the nerve below the elbow; only rarely is it necessary to transpose the nerve from its normal position behind the medial condyle of the humerus to a more relaxed position in front of the elbow.

THORACIC OUTLET SYNDROME

Neurological and vascular symptoms and signs in the upper limbs may be produced by compression of the lower trunk of the brachial plexus (C8 and T1) and subclavian vessels between the clavicle and the first rib. These neurovascular structures are made taut when the shoulders are braced back and the arms held tightly to the sides; an extra rib (or its fibrous equivalent extending from a large costal process) exaggerates this effect by forcing the vessel and nerve upwards. Such anomalies are present at birth, yet symptoms are rare before the age of 30. This is probably because, with increasing age, the shoulders sag, thus putting more traction on the neurovascular bundle.

Clinical features

The patient, typically a woman in her 30s, complains of pain and paraesthesia extending from the shoulder, down the ulnar aspect of the arm and into the medial two fingers. Symptoms tend to be worse at night and are also aggravated by bracing the shoulders (wearing a back-pack) or working with the arms above shoulder height. Examination may show weakness and slight wasting of the intrinsic muscles in the hand. Vascular signs are uncommon, but the patient may complain of cyanosis, coldness of the fingers and increased sweating.

Symptoms and signs can sometimes be reproduced by certain provocative manoeuvres. In *Adson's test* the patient's neck is extended and turned towards the affected side while he or she breathes in deeply; this compresses the interscalene space and may cause paraesthesia and obliteration of the radial pulse. In *Wright's test* the arms are abducted and externally rotated; again, the symptoms recur and the pulse disappears on the abnormal side.

Investigations

X-rays of the neck occasionally demonstrate a cervical rib or an abnormally long C7 transverse process. However, similar features are sometimes encountered as purely incidental findings in asymptomatic people, and the demonstration of a cervical rib should not be taken as 'proof positive' of a thoracic outlet problem. Equally important are x-rays of the lungs (is there an apical tumour?) and the shoulders (to exclude any local lesion).

Electrodiagnostic tests are helpful mainly to exclude peripheral nerve lesions such as ulnar or median nerve compression which may confuse the diagnosis.

Angiography and *venography* are reserved for the few patients with vascular symptoms.

Diagnosis

The diagnosis of thoracic outlet syndrome is not easy. Indeed, some clinicians doubt its very existence as a pathological entity!

Tumours of the lower cervical cord or cervical vertebrae and compressive lesions affecting the lower cervical nerve roots must always be excluded. The presence of Horner's syndrome is a valuable clue (see page 98).

Cervical spondylosis is sometimes discovered on x-ray. However, this seldom involves the T1 nerve root.

Pancoast's syndrome, due to apical carcinoma of the bronchus with infiltration of the structures at the root of the neck, includes pain, numbness and weakness of the hand. A hard mass may be palpable in the neck, and x-ray of the chest shows a characteristic opacity.

Ulnar nerve compression can be excluded by electromyography and nerve conduction studies.

Treatment

Conservative treatment suffices for most patients: exercises to strengthen the shoulder-girdle muscles, postural training and instruction in work practices and ways of preventing shoulder droop and muscle fatigue. Analgesics may be needed for pain.

Operative treatment is indicated if pain is severe, if muscle wasting is obvious or if there are vascular disturbances. The thoracic outlet is decompressed by removing the first rib (or the cervical rib). This can be accomplished by either a supraclavicular approach or a transaxillary approach.

CHAPTER 12

PRINCIPLES OF OPERATIVE TREATMENT

The art and skill of orthopaedic surgery are directed not to constructing a particular arrangement of parts but to restoring function to the whole. The operation is only part of this exercise; orthopaedic 'surgery' also involves careful preoperative preparation and planning, and postoperative rehabilitation.

PREOPERATIVE PREPARATION

General assessment of the patient

The need for general assessment of the patient and of his or her ability to tolerate the operation goes without saying. It is important also to evaluate the risk of complications such as thromboembolism and infection in the particular individual and, where necessary, to start prophylactic treatment before the operation.

Planning the operation

Operations must be carefully planned in advance, when accurate measurements can be made and the bones and joints can be compared for symmetry with those of the opposite side. X-rays, MRI and CT (if necessary with three-dimensional re-formation) are helpful; templates may be needed to help select the appropriate shape and size of a prosthetic implant; complex corrective osteotomies should ideally be simulated on paper cut-outs before the operation is undertaken; best of all is a rehearsal of the operation using artificial bones.

 Preoperative planning pays off. Something unexpected usually means something unprepared for.

The operating environment

Short operating times and limiting the number of people in the theatre will reduce the likelihood of infection. Long and complex operations, joint replacement procedures and all operations in which the risk of tissue contamination or infection is considered to be high should be performed in ultra-clean-air theatres and prophylactic antibiotics should be administered before, during and after the operation.

Equipment

The minimum requirements for orthopaedic operations are drills (for boring holes), osteotomes (for cutting cancellous bone), saws (for cutting cortical bone), chisels (for shaping bone), gouges (for removing bone) and plates, screws and screwdrivers (for fixing bone).

Operations such as joint replacement, spinal fusion and internal fixation require special implants and instruments. It is very unwise to attempt these operations without gaining familiarity with the equipment and practising on dry specimens. Equally important, it is the surgeon's responsibility to ensure that all the special equipment needed for the intended procedure is available in the theatre before starting the operation.

Intraoperative radiography

Intraoperative radiography, fluoroscopy and image intensification are often helpful and sometimes essential. Fracture reduction, osteotomy alignments and the positioning of implants and fixation devices can be checked during the operation and again at the end of the procedure.

Magnification

Magnification is an integral part of peripheral nerve and hand surgery. The improved view minimizes the trauma of surgery and allows more accurate apposition of tissues during reconstruction.

The 'bloodless field'

Many operations on limbs can be done more rapidly and accurately if bleeding is prevented by the application of a tourniquet. Only a *pneumatic cuff* is suitable. Rubber bandages are potentially dangerous: the pressure beneath the bandage cannot be controlled and there is a risk of damage to the underlying nerves and muscle. A layer of wool bandage beneath the pneumatic cuff will distribute the pressure and prevent wrinkling of the underlying skin.

Adequate exsanguination of the tissues can usually be achieved by elevating the limb for 1 minute before inflating the cuff. If a completely bloodless field is required, an Esmarch bandage wrapped from distal to proximal is effective.

Tourniquet pressure should not exceed 150 mmHg above systolic for the lower limb and 100 mmHg above systolic for the upper limb.

Tourniquet time should not exceed 2 hours. Time can be saved by ensuring that the limb is shaved, prepared, draped and marked before inflating the cuff. Whenever practicable, the tourniquet should be removed before the wound is closed, so that bleeding can be controlled and a 'silent' postoperative haematoma avoided. *Excessive or prolonged pressure can cause permanent nerve or muscle damage.* The time restriction is sometimes overcome by deflating and re-inflating the cuff during the operation; if this is done without allowing adequate perfusion of the tissues, it may aggravate ischaemic damage.

OPERATIONS ON BONES

FIXATION OF FRACTURES

Internal fixation

Fixation with screws, plates or intramedullary nails enables a reduced fracture to be held so securely that activity (although not necessarily weight-bearing) can begin immediately. It is particularly useful for fractures in elderly patients, for multiple injuries, and for fractures which are prone to displacement and malunion. Scrupulous asepsis and meticulous technique are imperative.

External fixation

Fractures associated with severe soft-tissue injuries are often best managed by external fixation. The principles are straightforward: metal pins or stiff wires are driven through the bone above and below the fracture; the fracture is reduced and the pins are attached to external bars which hold the system rigidly while leaving the soft tissues exposed and accessible for treatment. There are numerous variations in pin and frame configuration, aiming

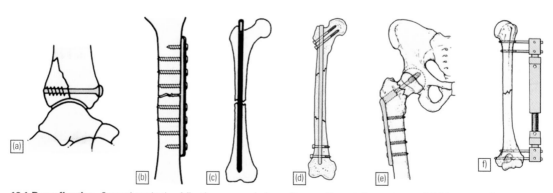

12.1 Bone fixation Several methods of fixation are used, depending on site and circumstances. (a) A lag screw for interfragmentary compression. (b) Plate and screws. (c) Intramedullary nail. (d) Locked intramedullary nail. (e) Dynamic hip screw. (f) External fixator.

to provide the best mechanical structure for the particular problem. Modifications in design have extended the use of external fixation to the management of non-union, bone elongation, repair of bone defects and correction of deformities (see pages 125–127).

OSTEOTOMY

Osteotomy may be used to correct deformity, to change the shape of the bone, or to relieve pain in arthritis by redirecting the load trajectories. Preoperative planning is essential, with precise measurements of the patient and the x-rays. The site of the osteotomy, the amount of bone to be removed (if any), the degree of angular and rotational correction and the proposed method of fixation should be firmly established beforehand.

To change an angular deformity, a wedge of bone may have to be removed ('closing wedge') or inserted ('opening wedge'). The size of the wedge should be calculated accurately and reproduced precisely by using suitable templates. The bone segments are then fixed in the new position, either with a plate and screws or (at the proximal and distal ends of the femur) with an angled blade-plate and screws. When correcting severe deformities, care should be taken not to put excessive tension on the soft tissues, as this may cause nerve damage. *Postoperatively, a careful watch should be kept for signs of compartment syndrome due to oozing from the cut bone surfaces into the surrounding tissues* (see page 294). Partial weight-bearing is allowed if fixation is stable; otherwise it is deferred until healing is sufficiently advanced.

An alternative approach is to divide the bone and then apply an adjustable external fixation device which will permit progressive correction over time (see page 127).

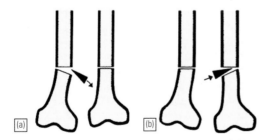

12.2 Osteotomy A bent bone can be straightened (a) by removing a wedge of bone and then placing the fragments in apposition (closing wedge osteotomy), or (b) by dividing the bone and inserting a wedge (opening wedge osteotomy).

BONE-GRAFTS

Bone-grafts are both *osteoinductive* and *osteoconductive,* i.e. they are able to stimulate osteogenesis, and they also provide linkage across defects and a scaffold upon which new bone can form. Osteogenesis is brought about partly by the activity of cells surviving on the surface of the graft, but mainly by the stimulation of osteoprogenitor cells in the host bed – an effect that is due to the presence of bone morphogenetic protein in the graft matrix. Cancellous grafts are more rapidly incorporated into host bone than cortical grafts, but sometimes the greater strength of cortical bone is needed to provide structural integrity.

Autografts (autogenous grafts)

In these, bone is transferred from one place to another in the same individual. This is the most commonly used form of bone-grafting, but it depends on there being sufficient donor bone of the sort required and a recipient site with a clean vascular bed. Most of the transplanted bone dies, but it continues to act as a scaffold, which is gradually replaced by a process of creeping substitution.

Cancellous autografts can be obtained from the thicker portions of the ilium, the greater trochanter, the proximal metaphysis of the tibia, the lower radius, the olecranon, or from an excised femoral head. Cortical grafts can be harvested from any convenient long bone or from the iliac crest; they usually need to be fixed with screws, sometimes reinforced by a plate, and can be placed on the host bone, or inlaid, or slid along the long axis of the bone.

The ideal autograft is one with an intact blood supply. Bone is transferred complete with its blood vessels, which are anastomosed to vessels at the recipient site. The technique is difficult and time consuming, requiring microsurgical skill. Available donor sites include the iliac crest (complete with one of the circumflex arteries), the fibula (with the peroneal artery) and the radial shaft. Vascularized grafts remain completely viable and become incorporated by a process analogous to fracture healing.

Allografts (homografts)

With these, bone is transferred from one individual (alive or dead) to another of the same species. The bone is harvested and stored until needed. The method is particularly useful when large defects have to be filled.

Fresh allografts, though dead, are not immunologically inert. They induce an inflammatory response in the host and this may lead to rejection. However, the antigenicity can be reduced by freezing or freeze-drying, or by ionizing radiation.

The process of incorporation (when it occurs) is similar to that with autografts but slower and less complete. Demineralization is another way of reducing antigenicity and it may also enhance the osteoinductive properties of the graft.

Allografts are plentiful and can be stored for long periods. However, sterility must be ensured. This can be done by exposure to ethylene oxide or by ionizing radiation, but their physical properties and potential for osteoinduction may be altered by doses that are high enough to ensure sterility. Freezing the grafts and storing them at −70°C is much less harmful, but the graft must then be harvested under sterile conditions and the donor must be cleared for malignancy, venereal disease, hepatitis and human immunodeficiency virus (HIV).

Other types of graft

Xenografts are obtained from another mammalian species, such as pigs or cows. After treatment for antigenicity, they should, theoretically, behave like allografts, but in practice they are much less effective unless host marrow is added to the graft. 'Artificial bone' made of *hydroxyapatite composites* can be used in the same way to fill a cavity or bridge a small gap. *Bioactive bone cements* (injectable calcium phosphate preparations) offer a simple alternative, e.g. for replacing bone loss in metaphyseal fractures.

Applications

Cancellous grafts are used for filling cavities, augmenting fracture healing and promoting arthrodesis.

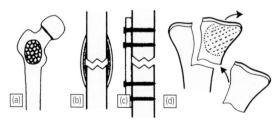

12.3 Bone-grafts Some of the more common applications are illustrated. (a) Chip grafts to fill a cavity. (b) Onlay strips of cancellous bone (Phemister technique). (c) Onlay cortical graft. (d) Cadaveric osteocartilaginous graft obtained fresh and sterile from an organ donor.

Cortical or *corticocancellous grafts* are needed where bone has been lost as a result of trauma or has been removed because it contained a tumour. When reinforced by metallic implants, large gaps can be filled.

Vascularized grafts tend to be used only in exceptional circumstances, such as treating large bone defects.

DISTRACTION HISTOGENESIS AND LIMB RECONSTRUCTION

Present-day limb reconstruction is founded on the principle that new-bone formation is stimulated in response to gradual increases in tension. This was originally discovered by Gavril Ilizarov in Russia and the application of this principle to bone reconstruction is widely referred to as *the Ilizarov method*.

Distraction histogenesis

Callotasis

Callus distraction, or *callotasis*, is perhaps the single most important application of the tension-stress principle. It is used for limb lengthening or the filling of large defects in bone, through either bone transport or other strategies. The basis of the technique is to produce a careful fracture through the bone, followed by a short wait (5–10 days) before the young callus is gradually distracted by traction on the bone via a circular or unilateral external fixator. Distraction proceeds at 1 mm a day, with small (usually 0.25 mm) increments spaced out evenly. New callus can be seen on the x-ray after 3 weeks; in optimum conditions, it forms an even column in the gap between the bone fragments (this is called the *regenerate*). If the distraction rate is too fast, or the osteotomy performed poorly, the regenerate may be thin with an hourglass appearance; conversely, if distraction is too slow, it may appear bulbous or, worse still, may consolidate prematurely, thereby preventing any further lengthening. When the desired length is reached, a second waiting period follows which allows the regenerate callus to consolidate and harden. Weight-bearing is permitted throughout this period. When cortices of even thickness appear in the regenerate, the fixator can be removed. Throughout treatment, physiotherapy is important to preserve joint movement and avoid contractures.

Patients should be warned that bone lengthening takes months rather than weeks and carries a risk of complications, such as pin-track infection, angulatory deformity, re-fracture and non-union.

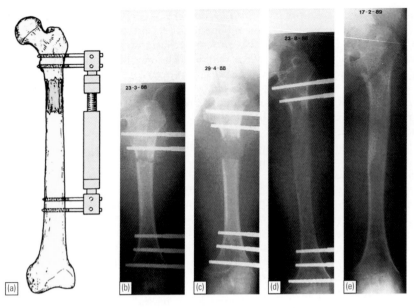

12.4 Callotasis Bone lengthening can be achieved by callotasis (callus 'stretching'). (a) A distracting external fixator is applied; the bone is then osteotomized and the fragments are gradually dragged apart over a period of months. (b–e) Serial x-rays show the progress over a period of 11 months. In this case, lengthening of 10 cm was achieved.

Ilizarov techniques should be employed only by surgeons who have undergone training in this method.

Chondrodiatasis

In children, bone lengthening can be achieved by distracting the physis (growth plate). No osteotomy is needed and the distraction rate is slower, usually 0.25 mm twice daily. Although a wide, even column of regenerate is usually seen, the fate of the physis is sealed: it frequently closes after the process, and for this reason the technique is best reserved for children close to the end of growth.

Bone transport

The principle of callotasis is used not only for limb lengthening but also as a means of treating nonunion and filling defects in bone. *Bone transport* allows a defect (or gap) to be filled in gradually by creating a 'floating' segment of bone through a corticotomy either proximal or distal to the defect, and slowly moving the isolated segment of bone across the gap. As the segment is transported from the corticotomy site to the new docking site, it leaves a trail of regenerate new bone behind it. An external fixator provides stability during this process.

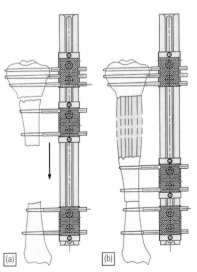

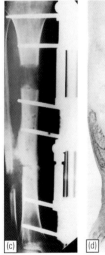

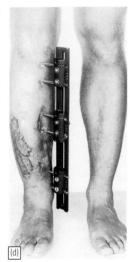

12.5 Bone transport (a) Bone loss may leave a gap in the shaft. Proximal osteotomy and callotasis allow a segment of the diaphysis to be moved distally until it 'docks' with the distal fragment (b). The resulting gap gradually fills, first with callus and then with new bone. (c) The x-ray shows the situation at the end of transport and docking. (d) The entire system is stabilized by some type of external fixation and the patient is able to walk about during the long transport period.

Correcting bone deformities and joint contractures

Angular bone deformities can usually be corrected by carefully planned closing or opening wedge osteotomies (see page 124). However, the degree of correction is limited by the effect on soft-tissue tension, especially nerves. With the Ilizarov method, it is now possible to undertake large corrections with much lower risk to the soft tissues. Length, rotation and translation deformities can be dealt with simultaneously by adjusting the traction wires and frame. Even intractable club-foot deformities can now be treated in this manner.

LEG-LENGTH EQUALIZATION

Inequality of leg length may result from many causes, including congenital anomalies, malunited fractures, epiphyseal and physeal injuries, infections and paralysis. Inequality of more than 2.5 cm needs treatment, either by providing a shoe-raise (usually rejected if the difference is more than 3 or 4 cm) or else by surgical measures – shortening the longer leg or lengthening the shorter leg.

In children the timing of surgery is vital. The rate of change in leg-length difference is charted and the discrepancy at the end of growth can then be predicted by reference to suitable charts or tables. This allows the surgeon to plan a timely intervention which will result in limb-length equality at skeletal maturity.

Shortening the longer leg

In children, growth in the normal leg can be stopped by arresting the activity of the growth plate; this can be either temporary, using removable staples fixed across the physis, or permanent (epiphysiodesis). In adults, a segment of bone can be excised and the approximated ends held by internal fixation.

Shortening should be advised only if the patient's residual height will still be acceptable. It should also be remembered that, since the longer leg is usually the normal one, if a serious complication such as non-union ensues, the patient may end up worse off than before.

Lengthening the shorter leg

Limb lengthening by the Ilizarov method is an appropriate solution for predicted length discrepancies of greater than 5 cm. Major length corrections can be tackled by staging the treatment process over several years. Patients should be warned that treatment will be prolonged and is often painful.

OPERATIONS ON JOINTS

INJECTIONS

It is often necessary to enter a joint with a sterile needle, either to aspirate fluid or to instil something into the joint. This barely qualifies as an 'operation'; however, it is an invasive procedure and it is well to remember that it carries some of the same risks as a 'real' operation, especially the risk of infection.

Aspiration may be purely diagnostic (e.g. in the management of suspected joint infection) or partly therapeutic (e.g. relief of a tense haemarthrosis).

Injection also is used for diagnostic purposes (e.g. the instillation of radio-opaque fluid for arthrography); usually, though, it means injection of an antibiotic or corticosteroid preparation into an infected or inflamed joint, or around neighbouring soft tissues. Corticosteroid injections should not be repeated more than three times over a period of 6 months. Although the

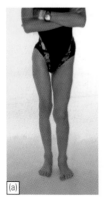
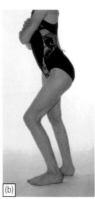
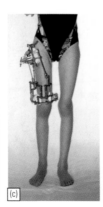
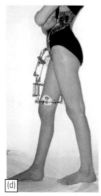

12.6 Leg lengthening
(a,b) Following a childhood infection of the right hip and destruction of the proximal femoral epiphysis, this patient ended up with marked shortening of the right femur and an awkward gait. (c,d) Here she is seen, markedly improved, after femoral lengthening by the Ilizarov method.

injected preparation is called a 'depot steroid', some of it is absorbed and systemic effects may occur. *All intra-articular injections should be performed with full aseptic precautions.*

ARTHROSCOPY

Arthroscopy is performed for both diagnostic and therapeutic purposes. Almost any joint can be reached, but the procedure is most usefully employed in the knee, shoulder, wrist, ankle and hip. If a definite abnormality is demonstrated, and is amenable to corrective surgery, it can often be dealt with at the same sitting without the need for an open operation. However, arthroscopy is an invasive procedure and its mastery requires skill and practice; it should not be used simply as an alternative to clinical examination and imaging.

The instrument is basically a rigid telescope fitted with fibreoptic illumination. Tube diameter ranges from about 2 mm (for small joints) to 4–5 mm (for the knee). It carries a lens system that gives a magnified image. The eyepiece allows direct viewing by the arthroscopist, but it is far more convenient to fit a small, sterilizable solid-state television camera which produces a picture of the joint interior on a television monitor.

The procedure is best carried out under general anaesthesia. The joint is distended with fluid and the arthroscope is introduced percutaneously. Instruments such as probes, curettes, forceps, nibblers, diathermy and powered abradors can be inserted through other skin portals and used to help expose less accessible parts of the joint, to obtain biopsies and to perform various operations. At the end of the procedure the joint is washed out and the small skin wounds are sutured. Patients are usually able to return home later the same day.

Arthroscopy is safe but not entirely free of complications, the commonest of which are haemarthrosis, thrombophlebitis, infection and joint stiffness. There is also a small risk of algodystrophy following arthroscopy.

ARTHROTOMY

Arthrotomy (opening a joint) may be indicated: (1) to inspect the interior or perform a synovial biopsy; (2) to drain a haematoma or an abscess; (3) to remove a loose body or damaged structure (e.g. a torn meniscus); and (4) to excise inflamed synovium. The intra-articular tissues should be handled with care, and if postoperative bleeding is expected (e.g. after synovectomy), a drain should be inserted. Following the operation, the joint should be rested for a few days, but thereafter movement should be encouraged.

JOINT RE-ALIGNMENT

Re-alignment osteotomy is a useful way of treating painful osteoarthritis of the hip or knee when the disease is too mild or the patient too young to consider total joint replacement. The bone is osteotomized close to the affected joint and the fragments are then re-aligned so that a less damaged part of the articular surface is exposed to load stresses. Often there is immediate pain relief, which may be because bone transection itself causes a reduction in intraosseous pressure.

Table 12.1 Applications of arthroscopic surgery

Knee		Wrist	
Knee	Meniscus repair	**Wrist**	Triangular cartilage repair
	Meniscectomy		Removal of loose bodies
	Synovectomy		
	Removal of loose bodies	**Ankle**	Treatment of osteochondritis dissecans
	Trimming of cartilage		Removal of loose bodies
	Division of synovial plica		
Shoulder	Rotator cuff decompression	**Hip**	Synovectomy
	Rotator cuff repair		Removal of loose bodies
	Glenoid labrum repair		

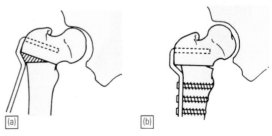

12.7 Joint realignment An incongruent joint can be re-aligned by osteotomizing the bone (a), changing the angle in one or more planes and then stabilizing the fragments by internal fixation (b).

An important part of the procedure is the preoperative planning – working out, from x-rays, the precise angles and wedges that will have to be cut in order to achieve the desired position of the joint surfaces. These geometric figures are reproduced during the operation with the aid of prepared templates or jigs; accuracy can also be checked by intraoperative x-rays.

After the bone is divided and repositioned, the fragments are held with internal fixation. Full weight-bearing should be avoided until bone union is complete, which usually takes 2–3 months.

JOINT FUSION (ARTHRODESIS)

The most reliable operation for a painful or unstable joint is arthrodesis; where stiffness does not seriously affect function, this is often the treatment of choice (e.g. in the spine, tarsus, wrist and ankle). Arthrodesis is useful also for a knee that is already fairly stiff (provided the other knee has good movement) and for a flail shoulder. More controversial is arthrodesis of the hip. Though it is a feasible alternative to arthroplasty or osteotomy for joint disease in young patients, there is an understandable resistance to sacrificing all movement in such an important joint. It is difficult to convey to the patient that a fused hip can still 'move' by virtue of pelvic tilting and rotation; the best approach is to introduce the patient to someone who has had a successful arthrodesis.

The operative principles are straightforward: the joint surfaces are denuded of cartilage and sometimes the subchondral bone is 'feathered' to increase the contact area; then the prepared surfaces are apposed in the optimum position and held rigidly by some form of internal or external fixation. Sometimes (especially in large joints) bone-grafts are added to promote osseous

bridging. The area is protected from excessive load stresses until union is complete (3–6 months).

The main *complication* is non-union and the formation of a pseudarthrosis. Rigid fixation lessens this risk; where feasible (e.g. the knee and ankle), the bony parts are squeezed together by compression–fixation devices.

Arthrodesis of the hip carries the risk of late 'secondary' complications due to abnormal loading of the knee (especially if the hip is fused in a little too much adduction or abduction) and chronic backache due to postural changes which compensate for the loss of hip extension and pelvic tilting while walking.

JOINT REPLACEMENT

Total joint replacement has been one of the triumphs of modern orthopaedic surgery. From the earliest development of total hip replacement in the 1950s by McKee and Farrar, and its perfection by Charnley 10 years later, this was envisaged as the ideal way of treating painful, destructive joint disorders. Several difficult problems had to be overcome: the prosthetic implants had to replicate a stable ball-and-socket joint; they had to be durable; they had to permit slippery movement at the articulation; they had to be firmly fixed to the skeleton; and they had to be made of inert materials which would not provoke any unwanted reaction in the tissues. The combination which Charnley designed had a stainless-steel femoral head articulating with a polyethylene socket. This is still the basis of modern designs, though there are now also prostheses made of titanium, cobalt–chrome alloy and ceramic materials.

Fixation is achieved in one of two ways. A putty-like bolus of methylmethacrylate cement is forced into the recipient bone cavity and the implant is then embedded in the cement and held there for

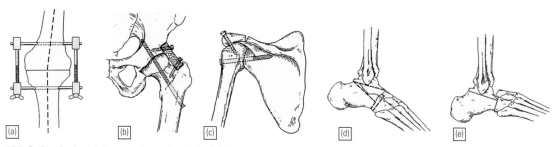

12.8 Arthrodesis (a) Compression arthrodesis. (b) Screw plus bone-graft; (c) similar technique using the acromion. (d,e) Subtalar and mid-tarsal fusion.

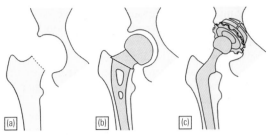

12.9 Arthroplasty The main varieties, as applied to the hip, are illustrated here. (a) Excision arthroplasty (Girdlestone); (b) partial replacement with an Austin–Moore prosthesis; (c) total replacement using a polyethylene implant for the socket and a metal implant for the femoral head and neck.

about 10 minutes while the methylmethacrylate polymerizes and hardens. The cement acts as a grouting material which fills the spaces between the implant and the bone and penetrates into interstices on the bone surface. The alternative method is to ream the bone cavity to a predetermined shape and size and then press-fit the implant snugly to the bone without cement. In neither case is there a true bond between implant and bone. Various modifications of implant design and surface coating have helped to reduce the long-term problem of implant loosening, but most important of all is sound technique.

Joint replacement has been most successful in the hip and knee. Similar principles have been applied to replacement operations for the shoulder, elbow and ankle, with less satisfactory long-term results.

Complications

Hip and knee replacements are usually performed on older patients, many of whom have generalized arthritis or systemic disorders. Consequently the *general complication rate* is by no means trivial; deep vein thrombosis is more common than with other types of surgery.

There are a number of *local complications* which are peculiar to total hip replacement. Factors that may contribute to their development include previous hip operations, severe deformity, lack of preoperative planning, inadequate 'bone stock', an insufficiently sterile operating environment and lack of experience or expertise on the part of the surgical team.

Intraoperative complications include perforation or even fracture of the femur or acetabulum. Special care should be taken in patients who are

very old or osteoporotic and in those who have had previous hip operations.

Sciatic nerve palsy (usually due to traction but occasionally caused by direct injury) occurs in about 2 per cent of patients undergoing total hip replacement. Most patients recover spontaneously, but if there is reason to suspect nerve damage, the area should be explored.

Postoperative dislocation is rare if the prosthetic components are correctly placed. Reduction is easy and traction in abduction usually allows the hip to stabilize. If there is malposition of either the femoral or the acetabular component, revision may be needed, or possibly augmentation of the socket.

Heterotopic bone formation around the hip is seen in about 20 per cent of patients 5 years after joint replacement. The cause is unknown, but patients with skeletal hyperostosis and ankylosing spondylitis are particularly at risk. In severe cases this is associated with pain and stiffness. Ossification can be prevented in high-risk patients by giving either a course of non-steroidal anti-inflammatory drugs for 3–6 weeks postoperatively or a single dose of irradiation to the hip.

Aseptic loosening of either the acetabular socket or the femoral stem is the commonest cause of long-term failure. Figures for its incidence vary widely, depending on the criteria used. With modern methods of implant fixation, there is likely to be radiographic evidence of loosening in about 10–20 per cent of patients 10 years after operation; at microscopic level, many stable implants show cellular reaction and membrane formation at the bone–cement interface; fortunately, only a fraction of these are symptomatic. Pain may be a feature, especially when first taking weight on the leg after sitting for a while, but the diagnosis usually rests on x-ray signs of progressively increasing radiolucency around the implant, fracturing of cement, movement of the implant or periprosthetic bone resorption. Radionuclide scanning shows increased activity in the bone around the implant. If symptoms are marked, and particularly if there is evidence of progressive bone resorption, the implant and cement should be painstakingly removed and a new prosthesis inserted – either cemented or uncemented, depending on the condition of the bone.

Aggressive osteolysis is sometimes seen. It is associated with granuloma formation at the interface between cement (or implant) and bone. This may be due to a severe histiocyte reaction stimulated by cement, polyethylene or metal particles that find their way into the boundary zone. Revision is usually necessary and this may have to be accompanied by impaction grafting with morsellized bone.

Infection is the most serious postoperative complication. With adequate prophylaxis, the risk should be less than 1 per cent, but it is higher in the very old, in patients with rheumatoid disease or psoriasis, and in those on immunosuppressive therapy (including corticosteroids). Other predisposing factors are prolonged wound exposure, tissue damage and local haematoma formation. Haematogenous spread from a distant site may cause late infection.

Early wound infection sometimes responds to antibiotics. Later infection does so less well and may need operative 'debridement' followed by irrigation with antibiotic solution for 3–4 weeks. Once the infection has cleared, a new prosthesis can be inserted, preferably without cement. An alternative, more applicable to 'mild' or 'dubious' infection, is a one-stage exchange arthroplasty using gentamicin-impregnated cement. The results of revision arthroplasty for infection are only moderately good. If all else fails, the implants and cement may have to be removed, leaving an excisional (Girdlestone) arthroplasty.

EXCISION ARTHROPLASTY

Sometimes the elected option is to excise the articular ends of the bones forming a joint, without implanting any type of prosthetic replacement. This sounds drastic, and in practice excision arthroplasty is reserved for situations where a more anatomical solution is either unnecessary (e.g. excision of the trapezium for trapeziometacarpal osteoarthritis – page 163) or inadvisable, perhaps because of intractable joint infection. Sufficient bone is excised to create a gap where movement can occur. In Girdlestone's arthroplasty of the hip (a 'last resort' when previous operations have failed or the joint has been irremediably destroyed), the femoral head and neck are excised, leaving a false articulation (pseudarthrosis) between the upper end of the femur and the side wall of the pelvis. The 'joint' is obviously unstable but, because of local fibrosis and the stabilizing effect of powerful surrounding muscles, the patient can still take weight on that side and can walk about, albeit with a marked limp.

MICROSURGERY

Microsurgical techniques are used in repairing nerves and vessels, transplanting bone with a vascular pedicle, and – occasionally – for reattaching a severed digit or part of a limb. Essential prerequisites are an operating microscope, special instruments, microsutures, a chair with arm supports and – not least – a surgeon well practised in microsurgical techniques.

For *replantation,* the severed part should be kept cool during transport. The more muscle in the amputated part, the shorter the period it will last; a fingertip may survive for 24 hours, a forearm only a few hours. Two teams dissect, identify and mark each artery, nerve and vein of the stump and the limb. Following careful debridement, the bones are shortened to reduce tension and fixed together by wires or plates. Next the vessels are sutured – arteries first and (if possible) two veins for each artery. A vessel of 1 mm diameter needs seven or eight circumferential sutures! Nerves and tendons next need suturing: only healthy ends of approximately equal diameter should be joined; tension, kinking and torsion must be prevented. Decompression of skin and fascia, as well as thrombectomy, may be needed in the post-operative period.

Replantation surgery is time consuming, expensive and often unsuccessful. It should be carried out only in specially equipped centres, and by teams specially trained for this work.

AMPUTATIONS

Indications
The indications for amputation are most easily remembered as the three Ds: *dead, dangerous* and *damned nuisance.*

Dead (or dying)
Peripheral vascular disease accounts for almost 90 per cent of all amputations. Other causes of tissue death are *severe trauma, burns* and *frostbite.*

Dangerous
'Dangerous' disorders are *malignant tumours, potentially lethal sepsis* and *crush injury.* In crush injury, releasing the compression may result in renal failure (the crush syndrome).

Damned nuisance
Retaining the limb may be worse than having no limb at all – because of *pain, gross malformation, recurrent sepsis* or *severe loss of function.*

Types of amputation
A *provisional amputation* may be necessary because primary healing is unlikely. The limb is amputated

as distal as seems appropriate; skin flaps sufficient to cover the deep tissues are cut and sutured loosely over a pack. Re-amputation is performed when the stump condition is favourable.

Definitive end-bearing amputation is performed when weight is to be taken through the end of a stump. Therefore the scar must not be terminal, and the bone end must be solid, not hollow, which means it must be cut through or near a joint. Examples are through-knee and through-ankle amputations.

Definitive non-end-bearing amputations are the commonest variety. All upper limb and most lower limb amputations come into this category. Because weight is not to be taken at the end of the stump, the scar can be terminal.

AMPUTATIONS AT THE SITES OF ELECTION

Most lower limb amputations are for ischaemic disease and are performed through the site of election below the most distal palpable pulse. The 'sites of election' are determined by the demands of prosthetic design and local function. Too short a stump may tend to slip out of the prosthesis. Too long a stump may have inadequate circulation and can become painful, or ulcerate; moreover, it complicates the incorporation of a joint in the prosthesis. For all that, the skill of the modern prosthetist has made it possible to amputate at almost any site.

Principles of technique

A tourniquet is used unless there is arterial insufficiency. Skin flaps are cut so that their combined length equals one and a half times the width of the limb at the site of amputation. As a rule, anterior and posterior flaps of equal length are used for the upper limb and for transfemoral (above-knee) amputations; below the knee, a long posterior flap is usual.

Muscles are divided distal to the proposed site of bone section; subsequently, opposing groups are sutured over the bone end to each other and to the periosteum *(myoplasty)*, thus providing better muscle control as well as better circulation. Nerves are divided proximal to the bone cut. Great care is taken to ensure that a raw nerve end will not bear weight.

The bone is sawn across at the proposed level. In transtibial amputations, the front of the tibia is usually bevelled and filed to create a smoothly rounded contour; the fibula is cut 3 cm shorter.

The main vessels are tied, the tourniquet is removed and every bleeding point meticulously ligated. The skin is sutured carefully without tension. Suction drainage is advised and the stump firmly bandaged.

Aftercare

If a haematoma forms, it is evacuated as soon as possible. Repeated elastic bandaging is applied to help shrink the stump and produce a conical limb-end. The muscles must be exercised, the joints kept mobile and the patient taught to use his or her prosthesis.

AMPUTATIONS OTHER THAN AT THE SITES OF ELECTION

Unusual sites of amputation – mainly for mutilating trauma, life-threatening sepsis or malignant disease – are sometimes chosen when there is no other option. Examples are *interscapulothoracic (forequarter) amputation; disarticulation at the shoulder; hemipelvectomy (hindquarter amputation); disarticulation through the hip; amputations leaving inconveniently short stumps; through-knee amputation (Stokes–Gritti); through-ankle amputation (Syme's); through the mid-tarsal joints (Chopart); and through the tarsometatarsal joints (Lisfranc).*

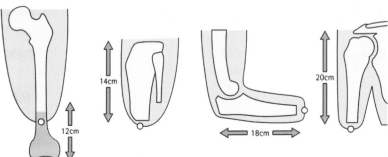

12.10 Amputations – sites of election The traditional sites of election are shown here. Where possible, the scar is made terminal because these are not end-bearing stumps.

PROSTHESES

All prostheses must fit comfortably; they should also function well and look presentable. The patient accepts and uses a prosthesis much better if it is fitted soon after operation; delay is unjustifiable now that modular components are available and only the socket need be made individually.

In the upper limb, the distal portion of the prosthesis is detachable and can be replaced by a 'dress hand' or by a variety of useful terminal devices. Electrically powered limbs are available for both children and adults.

In the lower limb, weight can be transmitted through the ischial tuberosity, the patellar tendon, the upper tibia or the soft tissues. Combinations are permissible; recent developments in silicone and gel materials provide improved comfort in total-contact self-suspending sockets.

COMPLICATIONS OF AMPUTATION STUMPS

Early complications

In addition to the complications of any operation (especially secondary haemorrhage or infection), there are two special hazards: breakdown of skin flaps and gas gangrene.

Breakdown of skin flaps

This may be due to ischaemia, to suturing under excessive tension or (in below-knee amputations) to an unduly long tibia pressing against the flap.

Gas gangrene

Clostridia and spores from the perineum may infect a high above-knee amputation (or re-amputation), especially if performed through ischaemic tissue.

Late complications

Skin

Eczema is common, and tender purulent lumps may develop in the groin. A rest from the prosthesis is indicated. Ulceration is usually due to poor circulation, and re-amputation at a higher level is then necessary. If, however, the circulation is satisfactory and the skin around an ulcer is healthy, it may be sufficient to excise 2.5 cm of bone and re-suture.

Muscle

If too much muscle is left at the end of the stump, the resulting unstable 'cushion' induces a feeling of insecurity which may prevent proper use of a prosthesis; the excess soft tissue should be excised.

Artery

Poor circulation gives a cold, blue stump which is liable to ulcerate. This problem chiefly arises with below-knee amputations, and often re-amputation is necessary.

Nerve

A cut nerve always forms a tiny 'neuroma' and occasionally this is painful and tender. Excising

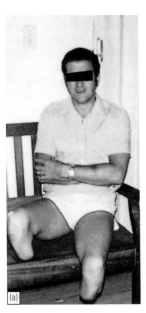
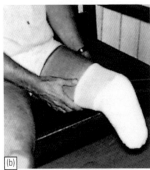
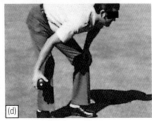
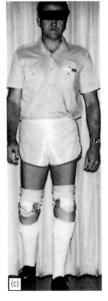

12.11 Amputations – fitting the prosthesis (a) This man had severe congenital deformities which necessitated bilateral below-knee amputations. (b) A cast was made of each stump; from this the stump socket was fashioned and fitted into a prosthesis. (c) The patient is shown wearing two patellar-tendon-bearing prostheses. (d) After rehabilitation, he had excellent balance and could resume a near-normal life.

3 cm of the nerve above the bulb sometimes succeeds. Alternatively, the epineural sleeve of the nerve stump is freed from nerve fascicles for 5 mm and then sealed with a synthetic tissue adhesive or buried within muscle or bone away from pressure points.

Phantom limb

This term is used to describe the feeling that the amputated limb is still present; the patient should be warned of this possibility. In most cases the feeling recedes and eventually disappears. A painful phantom limb is very difficult to treat. Intermittent percussion to the end of the stump has been recommended; it sounds brutal, but success is claimed.

GENERAL COMPLICATIONS OF ORTHOPAEDIC OPERATIONS

Five important complications which are common to most orthopaedic operations are:

- swelling,
- haematoma formation,
- delayed wound healing,
- infection, and
- thromboembolism.

SOFT-TISSUE SWELLING

Swelling is common after operations on the limbs and its effects are often aggravated by tight dressings or plaster casts. This may prove a threat to wound healing and will delay the recovery of joint movement. In the worst cases it may interfere with vascular perfusion and give rise to an ischaemic compartment syndrome (see page 294). Prevention is all-important: (1) dressings should be snug but not tight; (2) the limb should be elevated; (3) movements should be encouraged; and (4) if a cast is used, it should be well padded or split.

HAEMATOMA FORMATION

Postoperative bleeding or oozing from cut surfaces may be considerable. Haematoma formation is reduced by adequate suction drainage; however, this should not be too vigorous or prolonged, lest it encourage further bleeding.

DELAYED WOUND HEALING

Poor peripheral circulation may cause delayed healing or breakdown of the wound. The circulation should always be checked before any operation is undertaken.

INFECTION

Postoperative infection is always a nuisance; in joint replacement surgery it may be a disaster. The subject is dealt with in Chapter 2.

THROMBOEMBOLISM

Thromboembolism is the commonest complication of lower limb surgery; however, the incidence is different for different types of operation. Statistics are usually cited for three specific events: *deep vein thrombosis (DVT), pulmonary embolism (PE)* and *fatal pulmonary embolism (FPE)*. In addition, there is the late complication of *chronic venous insufficiency.*

In patients undergoing joint replacement surgery, the incidence of clinically detectable DVT and PE together is probably in the region of 5 per cent, and of FPE between 0.25 and 0.5 per cent.

Elderly patients with hip fractures are at considerably greater risk, the incidence of FPE being about 1 per cent. Following major trauma, the incidence of FPE is also about 1 per cent.

The most important *general risk factors* are a family history, increasing age, obesity, and a history of previous thrombosis.

Pathophysiology

Thrombosis results from an interaction between vessel wall damage, alterations in blood components and venous stasis. Following major orthopaedic operations, there is activation of the coagulation cascade and restricted fibrinolysis lasting for several days. During hip replacement, femoral vein blood flow is temporarily interrupted when the acetabulum and femoral medulla are exposed. There is also more prolonged stasis as the patient recovers from surgery and begins to mobilize. DVT occurs most frequently in the veins of the calf, and less often in the proximal veins of the thigh and pelvis. It is from the larger thrombi that fragments sometimes break off and get carried to the lungs, where they may give rise to PE, and both symptomatic and asymptomatic PE may result in sudden death (FPE).

Clinical features and diagnosis

Asymptomatic DVT is probably quite common. When clinical features appear, they usually consist of pain in the calf or thigh; however, following trauma or operation, even those patients who do not complain should be examined regularly for swelling, soft-tissue tenderness and a sudden slight increase in temperature and pulse rate. *Homans' sign – increased calf pain on passive dorsiflexion of the foot and toes – is often sought to clinch, or exclude, the diagnosis of DVT. This is regrettable as more accurate techniques have shown that the sign is unreliable.* The diagnosis can be confirmed by ascending venography. Duplex ultrasound scanning is highly accurate for proximal DVT, the usual prelude to PE.

Patients with symptomatic DVT, and also asymptomatic patients who develop pain in the chest, shortness of breath or haemoptysis, should be examined for signs of PE. The diagnosis can be confirmed by ventilation–perfusion (V/Q) scanning or spiral CT.

Chronic venous insufficiency occurs some years after the DVT. The patient presents with leg discomfort, swelling, skin changes and/or frank ulceration. The diagnosis is usually obvious. This is a debilitating condition which places huge demands on health resources.

 Early signs of postoperative DVT resemble those of compartment syndrome. Check for both.

Prevention

The risk of DVT and PE can be reduced by physical methods or prophylactic medication.

Physical methods

These vary from *simple routines* such as elevation of the foot of the bed, use of elastic stockings and early mobilization to more sophisticated contrivances like the application of *intermittent plantar venous compression by foot-pump* or *intermittent pneumatic compression of the leg.* The use of *spinal or epidural anaesthesia* also reduces the incidence of DVT by improving venous blood flow and possibly by a local fibrinolytic effect.

Prophylactic medication

Low-dose unfractionated heparin, by subcutaneous injection, was the usual choice for thromboprophylaxis in the past. Unfortunately, this carries a risk of increased bleeding after operation and it is contraindicated in elderly people. Moreover, there are doubts about its efficacy in preventing proximal DVT. *Low-molecular-weight heparin,* given preoperatively and postoperatively, is now the preparation of choice. Dose adjustment and monitoring are not required. Randomized studies have shown that it

effectively reduces the prevalence of venographic DVT in hip and knee replacement surgery. *Warfarin* has also been widely used; it reduces the prevalence of DVT after hip and knee replacement and FPE is extremely rare. Drawbacks are the difficulty in establishing appropriate dosage levels and the need for constant monitoring; there is also a risk of interaction with other drugs and alcohol. *Aspirin* probably provides a small reduction in the rate of PE after surgery; used alone it is inadequate.

The risk of thrombosis persists for at least 5 weeks after surgery and the death rate after hip replacement does not return to 'normal' until 3 months. Theoretically, therefore, thromboprophylaxis should be prolonged for some time after discharge from hospital; however, there is little agreement on the optimal duration of treatment.

Treatment of thromboembolism

Whenever possible, the clinical diagnosis of DVT or PE should be confirmed by imaging (venography or ultrasound for DVT, V/Q scanning, spiral CT or pulmonary angiography for PE) before treatment is started. This is important because the clinical diagnosis of these complications is notoriously unreliable and full therapeutic anticoagulation carries a high complication rate soon after major surgery.

Once the diagnosis of DVT has been confirmed, treatment is started with a loading dose of 5000 units of heparin intravenously. This is followed by a daily weight-adjusted dose of low-molecular-weight heparin subcutaneously. Warfarin is started with a loading dose of 10 mg daily for 3 days. Thereafter the dose is adjusted until the international normalized ratio (INR) is prolonged and stable at 2.0–3.0 times the control value, and the heparin is then discontinued. If low-molecular-weight heparin is not available, unfractionated heparin can be given by continuous intravenous infusion, or twice daily subcutaneously, adjusted to maintain the activated partial thromboplastin time (APPT) at 1.5–2 times normal.

Acute, severe PE demands cardiorespiratory resuscitation, vasopressors for shock, oxygen, and a large intravenous dose (15 000 units) of heparin. Streptokinase is used both to dissolve clots and to prevent more forming. Emergency pulmonary thrombectomy may be considered. Antibiotics should be given to prevent lung infection. Anticoagulant treatment is continued for at least 6 months.

PHYSICAL THERAPY

PHYSIOTHERAPY

Physiotherapy is a very important adjunct to orthopaedic surgery, (a) in postoperative rehabilitation and (b) in the non-operative management of bone and joint disorders.

Rest

This is the oldest and most natural form of treatment for arthritis. But 'rest' does not mean complete and continuous immobility of the patient, which may do more harm than good. Bed-rest should, whenever possible, be intermittent, and even then it should be accompanied by exercises for joints that are not affected. In local inflammatory disorders, and following injury or operation, individual joints can be rested by appropriate splintage while the patient is kept mobile.

Splintage

Splintage is often used as a form of treatment for painful arthritic joints and for unstable joints. *Static splints* hold the joint in a functional position which will permit useful movement in other, unaffected joints. *Dynamic splints* assist movement in the affected joint, for example while waiting for active movement to return after a nerve injury or tendon operation.

Exercise

Exercise is usually referred to as either *passive* or *active;* the former is directed at maintaining or improving the range of motion; the latter at maintaining or improving muscle strength (and thereby also joint stability).

Passive exercise

The therapist moves the patient's joint without the patient contributing any force whatever. In this way, the joint capsule and ligaments are maintained at normal length or even stretched to achieve an increased range of motion. This can be useful in the early stages of osteoarthritis when joint movement is restricted and the patient experiences pain only at the end of the range in any particular direction. Passive movement can also be achieved by using a mechanical device which applies *continuous passive motion (a CPM machine),* e.g. when stiffness is likely to occur after a tibial plateau fracture or operations on the knee. As pain subsides and the range improves, the patient gradually takes over with *active assisted exercises.*

Active exercise

The object here is to improve muscle power by teaching the patient to move the affected joint against resistance, at first relying only on the weight of the limb, but gradually increasing the resistance by applying additional weights (or some other resisting device) to the limb. Increased muscle strength brings increased joint stability and easier purposive movements. Even if the joint is immobilized, muscle tone and power can be maintained by performing repetitive muscle contractions in runs of about 20 contractions two or three times a day over a period of several weeks *(isometric exercise).*

Heat and cold

These are time-honoured methods of alleviating pain and muscle spasm. Warmth applied to the superficial tissues by hot packs, heat pads or simple radiation is often used to relieve pain and stiffness; the deeper tissues can be reached by short-wave diathermy or ultrasonic vibration. Ice packs have a more immediate analgesic effect and are recommended for patients with pain and swelling following joint and muscle injuries. These methods should obviously be avoided in patients with loss of sensibility, and heat must not be applied to bones or joints with metal implants.

Manipulation

Physiotherapists are skilled at moving or manipulating joints and small segments of the vertebral column. This is a useful technique for the treatment of stiffness and pain in the neck or back. Similar methods are employed for painful peripheral joints.

Electrical stimulation

Intermittent low-voltage nerve stimulation has a blocking effect on pain perception. This observation has been applied to the development of non-invasive, transcutaneous electrical nerve stimulation by small, portable, battery-operated 'TENS' machines. Patient response is variable, but many of those with chronic backache and cervicobrachial pain report good pain relief.

OCCUPATIONAL THERAPY

Physiotherapy aims to restore movement and power to a particular part; occupational therapy translates that movement into useful function as part of the individual's daily activity. This involves careful assessment of the patient's functional needs and their ability (or lack of it) to meet those needs. A programme of rehabilitation can then be devised, including the provision of such functional aids as will help the patient to return to independent living. Ideally, the occupational therapy department should be equipped to simulate all the common activities of daily living.

Diversional therapy – which keeps the patient happily occupied during convalescence – is itself a form of psychological rehabilitation.

ERGONOMIC TRAINING

'Hands-on' alone is not enough. Patients often have to be trained to use their bodies in ways that are ergonomically efficient and protective of the underlying pathology. Those with back pain need to be taught how to lift and carry. Posture and movements may have to be modified to suit individual patients.

FUNCTIONAL AIDS AND APPLIANCES

The walking stick or cane is the prototypical, universal functional aid. It does not take a degree in biomechanics to know instinctively that leaning on a stick will reduce the load on one side of the body and so diminish pain associated with weight-bearing. What is more difficult to recognize (and even doctors often miss the point) is that with hip disorders the stick must be used on the side opposite to the painful limb. Crutches provide even greater load reduction, and walking frames have the added advantage of stability.

Upper limb aids, limited in variety only by the ingenuity of their inventors, are available: handles that make cutlery, taps and door-knobs more manageable; extending 'slip-ons' that help with putting on socks and shoes; long pincers that can reach the floor for those who cannot bend down; and many more.

APPLIANCES

Gone are the days when struts, corsets and braces were the mainstay of orthopaedic treatment. Paralysed limbs are less common than before, and deformed or unstable joints can be managed by reconstructive surgery. Yet appliances are still useful where more radical methods are contraindicated, and in some parts of the world they are the only methods available.

Appliances are prescribed for four main purposes: (1) protection, (2) lengthening, (3) splintage and (4) stabilization. Usually they are employed as stand-ins while recovery or more definitive treatment is awaited. Often, though, they prove so useful that patients prefer them to operation. The most common examples are described below.

Collars

A soft collar can be used to provide rest or partial splintage for a painful neck; this is usually the first line of treatment for a suspected disc lesion. For severe injuries (including stable fractures), a rigid brace is preferable; it is usually worn for 6–8 weeks. Soft-tissue sprains (including 'whiplash' injuries) should be treated by movement and exercise.

Spinal supports

A rigid spinal brace may be used to alleviate pain and prevent deformity after stable vertebral injuries, in the management of infection or metastatic disease, or after spinal fusion. Specialized braces are also used in the management of scoliosis. Soft supports (corsets) are sometimes prescribed for disc lesions or non-specific low-back pain; they obviously cannot immobilize the spine, but they restrict movement by compressing the soft tissues into a less flexible tube. All of these should be regarded as temporary measures; if continued for too long, they weaken the muscles, reduce mobility and predispose to vertebral osteoporosis.

Footwear

Custom-made shoes and boots, capacious enough to accommodate severe toe deformities or misshapen feet, will protect against abnormal pressure and strain. They are particularly useful in the management of rheumatoid deformities and may avoid the need for operation.

Elevation of the sole and heel is the easiest way to correct asymmetrical shortening, but patients will rarely tolerate more than a 4 cm raise. Perhaps the commonest appliance of all is the insole, a thin platform with moulded elevations to support a flat-foot or dropped metatarsal heads.

Orthoses

Orthoses (Greek 'ortho' = straight or correct) are corrective splints, braces or calipers that are designed to stabilize an unstable joint or an incompletely united fracture. Above-knee metal calipers were frequently prescribed to provide stable knee extension for patients with paralysed quadriceps muscles, and below-knee calipers for ankle support. They are still used as temporary measures after injury or operation to protect a weak joint while awaiting full recovery, or where other methods are contraindicated or not available. Light-weight orthoses (e.g. polyethylene drop-foot splints or wrist braces) can be worn under normal clothing.

COMPLEMENTARY AND ALTERNATIVE TREATMENT

'Alternative treatment' comprises an array of remedies and physical techniques based on theories and beliefs outside the broad field of science-based medicine. Some of these remedies derive from traditional 'folk' medicine; some involve the use of dietary and herbal substances, which are considered to have 'natural' curative properties; copper bracelets are often worn as a 'cure' for arthritis; and homeopathic remedies are based on the belief that symptoms can be relieved, or 'cured', by administering substances that produce similar symptoms in healthy people, provided that these substances are given in a highly diluted form – sometimes so dilute that their molecules can no longer be detected. None of these 'cures' has stood the test of rigorous scientific investigation, including methods such as double-blind controlled trials. Those that have an effect on pain are only mildly analgesic compared to pharmacological analgesics and anti-inflammatory agents. Nevertheless, they have attracted millions of followers who claim to have benefited from them. Their most persuasive advocates are people with complaints of chronic back pain, fibromyalgia, arthralgia, weakness and fatigue, who usually have no demonstrable pathophysiological signs to account for their symptoms; but they are employed also by patients with unequivocal pathological conditions such as arthritis and intervertebral disc degeneration. Undoubted advantages are that they involve the patients in controlling their own cures, that the risks of unwanted side-effects are very small and – perhaps – that the healers engage with their patients more sympathetically than do professional physicians and surgeons, who often show little patience in dealing with complaints that are not backed up by 'real' pathology.

Chiropractic treatment and osteopathy

Chiropractic and osteopathy were developed in the USA during the latter part of the nineteenth century, when mainstream medicine was itself directed mainly at symptomatic treatment. These new forms of treatment were originally based on the belief that most chronic diseases were due to skeletal displacements or subluxations and their symptoms could, therefore, be relieved by various types of physical manipulation. In recent times these ideas have been refined, and both chiropractic and osteopathy now require a formal period of study and training which includes instruction in science-based physiology and pathology. In the UK, practitioners in these modalities are subject to statutory regulation by, respectively, the General Chiropractic Council and the General Osteopathic Council. Patients with 'orthopaedic' disorders such as chronic low-back pain and fibromyalgia often benefit from physical manipulative treatment, and several controlled studies have shown that the results are at least as good as those of 'traditional' orthopaedic methods such as exercise and wearing corsets or braces. Patients who choose to undergo these methods of treatment need not necessarily be discouraged, provided that they continue with any ongoing medical treatment, that all necessary steps are taken to exclude serious or progressive pathology, that the therapist is properly registered, and that the patients are advised that although complementary care may be useful in controlling symptoms, it will not cure any underlying pathology.

Other complementary techniques

Relaxation exercises and *massage* provide temporary benefit in painful conditions associated with psychological stress, tension or muscle spasm. *Postural re-training* and modification of work practices also are often helpful.

Acupuncture is one of the oldest and most widely practised forms of complementary treatment. It has been shown without doubt to be capable of relieving pain in certain chronic musculoskeletal disorders, probably due to release of endogenous endorphins and serotonin. Claims for its efficacy in curing disease are unfounded.

2 Regional Orthopaedics

CHAPTER 13

THE SHOULDER

CLINICAL ASSESSMENT

HISTORY

Pain from the shoulder or its surrounding tendons is felt anterolaterally and at the insertion of the deltoid; sometimes it radiates down the arm. Pain on top of the shoulder suggests acromioclavicular dysfunction or a cervical spine disorder. The entire shoulder is a common site of referred pain from the cervical spine, heart, mediastinum and diaphragm.

Stiffness may be progressive and severe – so much so as to merit the term 'frozen shoulder'.

Deformity may consist of prominence of the acromioclavicular joint or winging of the scapula.

Loss of function is expressed as inability to reach behind the back and difficulty with combing the hair or dressing.

The painful shoulder
Referred pain
Cervical spondylosis
Mediastinal pathology
Cardiac ischaemia
Joint disorders
Glenohumeral arthritis
Acromioclavicular arthritis
Rotator cuff disorders
Tendinitis
Rupture
Frozen shoulder

 Sudden shoulder pain plus winging of scapula: check for neuralgic amyotrophy.

EXAMINATION

The patient should always be examined from in front and from behind. Both upper limbs, the neck and the chest must be visible. Because shoulder and neck symptoms are often felt in the same areas, examination of the shoulder must include a full examination of the neck, and vice versa.

Look

Skin

Scars or sinuses are noted; don't forget the axilla!

Shape

Asymmetry of the shoulders, winging of the scapula, wasting of the deltoid or short rotators and acromioclavicular dislocation are best seen from behind; joint swelling or wasting of the pectoral muscles is more obvious from in front. A joint effusion may 'point' in the axilla.

Position

If the arm is held internally rotated, think of posterior dislocation of the shoulder.

Feel

Because the joint is well covered, inflammation rarely influences skin temperature. The soft tissues and bony points are carefully palpated, following a mental picture of the anatomy. Start with the sternoclavicular joint, then follow the clavicle laterally to the acromioclavicular joint, on to the anterior edge of the acromion and around the acromion to the back of the joint. The supraspinatus tendon lies just below the anterior edge of the acromion. Tenderness and crepitus can often be accurately localised to a particular structure.

Move

Active movements

The patient is asked to raise both arms sideways until the fingers point to the ceiling. Abduction may be: (1) difficult to initiate; (2) diminished in range; (3) altered in rhythm, the scapula moving too early and creating a shrugging effect.

If movement is painful, the arc of pain must be noted; pain in the mid-range of abduction suggests a rotator cuff tear or supraspinatus tendinitis; pain at the end of abduction is often due to acromioclavicular arthritis.

The patient is then asked to perform other active movements: flexion and extension by raising the arms forwards and then backwards as far as possible; adduction by moving each arm across the front of the body; and rotation by holding the arms close to the body, flexing the elbows to 90 degrees and first separating the hands as widely as possible (external rotation) and then folding the forearms across the front of the body (internal rotation). Three composite movements are essential for normal function: clasping the hands behind the neck; reaching high up on the back; and performing a circular ('pot-stirring') movement with each arm in turn.

Passive movements

These can be deceptive because even with a stiff shoulder the arm can be raised to 90 degrees by

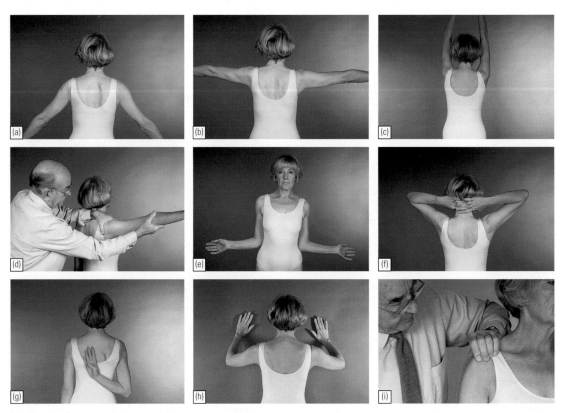

13.1 Examination Active movements are best examined from behind the patient, paying careful attention to symmetry and the co-ordination between scapulothoracic and glenohumeral movements. (a) Abduction; (b) limit of glenohumeral abduction; (c) full abduction and elevation, a combination of scapulothoracic and glenohumeral movement. (d) The range of true glenohumeral movement can be assessed by blocking scapular movement with a hand placed firmly on the top edge of the scapula. (e) External rotation. (f,g) Complex movements involving abduction, rotation and flexion or extension of the shoulder. (h) Testing for serratus anterior weakness. (i) Feeling for supraspinatus tenderness.

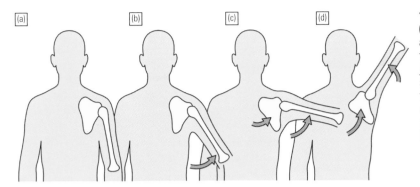

13.2 Abduction and elevation (a–c) During the early phase of abduction, most of the movement takes place at the glenohumeral joint. As the arm rises, the scapula begins to rotate on the thorax (c). In the last phase of abduction, the movement is almost entirely scapulothoracic (d).

scapulothoracic movement. To test true glenohumeral abduction, the scapula must first be anchored; this is done by pressing firmly down on the top of the shoulder with one hand while the other hand moves the patient's arm.

Power

The deltoid is examined while the patient abducts against resistance. To test serratus anterior (long thoracic nerve), ask the patient to push forcefully against a wall with both hands; if the muscle is weak, the scapula is not stabilized on the thorax and stands out prominently *(winged scapula)*. Pectoralis major is tested by the patient thrusting both hands firmly into the waist. Any difference in muscle bulk between the two sides is noted at the same time.

IMAGING

At least two x-ray views should be obtained: an anteroposterior (AP) view in the plane of the glenoid, and an axillary projection with the arm in abduction to show the relationship of the humeral head to the glenoid. Look for evidence of subluxation, or dislocation, joint-space narrowing, bone erosion and calcification in the soft tissues.

Double contrast arthrography, ultrasonography, CT and MRI are useful methods for diagnosing rotator cuff tears or atypical forms of shoulder instability.

ARTHROSCOPY

Arthroscopy is useful for diagnosing intra-articular lesions, detachment of the glenoid labrum and rotator cuff tears. In some cases the disorder can be dealt with surgically at the same time.

DISORDERS OF THE ROTATOR CUFF

The rotator cuff is a sheet of conjoint tendons closely applied over the shoulder capsule and inserting mainly into the greater tuberosity of the humerus (subscapularis is inserted into the lesser tuberosity). The cuff is made up of subscapularis in front, supraspinatus above and infraspinatus and teres minor behind – the 'rotator' muscles, which have an important function in stabilizing the head

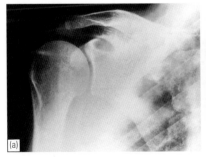
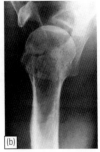
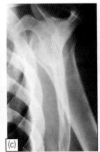
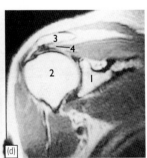

13.3 Imaging (a) Normal anteroposterior x-ray. (b) Axillary view showing the humeral head opposite the shallow glenoid fossa. (c) True lateral view; the head of the humerus should lie where the coracoid process, the spine of the scapula and the blade of the scapula meet. (d) MRI. Note (1) the glenoid, (2) the head of the humerus, (3) the acromion process and (4) the supraspinatus. The high signal in the supraspinatus suggests degenerative change.

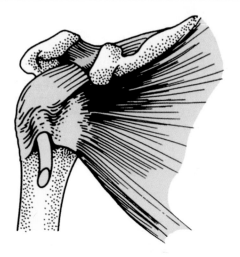

13.4 The rotator cuff The coracoacromial ligament (coloured green) stretches from the coracoid to the underside of the anterior third of the acromion process. The humeral head moves beneath this arch during abduction, guided and motorized by the rotator muscles (coloured brown).

of the humerus by pulling it firmly into the glenoid whenever the deltoid lifts the arm forwards or sideways.

Arching over the cuff is a fibro-osseous canopy – the coracoacromial arch – formed by the acromion process posterosuperiorly, the coracoid process anteriorly and the coracoacromial ligament joining them. Separating the tendons from the arch and allowing them to glide is the subacromial bursa.

Painful lesions of any of these structures will result in awkward or abnormal shoulder movement.

Pathology

The differing clinical pictures stem from three basic pathological processes: degeneration, trauma and vascular reaction.

Degeneration

With advancing age, the cuff degenerates; minute tears develop, and there may be scarring, fibrocartilaginous metaplasia or calcification. The common site is the 'critical zone' of the supraspinatus, the relatively avascular region near its insertion.

Trauma and impingement

The supraspinatus tendon is liable to injury if it contracts against firm resistance; this may occur when lifting a weight, or when the patient uses his arm to save himself from falling. This is much more likely if the cuff is already degenerate.

An insidious type of trauma is attrition of the cuff due to impingement against the coracoacromial arch during abduction. The long head of biceps also may be abraded to the point of rupture. Small tears of the cuff or the long head of biceps are found at autopsy in almost everyone aged over 60.

Vascular reaction

In an attempt to repair a torn tendon or to revascularize a degenerate area, new blood vessels grow in and calcium deposits are resorbed. This vascular reaction causes congestion and pain.

The three pathological processes described here may be summed up as *'wear', 'tear'* and *'repair'*. In the young patient, 'repair' is vigorous; consequently, healing is relatively rapid, but (because the repair process itself causes pain) it is accompanied by considerable distress. The older patient has more 'wear' but less vigorous 'repair'; healing will be slower but pain less severe. Thus acute tendinitis (which affects younger patients) is intensely painful but rapidly better; chronic tendinitis (a middle group) is only moderately painful but takes many months to recover and may be complicated by partial tears; and a complete

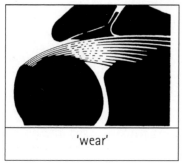
'wear'

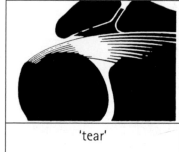
'tear'

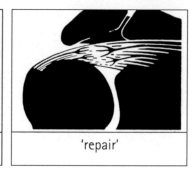
'repair'

13.5 Pathological progression of rotator cuff lesions

tear (which usually occurs in the elderly) becomes painless soon after injury, but never mends.

Clinical syndromes

Rotator cuff lesions present as five more or less distinct clinical syndromes:

1. acute tendinitis,
2. chronic tendinitis (impingement syndrome),
3. tears of the rotator cuff,
4. adhesive capsulitis (frozen shoulder),
5. biceps tendon lesions.

ACUTE CALCIFIC TENDINITIS

Deposits of calcium hydroxyapatite appear in the supraspinatus tendon. Calcification alone is probably not painful; symptoms, when they occur, are due to the florid vascular reaction which produces swelling and tension in the tendon. Resorption of the calcific material is rapid and it may soften or disappear entirely within a few weeks.

Clinical features

An adult, often young, complains of aching, sometimes following over-use. Hourly, the pain increases in severity, rising to an agonizing climax. After a few days, pain subsides and the shoulder gradually returns to normal. During the acute stage the arm is held immobile; the joint is usually too tender to permit palpation or movement.

X-ray

Calcification just above the greater tuberosity is always present. As pain subsides, the dense blotch gradually lightens and may disappear.

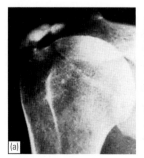 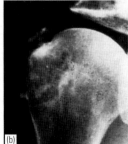

13.6 Acute calcification of supraspinatus The dense mass in the tendon (a) is gradually resorbed or dispersed into the subdeltoid bursa (b).

Treatment

If symptoms are not very severe, the arm is rested in a sling and the patient is given a short course of non-steroidal anti-inflammatory medication. If pain is more intense, a single injection of corticosteroid (methylprednisolone 40 mg) and local anaesthetic (lignocaine 1%) is given into the most painful area. If this is not rapidly effective, or if symptoms soon recur, relief can be obtained by an operation at which the calcific material is removed.

CHRONIC TENDINITIS (THE IMPINGEMENT SYNDROME)

Over-use or minor tears of the rotator cuff may initiate a subacute or chronic vascular response in the tendon. Impingement of the rotator cuff against the coracoacromial arch during abduction may play a part in this process. A more obvious cause of impingement is osteophyte formation on the under-surface of the acromioclavicular joint.

Clinical features

The patient, usually aged 40–60 years, complains of pain in the shoulder and over the deltoid muscle. It is characteristically worse at night and may be quite severe on attempting certain activities, such as putting on a jacket. The shoulder looks normal but is tender just below the anterior edge of the acromion. On abduction, scapulohumeral rhythm is disturbed and pain is aggravated as the arm traverses an arc between 60 and 120 degrees (the *painful arc*). Repeating the movement with the arm in full external rotation throughout may be much easier and relatively painless; this is virtually pathognomonic of supraspinatus tendinitis.

Crepitus or clicking during movement suggests a partial tear of the rotator cuff.

In long-standing cases there is wasting of the muscles and loss of power; movements, especially abduction and external rotation, are restricted.

Imaging

X-rays may show calcification just above the greater tuberosity – a legacy of former events. *Ultrasound scans* and *MRI* may show changes in the cuff.

Complications

In long-standing and refractory cases, the absence of the stabilizing effect of the rotator cuff may lead to the humeral head gradually subluxating upwards. With increasing joint incongruity,

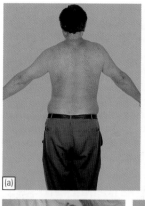
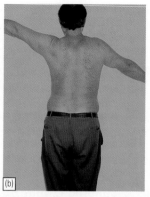
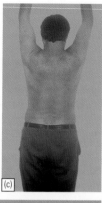
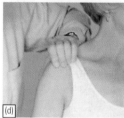
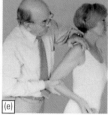
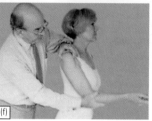

13.7 Supraspinatus tendinitis (a–c) The painful arc. During active abduction, the scapulohumeral rhythm is disturbed on the right and the patient starts to experience pain at about 60 degrees (b). As the arm passes beyond 120 degrees (c), the pain eases and the patient is able to abduct and elevate up to the full 180 degrees. (d–f) The tender spot is at the anterior edge of the acromion process. With the shoulder extended (e), tenderness is more acute. When the shoulder is flexed (f), the painful tendon disappears under the acromion process and tenderness disappears.

osteoarthritis of the shoulder may supervene and shoulder movements become restricted.

Treatment

Some patients improve with a short course of anti-inflammatory tablets. If this fails, local injection of methylprednisolone and lignocaine is tried.

If symptoms keep recurring, operation is advisable. The rotator cuff is 'decompressed' by excising the coracoacromial ligament and the antero-inferior part of the acromion. If acromioclavicular osteophytes are present, these also are removed. Small tears of the cuff are repaired at the same time.

Rotator cuff decompression is nowadays often performed by arthroscopic techniques.

ROTATOR CUFF TEARS

Partial tears of the rotator cuff frequently occur with supraspinatus tendinitis; indeed, it is possible that tendinitis is precipitated by a minor tear.

A complete tear may result from a sudden shoulder strain, or it may appear as a complication of tendinitis or partial rupture. With a partial tear, the intact tendon fibres provide continuity and allow vascular ingrowth and repair. With a complete tear, there is little or no reaction and no repair; the proximal fibres may retract and become stuck down.

Clinical features

The patient is usually aged 45–75. While lifting a weight or protecting himself from falling, he 'sprains' his shoulder. Pain is felt immediately and he is unable to lift his arm sideways.

Often the patient seeks no advice, or is given no effective treatment. If the tear is partial, he may gradually recover, although perhaps with a persistent painful arc of abduction. If the tear is complete, the pain soon subsides, but gross weakness of abduction persists.

The appearance is usually normal, but in long-standing cases there is supraspinatus wasting. Tenderness may be diffuse or may be localized to just below the tip of the acromion process. With a recent injury, active abduction is grossly limited and painful. To distinguish between partial and complete tears, pain is abolished by injecting a local anaesthetic; if active abduction is now possible, the tear must be only partial.

If some weeks have elapsed since the injury, the two types are easily differentiated. With a complete tear, pain has by then subsided and the clinical picture is unmistakable: active abduction is impossible and attempting it produces a characteristic shrug; but passive abduction is full and once the arm has been lifted above a right angle, the patient can keep it up by using his deltoid (the *abduction paradox*); when he lowers it sideways it suddenly drops (the *drop-arm sign*).

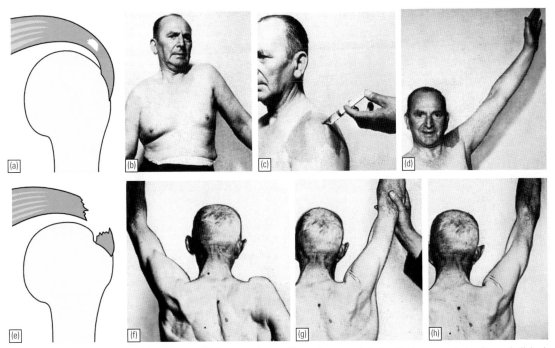

13.8 Torn supraspinatus (a–d) Partial tear of left supraspinatus. The patient can abduct actively once pain has been abolished with local anaesthetic. (e–h) Complete tear of right supraspinatus. Active abduction is impossible, even when pain subsides or is abolished by injection (f); but once the arm is passively abducted (g), the patient can hold it up with his deltoid muscle (h).

With a partial tear, abduction slowly recovers.

The diagnosis may be confirmed by ultrasonography, MRI or arthroscopy.

Treatment

In the acute phase

Treatment is conservative and consists of heat, exercises, and one or two injections of local anaesthetic into the tender area.

Later

After 3 weeks it is usually possible to assess the extent of the rupture. *Complete tears* in younger, active individuals should be repaired; operation is contraindicated in old or sedentary individuals, and in long-standing cases that are painless and accompanied by satisfactory function. *Partial tears* do not require operation unless they cause persistent pain.

ADHESIVE CAPSULITIS (FROZEN SHOULDER)

The term *frozen shoulder* should be reserved for a well-defined disorder characterized by progressive pain and stiffness which usually resolves spontaneously after about 18 months. The cause and pathogenesis are still topics of heated debate.

The process probably starts in the same way as a chronic tendinitis but it then spreads to involve the entire cuff and joint capsule.

Clinical features

The patient, aged 40–60, may give a history of trauma, often trivial, followed by pain. Gradually it increases in severity and often prevents sleeping on the affected side. After several months it begins to subside, but as it does so, stiffness becomes more and more of a problem. Untreated, stiffness persists for another 6–12 months. Gradually movement is regained, but may not return to normal.

Usually there is nothing to see except slight wasting; there may also be some tenderness, but movements are always limited and in a severe case the shoulder is extremely stiff.

X-rays show decreased bone density in the humerus; arthrography shows a contracted joint.

Differential diagnosis

Post-traumatic stiffness

After any severe shoulder injury, stiffness (without much pain) may persist for some months. It is maximal at the start and gradually lessens, unlike the pattern of a frozen shoulder.

147

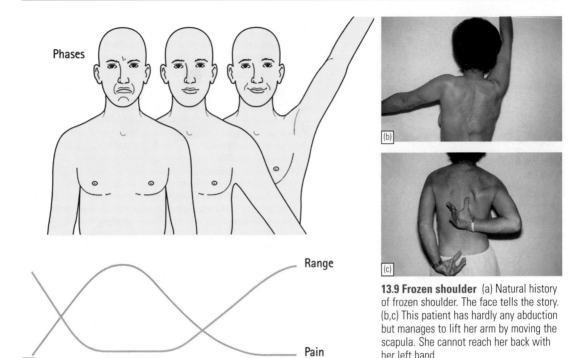

Phases

Range

Pain

(a)

13.9 Frozen shoulder (a) Natural history of frozen shoulder. The face tells the story. (b,c) This patient has hardly any abduction but manages to lift her arm by moving the scapula. She cannot reach her back with her left hand.

Disuse stiffness

If the arm is nursed over-cautiously (e.g. following a wrist fracture), the shoulder may stiffen. Again, the characteristic pain pattern of a frozen shoulder is absent.

Regional pain syndrome

This condition, formerly known as *reflex sympathetic dystrophy,* may follow acute trauma; it is also seen in patients with myocardial infarction or a stroke. The features are very similar to those of a frozen shoulder, and it has been suggested that the latter is a form of reflex sympathetic dystrophy.

Treatment

Conservative treatment with analgesics, anti-inflammatory drugs, local heat and exercise aims at relieving pain and preventing further stiffening while recovery is awaited. Injections of corticosteroid and local anaesthetic sometimes help. Once the acute pain has subsided, manipulation under anaesthesia often hastens recovery. Active exercises should recommence immediately afterwards.

Operative treatment is occasionally called for. Arthroscopic division of the interval between supraspinatus and infraspinatus may dramatically improve the range of movement.

BICIPITAL TENDINITIS

Though not part of the rotator cuff, the tendon of long head of biceps lies adjacent to the rotator cuff and may be involved in the impingement syndrome. Rarely, it presents as an isolated problem in young people after unaccustomed shoulder strain. Pain and tenderness are sharply localized to the bicipital groove.

Rest, local heat and deep transverse frictions usually bring relief; if recovery is delayed, a corticosteroid injection will help.

TORN LONG HEAD OF BICEPS

Degeneration and disruption of the tendon of long head of biceps are fairly common. The patient is usually middle-aged or elderly. While lifting a heavy object, he feels something snap; the shoulder, which previously felt normal, aches for a time and bruising appears over the front of the arm. Soon the ache subsides and good function returns, but when the elbow is flexed actively, the belly of the muscle contracts into a prominent lump. Sometimes the initial episode passes unremarked and the patient presents for the first time with a 'lump' in the arm, which is easily mistaken for a tumour. Ask the patient to flex the elbow against resistance; this will show

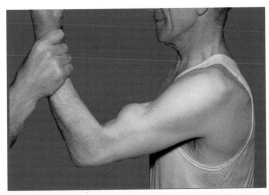

13.10 Ruptured long head of biceps The lump in the front of the arm becomes even more prominent when the patient contracts the biceps against resistance.

that the 'lump' is actually the bunched-up belly of biceps.

Function is usually so little disturbed that treatment is unnecessary.

CHRONIC INSTABILITY OF THE SHOULDER

The shoulder achieves its uniquely wide range of movement at the cost of stability. The glenoid socket is very shallow and the joint is held secure by the fibrocartilaginous glenoid labrum and the surrounding ligaments and muscles. If these structures give way, the shoulder becomes unstable and prone to recurrent dislocation or subluxation, which may be anterior, posterior or multidirectional.

Anterior dislocation usually follows an acute injury in which the arm is forced into abduction, external rotation and extension (see page 306). In *recurrent dislocation* the labrum and capsule are often detached from the anterior rim of the glenoid (the classic Bankart lesion).

Anterior subluxation may follow and alternate with episodes of dislocation.

Posterior dislocation is rare; when it occurs it is usually due to a violent jerk in an unusual position, following an epileptic fit or a severe electric shock. Recurrent posterior instability is almost always a *subluxation,* with the humeral head riding back on the posterior lip of the glenoid.

Multidirectional instability is associated with capsular and ligamentous laxity, and sometimes with weakness of the shoulder muscles.

ANTERIOR INSTABILITY

This is far and away the commonest type of instability, accounting for more than 95 per cent of cases. It usually occurs as a sequel to acute anterior dislocation of the shoulder, with detachment or stretching of the glenoid labrum and capsule (see page 306).

Clinical features

The typical patient is a young man who complains of the shoulder repeatedly 'going out of joint' during over-arm movements (lifting the arm in abduction, extension and external rotation), and each time having to have it manipulated back into position. An initial, acute episode of dislocation is followed by *recurrent dislocation* in more than 50 per cent of patients under the age of 25 years.

Recurrent subluxation is less obvious. The patient may describe a 'catching' sensation (rather than complete displacement), followed by 'numbness' or 'weakness' – the so-called dead arm syndrome – when attempting to throw a ball or serve at tennis.

Between episodes, the diagnosis rests on demonstrating the *apprehension sign.* With the patient seated, the examiner cautiously lifts the arm into abduction, external rotation and then extension; at the crucial moment, the patient senses that the humeral head is about to slip out anteriorly and his body tautens in apprehension.

Examination of the other joints may reveal generalized ligamentous laxity.

Imaging

The classic *x-ray* feature is a depression in the posterosuperior part of the humeral head (the Hill–Sachs lesion), where the bone has been damaged by repeated impact with the anterior rim of the glenoid. Subluxation is more difficult to demonstrate; an axillary view may show the humeral head riding on the anterior lip of the glenoid.

MRI may reveal a detached glenoid labrum (the Bankart lesion) and/or deformity of the humeral head.

Treatment

If dislocation recurs only at long intervals, the patient may choose to put up with the inconvenience. Indications for *operative treatment* are: (1) frequent dislocations, especially if these are painful; and (2) a fear of recurrent subluxation or dislocation sufficient to prevent participation in everyday activities, including sport.

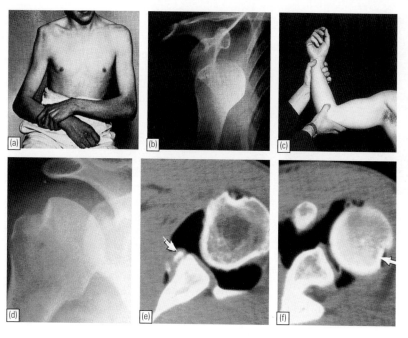

13.11 Anterior instability
(a,b) Anterior dislocation of the shoulder. If this is followed by recurrent dislocation, the apprehension test (c) will be positive. The plain x-ray (d) shows a large depression in the posterosuperior part of the humeral head (the Hill–Sachs lesion). (e,f) MRI showing a Bankart lesion with a flake of bone detached from the edge of the glenoid, and the Hill–Sachs lesion (arrows).

Three types of operation are used: (1) repair or re-attachment of the glenoid labrum (Bankart); (2) shortening and tightening of the anterior capsule and muscles (Putti–Platt); and (3) reinforcement of the antero-inferior capsule using adjacent muscles (Bristow).

POSTERIOR INSTABILITY

Posterior instability sometimes persists after an acute posterior dislocation (see page 307). It usually takes the form of recurrent subluxation rather than full-blown dislocation. The diagnosis is confirmed by x-rays and CT scans.

Treatment is usually conservative – muscle strengthening exercises and voluntary control of the joint. Operative reconstruction is indicated only if disability is marked and there is no gross joint laxity.

MULTIDIRECTIONAL INSTABILITY

In this condition, the patient complains of the shoulder going 'out of joint' with remarkable ease. Examination may show that these are alternating episodes of either anterior or posterior subluxation or dislocation. There is usually an association with generalized capsular and ligamentous hyperlaxity, and often the patient is able to dislocate (and re-locate) the joint voluntarily. Surgical treatment is seldom indicated; muscle strengthening exercises and training in joint control are helpful.

DISORDERS OF THE GLENOHUMERAL JOINT

TUBERCULOSIS

Tuberculosis of the shoulder is uncommon. It usually starts as an osteitis but is rarely diagnosed until arthritis has supervened. This may proceed to abscess and sinus formation; in some cases fibrous ankylosis develops. Patients are usually adults. They complain of a constant ache and stiffness lasting many months. The striking feature is wasting of the muscles around the shoulder. In neglected cases a sinus may be present. There is diffuse warmth and tenderness, and all movements are limited and painful. Axillary lymph nodes may be enlarged.

X-ray

Early signs are generalized rarefaction of bone on both sides of the joint and erosion of the joint surfaces. In late cases there may be 'cystic' destruction of the humeral head and/or glenoid.

Treatment

In addition to systemic treatment with anti-tuberculous drugs, the shoulder should be rested until acute symptoms have settled. Thereafter movement is encouraged and, provided the articular cartilage is not destroyed, the prognosis for painless function is good. If there are repeated flares, or if the articular surfaces are extensively destroyed, the joint should be arthrodesed.

RHEUMATOID ARTHRITIS

The acromioclavicular joint, the shoulder joint and the various synovial pouches around the shoulder are frequently involved in rheumatoid disease. Chronic synovitis leads to rupture of the rotator cuff and progressive joint erosion.

Clinical features

The patient, who usually has generalized arthritis, complains of pain in the shoulder and difficulty with tasks such as combing the hair or washing the back.

Active movements are limited, and passive movements are painful and accompanied by marked crepitus. If the supraspinatus is involved, the features are similar to those of post-traumatic cuff lesions.

X-ray

The characteristic features are progressive loss of the articular space with periarticular erosions. Often the acromioclavicular joint is involved. Although it may start on one side, the condition usually becomes bilateral.

Treatment

If general measures do not control the synovitis, methylprednisolone may be injected into the joint and the subacromial bursa. If synovitis persists, operative synovectomy is carried out and at the same time cuff tears are repaired. Excision of the lateral end of the clavicle may relieve acromioclavicular pain.

In advanced cases, pain and stiffness can be very disabling and may call for either arthroplasty or arthrodesis. Shoulder replacement gives good pain relief and improved function, even though the range of movement remains well below normal.

OSTEOARTHRITIS

Glenohumeral osteoarthritis is usually secondary to other fairly obvious disorders: congenital dysplasia, local trauma, long-standing rotator cuff lesions, rheumatoid disease or avascular necrosis of the head of the humerus.

Clinical features

Patients are usually in their fifties or sixties and the main complaint is of pain; they may give a history of previous shoulder problems. The most typical sign is progressive restriction of shoulder movements.

X-rays show the characteristic features of loss of the articular space, distortion of the joint, subchondral sclerosis and marginal osteophyte formation.

Treatment

Analgesics and anti-inflammatory drugs relieve pain, and exercises may improve mobility. Most patients manage to live with the restrictions imposed by stiffness, provided pain is not severe.

If pain and stiffness become intolerable, joint replacement is justified. It may not improve mobility much, but it does relieve pain.

MILWAUKEE SHOULDER

Occasionally a patient presents with swelling of the shoulder and x-rays show a bizarrely destructive form of arthritis. Similar conditions are encountered in other joints. It has been suggested that this is a crystal-induced, rapidly progressive

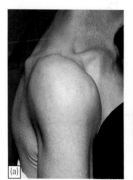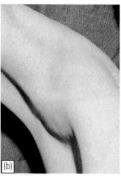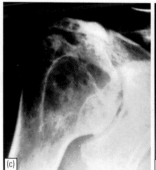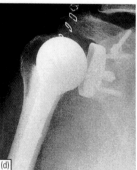

13.12 Rheumatoid arthritis (a) Large synovial effusions cause easily visible swelling; small ones are likely to be missed, especially if they are present in the axilla (b). (c) X-rays show progressive erosion of the joint. (d) X-ray appearance after total joint replacement.

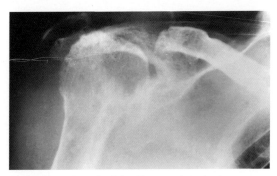

13.13 Milwaukee shoulder The x-ray features are arresting. There is gross destruction of the joint and calcification in the soft tissues around the shoulder.

arthropathy; it is sometimes associated with massive tears of the rotator cuff. The name 'Milwaukee shoulder' was suggested in an early description of the condition by McCarty, who hailed from the city of that name.

There is no satisfactory treatment. Arthroplasty may relieve pain but will not improve function because the joint is unstable.

DISORDERS OF THE SCAPULA AND CLAVICLE

CONGENITAL ELEVATION OF THE SCAPULA (SPRENGEL'S SHOULDER)

The scapulae normally complete their descent from the neck by the third month of fetal life; occasionally one remains unduly high. The shoulder on the affected side is elevated; the scapula looks and feels abnormally high, smaller than usual and somewhat prominent. Movements are painless, but abduction may be limited. Associated deformities such as fusion of cervical vertebrae, kyphosis or scoliosis may be present.

Treatment

Mild cases are best left untreated. Marked limitation of abduction or severe deformity may necessitate operation to lower the scapula.

KLIPPEL–FEIL SYNDROME

This rare congenital disorder comprises bilateral failure of scapular descent and fusion of several cervical vertebrae. The neck is unusually short and may be webbed; cervical mobility is restricted. The condition is usually left untreated.

WINGED SCAPULA

In this condition the scapula juts out under the skin, like a small wing. It is due to weakness of the serratus anterior, the muscle which stabilizes the scapula on the thoracic cage. It may cause asymmetry of the shoulders, but it is often not apparent until the patient tries to contract the serratus anterior against resistance (e.g. pushing hard against a wall).

Weakness of the serratus anterior may arise from (1) damage to the long thoracic nerve, (2) injury to the brachial plexus, (3) injury or viral infections of the 5th, 6th and 7th cervical nerve roots, and (4) certain types of muscular dystrophy.

A less obvious form of scapular instability may be caused by weakness of the trapezius following injury to the spinal accessory nerve.

Treatment

Some of the disorders causing winged scapula are self-limiting and the condition gradually improves. Even if it does not, disability is usually slight and is best accepted. However, if function is markedly impaired, the scapula can be stabilized by tendon transfer.

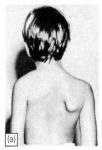 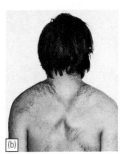 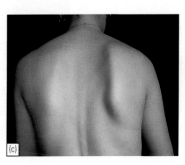

13.14 Scapular disorders
(a) Sprengel shoulder;
(b) Klippel–Feil syndrome;
(c) winged scapula.

ACROMIOCLAVICULAR INSTABILITY

This is a common condition, resulting from dislocation of the acromioclavicular joint and rupture of the ligaments which tether the outer end of the clavicle (see page 304). The patient may complain of discomfort and weakness during strenuous activities with the arm above shoulder height. On examination there is a fairly obvious bump over the acromioclavicular joint, and pressure on the joint may be painful. If the diagnosis is not obvious on plain x-ray, re-examination with the patient standing up and holding a heavy weight (to drag the shoulder downwards) will show the displacement.

Treatment

The condition causes little disability during non-strenuous activities and treatment is therefore unnecessary. However, certain types of work activity may be seriously curtailed, and in such cases reconstructive surgery should be considered.

OSTEOARTHRITIS OF THE ACROMIOCLAVICULAR JOINT

Clinical features

Acromioclavicular osteoarthritis is common in old people. When it occurs in younger individuals it is usually due to previous injury or repetitive stress (for example habitually carrying weights on the shoulder, or working with pneumatic hammers or drills).

The patient complains of pain over the top of the shoulder, particularly while using the arm above shoulder height. Tenderness and swelling are localized to the acromioclavicular joint.

X-rays show the characteristic features of osteoarthritis.

Treatment

If analgesics and corticosteroid injections are ineffectual, pain may be relieved by excision of the lateral end of the clavicle.

THE ELBOW

CLINICAL ASSESSMENT

HISTORY

Pain may be felt diffusely on the medial side of the joint (ulnohumeral), the posterolateral side (radiohumeral), or acutely localized to one of the humeral epicondyles ('tennis elbow' on the lateral side and 'golfer's elbow' on the medial side). Pain over the back of the elbow is often due to an olecranon bursitis.

Stiffness, if severe, can be very disabling; the patient may be unable to reach to the mouth (loss of flexion) or the perineum (loss of extension); limited supination makes it difficult to hold something in the palm or to carry large objects.

Swelling may be due to injury or inflammation; a soft lump on the back of the elbow suggests an olecranon bursitis.

Deformity is usually the result of previous trauma: (a) *cubitus varus* due to a malunited supracondylar fracture, or (b) *cubitus valgus* due to an old displaced and malunited fracture of the lateral condyle.

Instability is not uncommon in the late stage of rheumatoid arthritis.

Ulnar nerve symptoms (tingling, numbness and weakness of the hand) may occur in elbow disorders because the nerve is so near the joint.

Loss of function is noticed in grooming activities, carrying and hand work.

EXAMINATION

Both upper limbs must be completely exposed and it is essential to look at the back as well as the front. The neck, shoulders and hands should also be examined.

Look

Looking at the patient from the front, with his or her arms outstretched alongside the body and the palms facing forwards, the elbows are seen to be held in 5–10 degrees of valgus; this is the normal 'carrying angle'. Anything more, especially if unilateral, is regarded as a valgus deformity. Varus deformity is less obvious, but if the patient raises the arms to shoulder height, it is easily seen.

The most common swelling is in the olecranon bursa at the back of the elbow.

Feel

Important bony landmarks are the medial and lateral condyles and the tip of the olecranon. These are palpated to determine whether the joint is correctly positioned.

Superficial structures are examined for warmth and subcutaneous nodules. The joint line (including the radioulnar joint depression) is located and palpated for synovial thickening. Tenderness can usually be localized to a particular structure.

The ulnar nerve is fairly superficial behind the medial condyle and here it can be rolled under

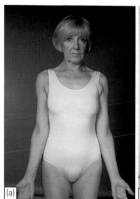
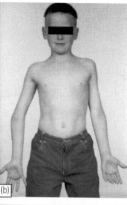
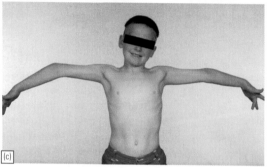

14.1 Examination (a) Note that the elbows are normally held in 5–10 degrees of valgus (the carrying angle). (b) This young boy ended up with slight varus angulation after a supracondylar fracture of the distal humerus. The deformity is much more obvious (c) when he raises his arms (the gun-stock deformity).

the fingers to feel if it is thickened or hyper-sensitive.

Move

Flexion and extension are compared on the two sides. Then, with the elbows tucked into the sides and flexed to a right angle, the radioulnar joints are tested for pronation and supination.

General examination

If the symptoms and signs do not point clearly to a local disorder, other parts are examined: the neck (for cervical disc lesions), the shoulder (for cuff lesions) and the hand (for nerve lesions).

X-RAY

The position of each bone is noted, then the joint line and space. Next, the individual bones are inspected for evidence of old injury or bone destruction. Finally, loose bodies are sought.

ELBOW DEFORMITIES

CUBITUS VARUS

Varus (or 'gun-stock') deformity is most obvious when the elbows are extended and the arms are elevated. The most common cause is malunion of a supracondylar fracture. The deformity can be corrected by a wedge osteotomy of the lower humerus.

CUBITUS VALGUS

The most common cause is non-union of a fractured lateral condyle; this may give gross deformity and a bony knob on the inner side of the joint. The importance of valgus deformity is the liability for delayed ulnar palsy to develop; years after the causal injury, the patient notices weakness of the hand with numbness and tingling of the ulnar fingers. The deformity itself needs no treatment, but for delayed ulnar palsy the nerve should be transposed to the front of the elbow.

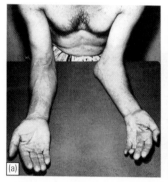
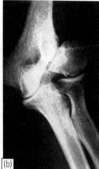

14.2 Cubitus valgus This man's valgus deformity, the sequel to an un-united fracture of the lateral condyle, has resulted in an ulnar nerve palsy.

TUBERCULOSIS

Clinical features

Although the disease begins as synovitis or osteomyelitis, tuberculosis of the elbow is rarely seen until arthritis supervenes. The onset is insidious, with a long history of aching and stiffness. The most striking physical sign is the marked wasting. While the disease is active, the joint is held flexed, looks swollen, feels warm and diffusely tender; movement is considerably limited and accompanied by pain and spasm.

X-rays

Typical features are generalized rarefaction and an apparent increase of joint space because of bone erosion.

Treatment

In addition to anti-tuberculous drugs, the elbow is rested, at first in a splint, but later simply by applying a collar and cuff. Surgical debridement is rarely needed.

RHEUMATOID ARTHRITIS

Clinical features

The elbow is involved in more than 50 per cent of patients with rheumatoid arthritis. Rheumatoid nodules can often be detected over the olecranon. There is pain and tenderness, especially around the head of the radius. Eventually the whole elbow may become swollen and unstable. Often both elbows are affected.

X-rays

Bone erosion, with gradual destruction of the radial head and widening of the trochlear notch of the ulna, is typical of chronic inflammatory arthritis.

Treatment

In addition to general treatment, the elbow should be splinted during periods of active synovitis. For chronic, painful arthritis of the radiohumeral joint, resection of the radial head and partial synovectomy gives good results. If the joint is diffusely involved, joint replacement should be considered. The result is often excellent, at least compared to the preoperative situation; however, the complication rate is fairly high.

OSTEOARTHRITIS

The elbow is an uncommon site for osteoarthritis; when it does occur, it is usually secondary to trauma. 'Primary' osteoarthritis of the elbow should suggest an underlying disorder such as pyrophosphate arthropathy or congenital dysplasia.

There may be pain and stiffness, but the symptoms are usually not severe. Occasionally ulnar palsy is the presenting feature. The joint may

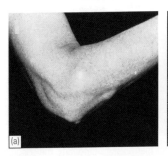
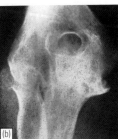
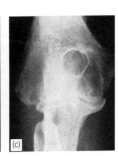

14.3 Rheumatoid arthritis
(a) This patient has a painful elbow as well as the typical rheumatoid nodules over the olecranon. (b) His x-rays show deformity of the radial head and marked erosion of the rest of the elbow joint. (c) Excision of the radial head combined with synovectomy relieved the pain.

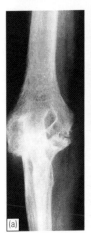
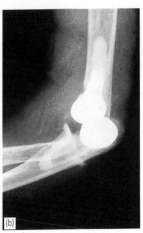
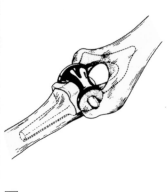

14.4 Total elbow replacement
(a) Severe rheumatoid arthritis of the elbow. (b) X-ray after joint replacement. (c) The Souter arthroplasty: a metal humeral prosthesis and polyethylene ulnar implant.

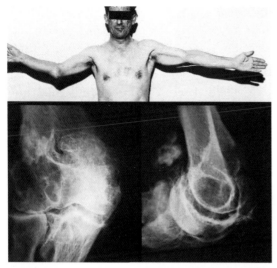

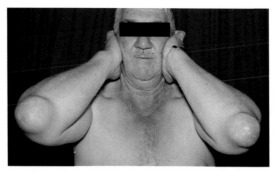

14.6 Olecranon bursitis The enormous red lumps over the points of the elbows are due to swollen olecranon bursae; the patient's ruddy complexion completes the typical picture of gout.

14.5 Osteoarthritis This patient has osteoarthritis and loose bodies in the elbow.

look and feel enlarged, and movements are somewhat limited.

X-rays

X-rays show diminution of the joint space with subchondral sclerosis and marginal osteophytes; one or more loose bodies may be seen.

Treatment

Osteoarthritis of the elbow rarely requires more than symptomatic treatment; loose bodies, however, should be removed if they cause locking. If stiffness is sufficiently disabling, removal of osteophytes (by either open or arthroscopic surgery) can improve the range of movement. If there are signs of ulnar neuritis, the nerve may have to be transposed to the front of the elbow.

LOOSE BODIES

The commonest cause of a single loose body in the elbow is osteochondritis dissecans of the capitulum. Multiple loose bodies may occur with osteoarthritis or synovial chondromatosis.

The cardinal clinical feature is sudden locking of the elbow. If this is troublesome, the loose bodies can be removed by arthroscopic methods.

OLECRANON BURSITIS

The olecranon bursa sometimes becomes enlarged as a result of pressure or friction. When it is also painful, the cause is more likely to be infection, gout or rheumatoid arthritis.

Gout is suspected if there is a history of previous attacks, if the condition is bilateral, if there are tophi, or if x-ray shows calcification in the bursa. Even then it is not easy to distinguish from acute infection, unless pus is aspirated.

Rheumatoid arthritis causes both swelling and nodularity over the olecranon. In almost all cases this will be associated with a typical symmetrical polyarthritis. In the late stages, erosion of the elbow joint may cause marked instability.

Treatment

The underlying disorder must be treated. Septic bursitis may need local drainage. Occasionally a chronically enlarged bursa has to be excised.

'TENNIS ELBOW' AND 'GOLFER'S ELBOW'

The cause of these common disorders is unknown, but they are seldom due to either tennis or golf. Most cases follow minor trauma or repetitive strain on the tendon aponeuroses attached to either the lateral or medial humeral epicondyle. Pain is probably due to a vascular repair process similar to that of rotator cuff tendinitis around the shoulder. Often there is a history of occupational stress or unaccustomed activity, such as house painting, carpentry or other activities that involve strenuous wrist movements and forearm muscle contraction.

Clinical features

In *'tennis elbow'*, pain is felt over the outer side of the elbow, but in severe cases it may radiate widely. It is initiated or aggravated by movements such as pouring out tea, turning a stiff door-handle, shaking hands or lifting with the forearm

157

pronated. The elbow looks normal and flexion and extension are full and painless. Tenderness is localized to a spot just below the lateral epicondyle, and pain is reproduced by getting the patient to extend the wrist against resistance, or simply by passively flexing the wrist so as to stretch the common extensors.

In *golfer's elbow*, similar symptoms occur around the medial epicondyle and, owing to involvement of the common tendon of origin of the wrist flexors, pain is reproduced by passive extension of the wrist.

Treatment

Rest, or avoiding the precipitating activity, may allow the lesion to heal. If pain is severe, the area of maximum tenderness is injected with a mixture of corticosteroid and local anaesthetic.

Persistent pain which fails to respond to conservative measures may call for operative treatment. The affected common tendon on the lateral or medial side of the elbow is detached from its origin at the humeral epicondyle.

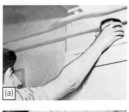
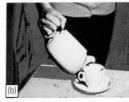
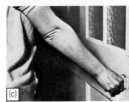
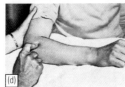
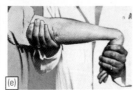
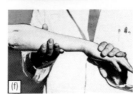

14.7 Tennis elbow
(a–c) Typical movements causing pain more or less over the head of the radius. (d) The tender spot. (e,f) Pain on passive stretching of the common extensor muscles and on resisted extension of the wrist.

CHAPTER 15

THE WRIST

CLINICAL ASSESSMENT

History

Pain may be localized to the radial side (especially in tenovaginitis of the thumb tendons), to the ulnar side (possibly from the radioulnar joint) or to the dorsum (the usual site in disorders of the carpus).

The painful wrist
Joint disorders
Infection
Kienböck's disease
Carpal instability
Rheumatoid arthritis
Osteoarthritis
Periarticular disorders
de Quervain's disease
Tenosynovitis
Referred pain
Cervical spondylosis

   Stiffness is often not noticed until it is severe.
   Swelling may signify involvement of either the joint or the tendon sheaths.
   Deformity is a late symptom except after trauma.
   Loss of function affects both the wrist and the hand. Firm grip is possible only with a strong,

stable, painless wrist that has a reasonable range of movement.

EXAMINATION

Examination of the wrist is not complete without also examining the elbow, forearm and hand. Both upper limbs should be completely exposed.

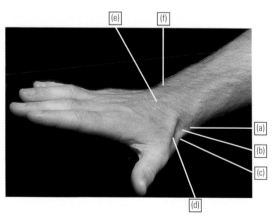

15.1 Tender points at the wrist (a) Tip of the radial styloid process; (b) anatomical snuff-box, bounded on the radial side by (c) the extensor pollicis brevis and on the ulnar side by (d) the extensor pollicis longus; (e) the extensor tendons of the fingers; and (f) the head of the ulna.

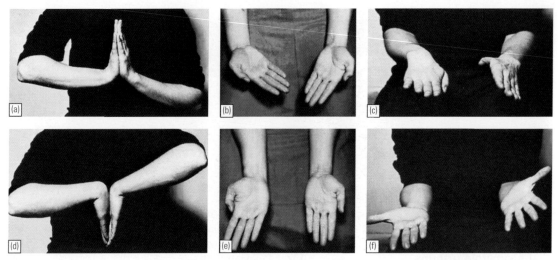

15.2 Examination All movements of the left wrist are limited: (a) extension (dorsiflexion), (b) flexion (palmarflexion), (c) ulnar deviation, (d) radial deviation, (e) pronation, (f) supination.

Look

The skin is inspected for scars. Both wrists and forearms are compared to see if there is any deformity. If there is swelling, note whether it is diffuse or localized to one of the tendon sheaths.

Feel

Undue warmth is noted. Tender areas must be accurately localized and the bony landmarks compared with those of the normal wrist.

Move

Passive flexion and extension of the wrist can be measured on each side in turn. To view both sides simultaneously and compare them, ask the patient first to place his or her palms together in a position of prayer, elevating the elbows, then to repeat the manoeuvre with the wrists back-to-back. The normal range for both flexion and extension is 80–90 degrees. Radial deviation and ulnar deviation are measured in the palms-up position; ulnar deviation is considerably greater than radial deviation.

Pronation and supination are included in wrist movements. The patient holds his or her elbows at right angles and tucked in to the sides, fingers extended and palms facing each other; the hands are then turned first palms downwards and then palms upwards.

Active movements should be tested against resistance; loss of power may be due to pain, tendon rupture or muscle weakness. Grip strength can be gauged by having the patient squeeze the examiner's hand; mechanical instruments allow more accurate assessment.

INVESTIGATIONS

X-rays are routinely obtained; often both wrists must be examined for comparison. Special oblique views are necessary to show up difficult scaphoid fractures. Note the position of the carpal bones and look for evidence of joint-space narrowing, especially at the carpometacarpal joint of the thumb.

MRI is useful for demonstrating the early features of avascular necrosis or detecting soft-tissue lesions such as an occult ganglion.

Arthroscopy is the most reliable way of diagnosing tears of the triangular fibrocartilage complex (TFCC). It will also reveal the early changes of osteoarthritis.

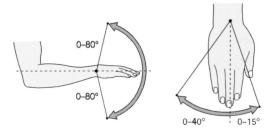

15.3 Normal range of movement From the neutral position extension is slightly less than flexion. Most hand functions are performed with the wrist in slight ulnar deviation.

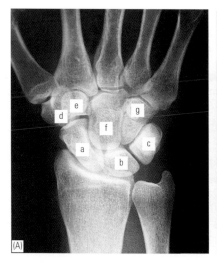

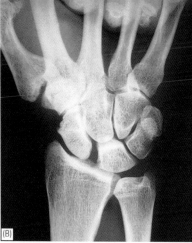

15.4 X-rays A. Note the shape and position of the bones which make up the normal carpus: (a) scaphoid, (b) lunate, (c) triquetrum overlain by pisiform, (d) trapezium, (e) trapezoid, (f) capitate, (g) hamate. **B** Compare this x-ray with **A**. The scaphoid is foreshortened and there is an abnormally large space between the scaphoid and the lunate. These are the classic signs of carpal instability.

WRIST DEFORMITIES

CONGENITAL DEFORMITIES

Radial club-hand

The infant is born with the wrist in marked radial deviation. There is absence of the whole or part of the radius, and usually also the thumb. Treatment in the neonate consists of gentle manipulation and splintage. If function deteriorates, centralization of the carpus over the ulna is recommended, preferably before the age of 3 years.

Madelung's deformity

The carpus is deviated forwards, leaving the ulnar head projecting on the back of the wrist. Deformity is seldom marked before the age of 10 years and function is usually excellent. In the worst cases the deformity may have to be corrected by osteotomy.

ACQUIRED DEFORMITY

Post-traumatic deformities are fairly common, as a consequence of physeal injuries, malunited fractures or subluxation of the distal radioulnar

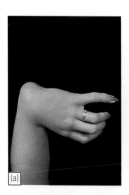

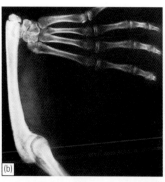

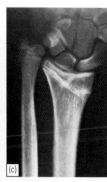

15.5 Congenital deformities (a,b) Radial club-hand. (c) X-ray of Madelung's deformity.

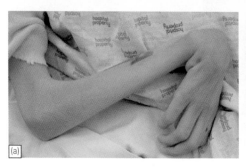

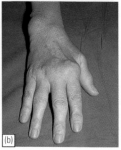

15.6 Acquired deformities (a) Flexion deformity in cerebral palsy. (b) Typical deformities in rheumatoid arthritis.

161

joint. Osteotomy of the radius or stabilization of the ulna may be needed.

Non-traumatic deformities are seen typically in rheumatoid arthritis and cerebral palsy. These disorders are discussed in Chapters 3 and 10, respectively.

TUBERCULOSIS

At the wrist, tuberculosis is rarely seen until it has progressed to a true arthritis. Pain and stiffness come on gradually and the hand feels weak. The forearm looks wasted; the wrist is swollen and feels warm. Involvement of the flexor tendon compartment may give rise to a large fluctuant swelling that crosses the wrist into the palm (compound palmar ganglion). In a neglected case there may be a sinus. Movements are restricted and painful.

X-rays

X-ray examination shows localized osteoporosis and irregularity of the radiocarpal and intercarpal joints, and sometimes bone erosion.

Diagnosis

The condition must be differentiated from rheumatoid arthritis. Bilateral arthritis of the wrist is nearly always rheumatoid in origin, but when only one wrist is affected, the signs resemble those of tuberculosis. X-rays and serological tests may establish the diagnosis, but sometimes a biopsy is necessary.

Treatment

Anti-tuberculous drugs are given and the wrist is splinted. If an abscess forms, it must be drained. If the wrist is destroyed, systemic treatment should be continued until the disease is quiescent and the wrist is then arthrodesed.

RHEUMATOID ARTHRITIS

Clinical features

After the metacarpophalangeal joints, the wrist is the most common site of rheumatoid arthritis. Pain, swelling and tenderness may at first be localized to the radioulnar joint, or to one of the tendon sheaths. Sooner or later the whole wrist becomes involved and tenderness is much more ill-defined. In late cases the wrist is deformed and unstable. Extensor tendons may rupture where they cross the dorsum of the wrist, causing one or more of the fingers to drop into flexion.

X-rays

The characteristic features are osteoporosis and bony erosions. Tell-tale signs are usually more obvious in the metacarpophalangeal joints.

Treatment

Management in the early stage consists of splintage and local injection of corticosteroids, combined with systemic treatment. Persistent synovitis may call for synovectomy and excision of the distal end of the ulna. If deformity has commenced, the wrist

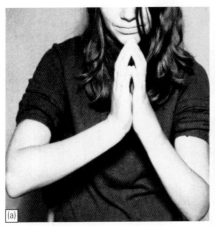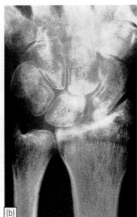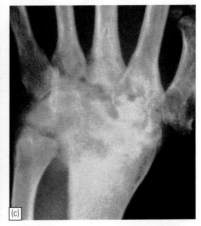

15.7 Tuberculosis (a) This girl developed a painful, swollen left wrist followed by progressive restriction of movement; her x-ray (b) shows marked osteoporosis in the distal radius and the carpus. (c) A much more advanced case of tuberculous arthritis giving rise to extensive bone destruction.

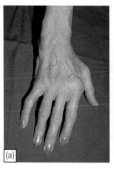
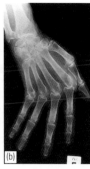
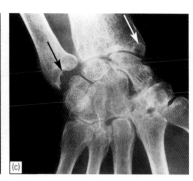

15.8 Rheumatoid arthritis
(a) Typical zig-zag deformity in established rheumatoid arthritis. The wrist is deviated radialwards and the fingers ulnarwards. (b) X-ray of the same patient. (c) Enlarged x-ray view – note the characteristic erosions at the distal ends of the radius and ulna (arrows).

should be stabilized by soft-tissue reconstruction. In the late stage, joint destruction may require either arthroplasty or arthrodesis.

OSTEOARTHRITIS

Osteoarthritis of the wrist joint proper is unusual except as a sequel to injury or Kienböck's disease (avascular necrosis of the lunate). The patient may have forgotten the old injury. Some years later, he or she begins to complain of pain, progressive loss of movement and weakness of grip. The appearance is usually normal, but the wrist is tender and movements are restricted and painful.

X-rays

Characteristic features are narrowing of the radiocarpal joint, bone sclerosis and irregularity of one or more of the proximal carpal bones. There may also be signs of an old injury.

Treatment

Rest, in a polythene splint, is often sufficient treatment. Painful but limited osteoarthritis following a scaphoid fracture can be alleviated by excision of the radial styloid process. Widespread osteoarthritis may require more extensive surgery, including partial or complete arthrodesis of the wrist.

CARPOMETACARPAL OSTEOARTHRITIS

Osteoarthritis of the thumb carpometacarpal joint is common in postmenopausal women. The patient complains of pain and swelling around the proximal end of the thumb metacarpal. Careful examination will show that tenderness is sharply localized to the carpometacarpal joint, about 1 cm distal to the radial styloid process. The condition is often bilateral, and Heberden's nodes of the finger joints are common. In late cases, fixed adduction of the first metacarpal produces a characteristic deformity. *X-ray* examination shows the usual features of joint-space narrowing, sclerosis and osteophyte formation.

Treatment

Local injection of corticosteroid usually relieves pain, and movements may improve. If this fails, operation may be advisable. The surest way of abolishing pain is to arthrodese the joint. The patient should be warned that this will result in further loss of movement; if this is unacceptable, function may be better preserved by excising the

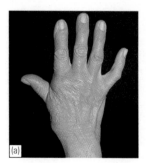
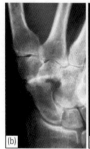
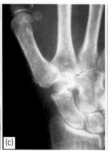
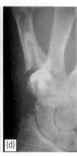
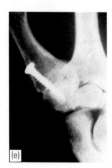

15.9 Osteoarthritis of the first carpometacarpal (CMC) joint (a) Typical deformity; note the swelling over the first CMC joint. (b) X-ray changes. Choice of treatment is between (c) trapeziectomy, (d) replacement arthroplasty and (e) arthrodesis.

trapezium. A more sophisticated, but less reliable, option is joint replacement.

KIENBÖCK'S DISEASE

After injury or stress, the lunate bone may develop a patchy avascular necrosis. A predisposing factor may be relative shortening of the ulna (negative ulnar variance), which could result in excessive stress being applied to the lunate where it is squeezed between the distal surface of the (over-long) radius and the second row of carpal bones.

The patient, usually a young adult, complains of ache and stiffness. Tenderness is localized to the centre of the wrist on the dorsum; wrist extension may be limited.

Imaging

The earliest signs of osteonecrosis can be detected only by MRI. Typical x-ray signs are increased density in the lunate and, later, flattening and irregularity of the bone. Ultimately there may be features of osteoarthritis of the wrist.

Treatment

During the early stage, while the shape of the lunate is more or less normal, osteotomy of the distal end of the radius may reduce pressure on the bone and thereby protect it from collapsing. Microsurgical revascularization of the bone is also worth considering if the necessary expertise is available. In late cases, partial wrist arthrodesis may be the only option.

TEARS OF THE TRIANGULAR FIBROCARTILAGE

The TFCC fans out from the base of the ulnar styloid process to the medial edge of the distal radius, acting somewhat like a meniscus in the wrist joint. Chronic pain in the wrist may be related to an old 'sprain' in which a more serious injury to the TFCC was overlooked. In addition to pain, there may be loss of grip strength and clicking on supination of the forearm.

The diagnosis can be confirmed by arthroscopy. Peripheral tears can be repaired, or ragged fragments removed, during the same arthroscopic procedure.

CHRONIC CARPAL INSTABILITY

The wrist functions as a system of intercalated segments stabilized by ligaments and by the scaphoid, which bridges the two rows of carpal bones. Following trauma to the carpus, there may be partial collapse of this structure, a condition which is not always recognized at the time. Some years later, the patient complains of progressive pain and weakness in the wrist.

Diagnosis

There are no defining clinical features. The diagnosis hinges on the x-ray appearances, which are shown on page 330. There may also be features of previous disorders, such as Kienböck's disease or osteoarthritis.

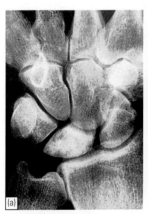 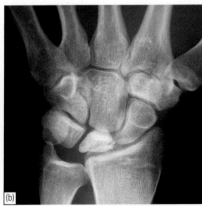 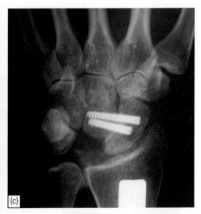

15.10 Kienböck's disease (a) Typical x-ray features of avascular necrosis of the lunate. (b) Late changes – marked distortion of the lunate. (c) Treatment, in this case, was first by osteotomy and shortening of the radius (the plate is still present) and then, when this failed to relieve pain, by lunate excision and scaphocapitate fusion.

Treatment

The best form of treatment is prevention. Acute 'wrist sprains' should be carefully assessed for signs of carpal displacement and instability (see page 332). Carpal displacement must be reduced and the bones held in position in plaster or with Kirschner wires.

Patients with chronic instability can usually be treated by splintage, analgesics and corticosteroid injections. Occasionally operative treatment is indicated: soft-tissue augmentation or partial fusion of the wrist.

TENOSYNOVITIS AND TENOVAGINITIS

The extensor retinaculum contains six compartments which transmit tendons lined with synovium. Tenosynovitis can be caused by unaccustomed movement, over-use or repetitive minor trauma; sometimes it occurs spontaneously. The resulting synovial inflammation causes secondary thickening of the sheath and stenosis of the compartment, which further compromises the tendon. Early treatment, including rest, anti-inflammatory medication and injection of corticosteroids, may break this vicious circle.

The first dorsal compartment (enclosing abductor pollicis longus and extensor pollicis brevis) and the second dorsal compartment (extensor carpi radialis longus and brevis) are the ones most commonly affected.

DE QUERVAIN'S DISEASE

Tenovaginitis of the first dorsal compartment is usually seen in women between the ages of 30 and 50 years. There may be a history of unaccustomed activity, such as pruning roses, cutting with scissors or wringing out clothes.

Clinical features

Pain, and sometimes swelling, is localized to the radial side of the wrist. The tendon sheath feels thick and hard. Tenderness is most acute at the very tip of the radial styloid.

The pathognomonic sign is elicited by *Finkelstein's test*. Hold the patient's hand firmly, keeping the thumb tucked in close to the palm, then turn the wrist sharply towards the ulnar side. A stab of pain over the radial styloid is a positive sign. Repeating the movement with the thumb left free is relatively painless.

Treatment

In early cases, symptoms can be relieved by ultrasound therapy or a corticosteroid injection into the tendon sheath, sometimes combined with splintage of the wrist. Resistant cases need an operation, which consists of slitting the thickened tendon sheath. Care should be taken to prevent injury to the dorsal sensory branches of the radial nerve, which may cause intractable dysaesthesia.

OTHER SITES OF EXTENSOR TENOSYNOVITIS

Over-use tenosynovitis of *extensor carpi radialis brevis* (the most powerful extensor of the wrist) or *extensor carpi ulnaris* may cause pain and point tenderness just medial to the anatomical snuffbox or immediately distal to the head of the ulna, respectively (see Figure 15.1). Splintage and corticosteroid injections are usually effective.

GANGLION

The ubiquitous ganglion is seen most commonly on the back of the wrist. It arises from cystic degeneration in the joint capsule or tendon sheath. The distended cyst contains a glairy fluid.

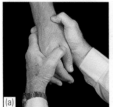 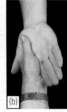 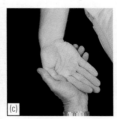 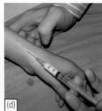

15.11 De Quervain's disease (a) There is point tenderness at the tip of the radial styloid process. (b,c) Finkelstein's test: Ulnar deviation with the thumb left free is relatively painless (b), but if the movement is repeated with the thumb held close to the palm (c), the pull on the thumb tendons causes intense pain. (d) Injecting the tendon sheath.

The patient, often a young adult, presents with a painless lump, usually on the back of the wrist. Occasionally there is a slight ache. The lump is well defined, cystic and not tender. It may be attached to one of the tendons.

Treatment

The ganglion often disappears after some months, so there should be no haste about treatment. If the lesion continues to be troublesome, it can be aspirated; if it recurs, excision is justified, but the patient should be told that there is a 30 per cent risk of recurrence, even after careful surgery.

CARPAL TUNNEL SYNDROME

This is the commonest and best known of all the nerve entrapment syndromes. In the normal carpal tunnel there is barely room for all the tendons and the median nerve; consequently, any swelling is likely to result in compression and ischaemia of the nerve. Usually the cause eludes detection; the syndrome is, however, common in women at the menopause, in rheumatoid arthritis, in pregnancy and in myxoedema. The usual age group is 40–50 years.

Clinical features

The history is most helpful in making the diagnosis. Pain and paraesthesia occur in the distribution of the median nerve in the hand. Night after night the patient is woken with burning pain, tingling and numbness. Patients tend to seek relief by hanging the arm over the side of the bed or shaking the arm; however, merely changing the position of the wrist will usually help.

Early on there is little to see, but there are two helpful tests: sensory symptoms can often be reproduced by percussing over the median nerve *(Tinel's sign)* or by holding the wrist fully flexed for a minute or two *(Phalen's test)*. In late cases there is wasting of the thenar muscles, weakness of thumb abduction and sensory dulling in the median nerve territory.

Electrodiagnostic tests, which show slowing of nerve conduction across the wrist, are reserved for those with atypical symptoms.

Radicular symptoms of cervical spondylosis may confuse the diagnosis and may coincide with carpal tunnel syndrome.

Treatment

Light splints that prevent wrist flexion can help those with night pain or with pregnancy-related symptoms. Steroid injection into the carpal canal, likewise, provides temporary relief.

Open surgical division of the transverse carpal ligament usually provides a quick and simple cure. The incision should be kept to the ulnar side of the thenar crease so as to avoid accidental injury to the palmar cutaneous (sensory) and thenar motor branches of the median nerve. Endoscopic carpal tunnel release offers an alternative with slightly quicker postoperative rehabilitation.

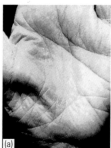
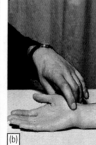
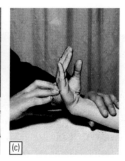
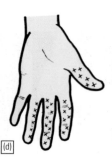
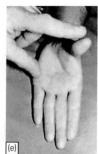

15.12 Carpal tunnel syndrome (a) Wasting of the thenar eminence is not usually as obvious as this. (b) Tinel's sign and (c) Phalan's test may be positive. (d) Area of paraesthesia and diminished sensibility. (e) Testing for thumb abductor weakness.

CHAPTER 16

THE HAND

CLINICAL ASSESSMENT

The hand is (in more senses than one) the medium of introduction to the outside world. Deformity and loss of function are quickly noticed – and often bitterly resented.

HISTORY

Pain is usually felt in the palm or in the finger joints. A poorly defined ache may be referred from the neck, shoulder or mediastinum.

Deformity can appear suddenly (due to tendon rupture) or slowly (suggesting bone or joint pathology).

Swelling may be localized, or may occur in many joints simultaneously. Characteristically, rheumatoid arthritis causes swelling of the proximal joints and osteoarthritis the distal joints.

Loss of function is particularly troublesome in the hand. The patient may have difficulty handling eating utensils, holding a cup or glass, grasping a doorknob (or a crutch), dressing or (most trying of all) attending to personal hygiene.

Sensory symptoms and motor weakness provide clues to neurological disorders affecting the lower cervical nerve roots and their peripheral extensions.

EXAMINATION

Both upper limbs should be bared for comparison. Examination of the hand needs patience and meticulous attention to detail.

Look

The skin may be scarred, altered in colour, dry or moist, and hairy or smooth. Wasting and deformity, and the presence of any lumps, should be noted. The resting posture is an important clue to nerve or tendon damage. Swelling may be in the subcutaneous tissue, in a tendon sheath or in a joint.

Feel

The temperature and texture of the skin are noted. If a nodule is felt, the underlying tendon should be moved to discover if it is attached. Swelling or thickening may be in the subcutaneous tissue, a tendon sheath, a joint or one of the bones. Tenderness should be accurately localized to one of these structures.

Move

Passive movements

It is useful to test first for passive movements; this will tell you whether the joints are 'movable' before you ask the patient to move them actively. The range of movement is recorded, starting with the metacarpophalangeal (MCP) joints and then going on to the proximal interphalangeal (PIP) and distal interphalangeal (DIP) joints.

Active movements

With palms facing upwards, the patient is asked to curl the fingers into full flexion; a 'lagging finger' is immediately obvious. Individual movements are then examined.

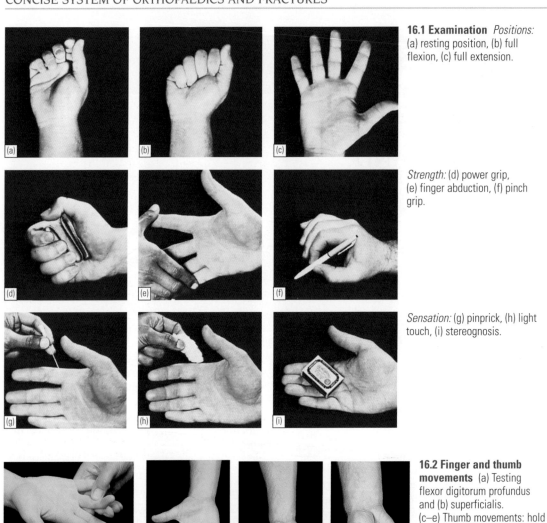

16.1 Examination *Positions:* (a) resting position, (b) full flexion, (c) full extension.

Strength: (d) power grip, (e) finger abduction, (f) pinch grip.

Sensation: (g) pinprick, (h) light touch, (i) stereognosis.

16.2 Finger and thumb movements (a) Testing flexor digitorum profundus and (b) superficialis. (c–e) Thumb movements: hold the patient's hand flat on the table and ask him/her to stretch the thumb (c) to the side (extension), (d) towards the ceiling (abduction) and then (e) across the palm to touch the little finger (opposition).

Testing for *flexor digitorum profundus* is straightforward: the PIP joint is immobilized and the patient is then asked to bend the tip of the finger.

To test *flexor digitorum superficialis,* the flexor profundus must first be inactivated, otherwise one cannot tell which of the two tendons is flexing the PIP joint. This is done by grasping all the fingers, except the one being examined, and holding them firmly in full extension; because the profundus tendons share a common muscle belly, this manoeuvre automatically prevents *all* the profundus tendons from participating in finger flexion. The patient is then asked to flex the isolated finger which is being examined; this movement must be activated by flexor digitorum superficialis. There are two exceptions to this rule: first, the little finger sometimes has no independent flexor digitorum superficialis; second, the index finger often has an entirely separate flexor profundus, which cannot be inactivated by the usual mass action manoeuvre. Instead, flexor superficialis is tested by asking the patient to pinch hard with the DIP joint in full extension and the PIP joint in full flexion; this position can be maintained only if the superficialis tendon is active and intact.

The *long extensors* are tested by asking the patient to extend the MCP joints. Inability to do this does not necessarily signify either paralysis or tendon rupture: the long extensor tendon may simply have slipped off the knuckle into the interdigital gutter (a common occurrence in rheumatoid arthritis).

MCP flexion and IP extension are activated by the *intrinsic muscles (lumbricals* and *interossei)*. Ask the patient to extend the fingers with the MCP joints flexed (the 'duckbill' position). The interossei also motivate finger abduction and adduction.

Thumb movements are somewhat confusing as they also involve the carpometacarpal (CMC) joint. With the hand lying flat, palm upwards, five types of movement are possible: *extension* (sideways movement in the plane of the palm); *flexion* (sideways movement towards the palm in the plane of the palm); *abduction* (upward movement at right angles to the palm); *adduction* (pressing downwards against the palm); and *opposition* (touching the tips of the fingers). Since the thumb has only a single IP joint, the *flexor pollicis longus* is tested by immobilizing the thumb MCP joint.

Grip strength

Grip strength is assessed (rather crudely) by asking the patient to squeeze the examiner's fingers; it may be diminished because of muscle weakness, tendon damage, finger stiffness or wrist instability. Strength can be measured more accurately with a mechanical dynamometer. Pinch grip also should be measured.

Neurological assessment

If symptoms such as numbness, tingling or weakness exist – and in all cases of trauma – a full neurological examination of the upper limbs should be carried out, testing power, reflexes and sensation. Further refinement is achieved by testing two-point discrimination, sensitivity to heat and cold and stereognosis.

CONGENITAL VARIATIONS

The hand and foot are much the most common sites of congenital deformities of the locomotor system; the incidence is about 1:1000 live births. Early recognition is important, and definitive treatment should be timed to fit in with the functional demands of the child. There are seven types of malformation.

Failure of formation

Total or partial absence of parts may be transverse ('congenital amputations') or axial (missing rays).

Failure of differentiation

Fingers may be partly or wholly joined together (syndactyly). This may be corrected by separating the fingers and repairing the defects with skin-grafts.

Duplication

Polydactyly (extra digits) is the most common hand malformation. The extra finger should be amputated, if only for cosmetic reasons.

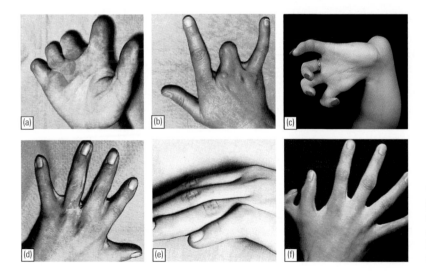

16.3 Congenital variations (a,b) Congenital absence of part or all of some digits. (c) Radial club-hand. (d) Syndactyly. (e) Camptodactyly. (f) Extra digits.

Undergrowth

The thumb can be very small or even absent.

Overgrowth

A giant finger is unsightly, but attempts at operative reduction are fraught with complications.

Constriction bands

These have the appearance of an elastic band constricting the finger. In the worst cases this may lead to amputation.

Generalized malformations

The hand may be involved in generalized disorders such as Marfan's syndrome ('spider hands') or achondroplasia ('trident hand').

ACUTE INFECTIONS OF THE HAND

Infection of the hand is frequently limited to one of several well-defined compartments: under the nailfold (paronychia); the pulp space (whitlow); subcutaneous tissues elsewhere; a tendon sheath; one of the deep fascial spaces or a joint. Almost invariably the cause is a *Staphylococcus* which has been implanted by trivial or unobserved injury.

Pathology

Acute inflammation and suppuration in small closed compartments (e.g. the pulp space or tendon sheath) may cause an increase in pressure to levels at which the local blood supply is threatened. In neglected cases tissue necrosis is an immanent risk. Even if this does not occur, the patient may end up with a stiff and useless hand unless the infection is rapidly brought under control.

Clinical features

Usually there is a history of trauma, but it may have been so trivial as to pass unnoticed. A thorn prick can be as dangerous as a cut. Within a day or two, the finger (or hand) becomes painful and tensely swollen. The patient may feel ill and feverish and the pain becomes throbbing. There is obvious redness and tension in the tissues, and exquisite tenderness over the site of infection. Finger movements may be markedly restricted.

Principles of treatment

Antibiotics

As soon as the diagnosis is made and specimens have been taken for microbiological investigation, antibiotic treatment is started – usually with

flucloxacillin and, in severe cases, with fusidic acid or a cephalosporin as well. This may later be changed when bacterial sensitivity is known.

Rest and elevation

In a mild case the hand is rested in a sling. In a severe case the arm is elevated in a roller towel while the patient is kept in hospital under observation. Analgesics are given for pain.

Drainage

If there are signs of an abscess (throbbing pain, marked tenderness and toxaemia), the pus should be drained. A tourniquet and either general or regional block anaesthesia are essential. The incision should be made at the site of maximal tenderness, *but never across a skin crease.* Necrotic tissue is excised and the area thoroughly washed and cleansed. The wound is either left open or lightly sutured and then covered with non-stick dressings. A pus specimen is sent for microbiological investigation.

Splintage

After draining tendon sheath or fascial space infections or, if conservative treatment is likely to be prolonged, a removable splint should be applied – *always with the joints in the position of safe immobilization,* that is with the wrist slightly extended, the MCP joints in full flexion, the IP joints extended and the thumb in abduction (see Fig. 16.5c).

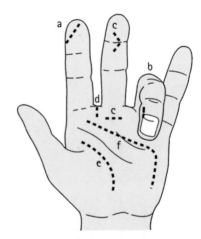

16.4 Incisions for infection The incisions for surgical drainage are illustrated here: (a) pulp space (directly over the abscess); (b) nailfold (it may also be necessary to excise the edge of the nail); (c) tendon sheath (two incisions, one distal and one proximal); (d) web space; (e) thenar space; (f) mid-palmar space.

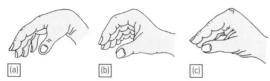

16.5 Three positions of the hand (a) The position of relaxation; (b) position of function (ready for action) and (c) position of safe immobilization (wrist slightly extended, metacarpophalangeal joints in flexion, interphalangeal joints extended and thumb in abduction). *If the hand has to be splinted, it should always be splinted in the position of safe immobilization, in which the ligaments are at their greatest length. This will reduce the likelihood of irreversible stiffness.*

Physiotherapy

Once the acute inflammation subsides, movements are encouraged. Ideally this should be done under the direction of a physiotherapist specialized in 'hand therapy'. The splint is reapplied between exercise sessions.

SPECIFIC TYPES OF INFECTION

Paronychia

Infection under the nailfold is common. The area is swollen, red and tender. At the first sign of infection, antibiotic treatment alone may be effective. If pus is present, it can often be released simply by lifting the nailfold from the nail; otherwise the nailfold must be incised. Occasionally a portion of the nail needs to be removed.

Pulp-space infection (felon)

Pulp-space infection (usually due to a prick or splinter) causes throbbing pain. The fingertip is swollen, red and acutely tender. Antibiotic treatment is started immediately. However, if pus has formed, it must be released through a small incision over the site of maximal tenderness.

Other subcutaneous infections

Anywhere in the hand, a blister or superficial cut may become infected, causing redness, swelling and tenderness. A local collection of pus should be drained through a small incision over the site of maximal tenderness. It is important to exclude a deeper pocket of pus in a nearby tendon sheath or in one of the deep fascial spaces.

Tendon-sheath infection

Suppurative tenosynovitis is uncommon but dangerous. Unless treatment is swift and effective, there is a risk of tendon necrosis and the patient may end up with a useless finger.

The affected digit is painful and swollen; it is held bent, is very tender, and the patient will not move it or permit it to be moved.

Treatment

Treatment must be started as soon as the diagnosis is suspected. The hand is splinted and elevated and antibiotics are administered intravenously – initially a broad-spectrum penicillin or a systemic cephalosporin, to be modified if necessary once the organism has been cultured and tested for antibiotic sensitivity. If there is no improvement

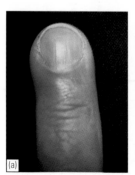
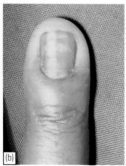
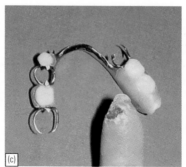
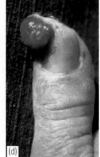

16.6 Fingertip infections (a) Acute nailfold infection (paronychia). (b) Chronic paronychia; (c) Pulp-space infection due to a prick injury on the patient's own denture. (d) Septic granuloma.

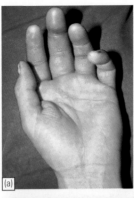
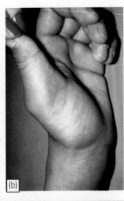
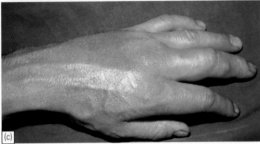

16.7 Tendon-sheath infections (a) Flexor tenosynovitis of the middle finger following a cortisone injection.
(b) Tuberculous synovitis of flexor pollicis longus. (c) Septic extensor tenosynovitis.

after 24 hours, surgical drainage is essential. Two incisions are needed, one at the proximal end of the sheath and one at the distal end; using a fine catheter, the sheath is then irrigated with saline or Ringer's lactate solution (always from proximal to distal). The catheter is left in place for postoperative irrigation during the next 2 days.

Tendon-sheath infection in the thumb or little finger may spread proximally to the synovial bursa. This has to be drained through a further incision just above the wrist.

At the end of the operation, the hand is swathed in absorbent dressings and splinted in the position of safe immobilization.

Deep fascial space infection

Infection from a web space or from an infected tendon sheath may spread to either of the deep fascial spaces of the palm. The palm is ballooned, so its normal concavity is lost. There is extensive tenderness and the whole hand is held still.

For drainage, an incision is made directly over the abscess and sinus forceps inserted; if the web space is also infected, it too should be incised. Postoperatively the hand is dressed and splinted as described above.

Joint infection

Any of the joints may be infected, either directly by a penetrating injury on injection, or indirectly from adjacent structures. At the onset, the clinical features may be hard to distinguish from those of acute gout. Joint aspiration will provide the answer.

Intravenous antibiotics are administered and the hand is splinted. If symptoms and signs do not improve within 24 hours, open drainage is needed.

Bites

Animal bites are usually inflicted by cats, dogs or farm animals. Many become infected and, although the common pathogens are staphylococci and streptococci, unusual organisms are also encountered.

Human bites and lacerations sustained during fist-fights are generally thought to be even more prone to infection. A variety of organisms (including anaerobes) are encountered, the commonest being *Staphylococcus aureus, Streptococcus group A* and *Eikenella corrodens*. All such wounds should be assumed to be infected. X-rays should be obtained, to exclude a fracture or foreign body.

Treatment

Fresh wounds should be carefully examined in the operating theatre. Swab samples are taken for bacterial culture and sensitivity. If necessary, the wound should be extended and debrided; search for a fragment of tooth or a divit of articular cartilage from the joint. The hand is then splinted and elevated and antibiotics are given prophylactically until the laboratory results are obtained.

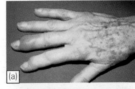
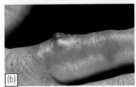
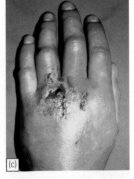

16.8 Joint infections (a) Septic arthritis of the terminal interphalangeal joint following a cortisone injection.
(b) Infected insect bite. (c) Septic human bite resulting in acute infection of the fourth metacarpophalangeal joint.

Infected bites will need debridement, wash-outs and intravenous antibiotic treatment. The common infecting organisms are all sensitive to broad-spectrum penicillins and cephalosporins. With animal bites one should also consider the possibility of rabies.

Postoperative treatment consists, as usual, of copious wound dressings, splintage in the 'safe' position and encouragement of movement once the infection has resolved. Tendon lacerations can be dealt with when the tissues are completely healed.

 Bites are considered to be infected until proved otherwise.

RHEUMATOID ARTHRITIS

The hand, more than any other part of the body, is where rheumatoid arthritis carves its story. Early on, there is synovitis of the proximal joints and tendon sheaths; later, joint and tendon erosions prepare the ground for mechanical derangement; in the final stage, joint instability and tendon rupture cause progressive deformity and loss of function.

Clinical features

Pain and stiffness of the fingers are early symptoms; often the wrist also is affected. Examination may show swelling of the MCP and PIP joints; both hands are affected, more or less symmetrically. Joint mobility and grip strength are diminished.

As the disease progresses, deformities begin to appear (and are increasingly difficult to correct). In the late stage one sees the characteristic ulnar deviation of the fingers and subluxation of the MCP joints, often associated with swan-neck or

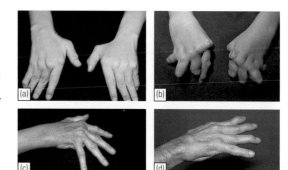

16.9 Rheumatoid arthritis (a) Typical deformities in established rheumatoid arthritis. The proximal joints are the ones most severely affected; there is subluxation of the metacarpophalangeal joints and the fingers are deviated ulnarwards. (b) Severe rheumatoid deformities with dislocation of the metacarpophalangeal joints and ulceration of the skin over the knuckles. (c) 'Dropped fingers' due to rupture of extensor tendons where they cross the back of the wrist. (d) Swan-neck deformities of the fingers.

boutonnière deformities. When these abnormalities become fixed, functional loss may be so severe that the patient needs help with washing, dressing and feeding.

X-rays

During the initial stages, x-rays show only soft-tissue swelling and osteoporosis around the joints. Later there is narrowing of the joint spaces and small periarticular erosions appear. In the last stage, articular destruction may be marked, with joint deformity and dislocation.

Treatment

In early cases, treatment is directed at controlling the systemic disease and the local synovitis. In addition to general measures, splints may reduce pain and swelling and improve mobility.

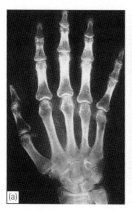
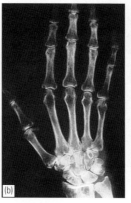
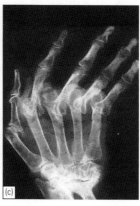

16.10 Rheumatoid arthritis – x-ray changes (a) Early on, the x-rays may show no more than soft-tissue swelling and juxta-articular osteoporosis. (b) A later stage showing characteristic punched-out juxta-articular erosions at the second and third metacarpophalangeal joints. The wrist is now also involved. (c) In the most advanced stage, the metacarpophalangeal joints are dislocated and the hand is severely deformed.

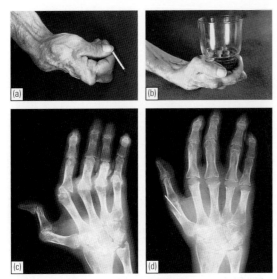

16.11 Rheumatoid arthritis – treatment (a,b) Even with severe deformities, the patient may regain good function. Why interfere if the disease is quiescent and the hand works well? (c,d) If function is markedly restricted, reconstructive surgery has a useful role. X-rays before and after metacarpophalangeal joint replacement with Silastic spacers and fusion of the thumb metacarpophalangeal joint.

Persistent synovitis may benefit from local injections of methylprednisolone, but sometimes surgical synovectomy is needed.

As the disease progresses, it becomes increasingly important to prevent deformity. Uncontrolled synovitis requires synovectomy followed by physiotherapy. Isolated tendon ruptures are repaired or bypassed by appropriate tendon transfers. Joint instability may require stabilization or arthroplasty.

In late cases with established deformities, reconstructive surgery may be needed, but treatment should be directed at restoring function rather than merely correcting deformity.

OSTEOARTHRITIS

Osteoarthritis of the DIP joints is very common in postmenopausal women and is usually a manifestation of polyarticular osteoarthritis. It often starts with pain in one or two fingers; the distal joints become swollen and tender, the condition usually spreading to all the fingers of both hands. On examination, there is bony thickening around the DIP joints (Heberden's nodes) and some restriction of movement. Not infrequently, some of the PIP joints are involved (Bouchard's nodes) and the CMC joint of the thumb may show similar changes.

The distinction from rheumatoid arthritis is very important. In both conditions, the finger joints are swollen and stiff. However, whereas rheumatoid arthritis affects the proximal joints (particularly the MCP joints), osteoarthritis affects mainly the terminal IP joints.

Treatment is symptomatic; pain and tenderness gradually subside and the patient is left with painless, knobbly fingers. Occasionally (if pain or deformity is particularly marked), fusion of the IP joint may be called for.

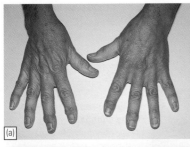

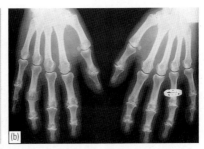

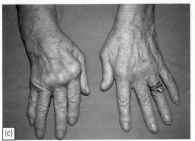

16.12 Osteoarthritis (a,b) Osteoarthritis affects mainly the distal interphalangeal joints. The knobbly joints are called Heberden's nodes. (c) Rheumatoid arthritis can look similar, but here it is mainly the proximal joints that are affected.

ACQUIRED DEFORMITIES

Deformity of the hand may be due to disorders of the skin, subcutaneous tissues, muscles, tendons, joints, bones or neuromuscular function.

SKIN CONTRACTURE

Cuts and burns of the palmar skin are liable to heal with contracture; this may cause puckering of the palm or fixed flexion of the fingers. Surgical incisions should never cross flexor creases. Established contractures may require excision of the scar and Z-plasty of the overlying skin.

DUPUYTREN'S CONTRACTURE

This is a nodular hypertrophy and contracture of the palmar aponeurosis. The condition is familial, but there is a higher than usual incidence in patients with diabetes and acquired immunodeficiency syndrome (AIDS) and in people with epilepsy receiving phenytoin therapy. Smoking and heavy alcohol consumption are also risk factors.

Clinical features

The patient – usually a middle-aged man – complains of a nodular thickening in the palm. Gradually this progresses distally to involve the ring or little finger. Pain is unusual. Often both hands are involved, one more than the other. The palm is puckered, nodular and thick. If the subcutaneous cords extend into the fingers, they may produce flexion deformities at the MCP and PIP joints. Sometimes the dorsal knuckle pads are thickened.

Similar nodules may be seen on the soles of the feet. There is a rare, curious association with fibrosis of the corpus cavernosum (*Peyronie's disease*).

Diagnosis

Dupuytren's contracture must be distinguished from skin contracture (where a previous laceration is usually obvious) and tendon contracture (where the 'cord' moves on passive flexion of the finger).

Treatment

Operation is indicated if the deformity is progressive and interferes with function. By careful dissection, the thickened part of the aponeurosis is excised. A Z-plasty or skin-graft may be needed to permit adequate skin closure. Postoperative splintage and physiotherapy are rewarded by the restoration of painless hand function.

NEUROMUSCULAR DISORDERS

Ulnar claw-hand

The characteristic deformity following an ulnar nerve lesion is hyperextension of the MCP joints and flexion of the IP joints (see Chapter 11). This is due to paralysis of the intrinsic muscles which normally activate flexion at the MCP joints and extension at the IP joints. Thus the deformity is sometimes called *intrinsic minus*.

Shortening of the intrinsic muscles

Intrinsic muscle shortening produces a characteristic deformity: flexion at the MCP joints with extension of the IP joints and adduction of the thumb. Anatomically speaking, this is the opposite of an intrinsic minus deformity and, not surprisingly, is referred to as *intrinsic plus*. The

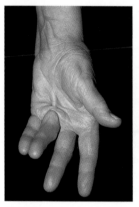
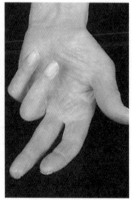

16.13 Dupuytren's contracture (a) Moderately severe contracture of the fourth finger. (b) Severe contractures affecting the interphalangeal joints as well.

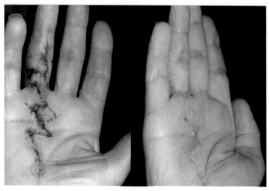

16.14 Z-plasty Z-plasty in the hand shortly after operation, and several months later when healing is almost complete.

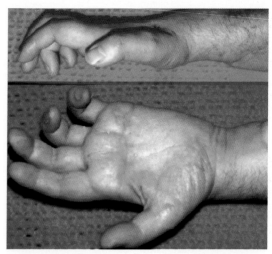

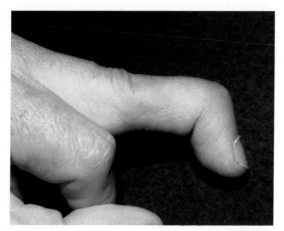

16.17 'Mallet' finger Disruption of the distal attachment of the finger extensor mechanism causes the distal phalanx to 'drop'.

16.15 Ulnar claw-hand This typical deformity followed a low ulnar nerve injury.

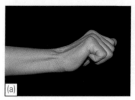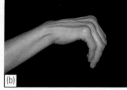

(a)　(b)

16.16 Contracture of the long flexors (a) When the wrist is extended, the fingers involuntarily curl into tight flexion. (b) When the wrist is flexed, tension on the long flexor muscles is relaxed and the fingers can uncurl to a certain extent.

main causes are spasticity (e.g. in cerebral palsy) and scarring (after trauma or infection). Moderate contracture can be treated by releasing the intrinsic muscles where they cross the MCP joints.

Ischaemic contracture of the forearm muscles

This follows circulatory insufficiency due to injuries at or below the elbow (Volkmann's ischaemic contracture: see page 300). There is shortening of the long flexors; the fingers are held in flexion and can be straightened only when the wrist is flexed. Sometimes the picture is complicated by associated damage to the ulnar or median nerve (or both). If disability is marked, some improvement may be obtained by releasing the shortened muscles at their origin above the elbow, or else by excising the dead muscles and restoring finger movement with tendon transfers.

TENDON LESIONS

'Mallet' finger ('baseball' finger)

This results from injury to the extensor tendon of the terminal phalanx. The patient cannot actively straighten the terminal joint, but passive movement is normal. The DIP joint should be splinted for 8 weeks, with the proximal joint free (see page 338).

Ruptured extensor pollicis longus

The long thumb extensor may rupture after fraying where it crosses the wrist (e.g. after a Colles' fracture, or in rheumatoid arthritis). Direct repair is unsatisfactory and a tendon transfer, using the extensor indicis, is needed.

Dropped finger

The patient finds that he or she is suddenly unable to hold the finger in extension at the MCP joint (see Fig. 16.9c). The cause usually lies not at the MCP joint but at the wrist, where one of the extensor tendons has ruptured (e.g. in rheumatoid arthritis). If direct repair is not possible, the distal portion of the tendon can be attached to an adjacent finger extensor.

Boutonnière

This is a flexion deformity of the PIP joint, due to interruption of the central slip of the extensor tendon. The lateral slips separate and the head of the proximal phalanx pops through the gap like a finger through a buttonhole. It is seen after trauma or in rheumatoid disease. Post-traumatic rupture can sometimes be repaired; the chronic deformity in rheumatoid disease usually defies correction.

Swan-neck deformity

This is the reverse of boutonnière: the PIP joint is hyperextended and the DIP joint flexed (Fig.

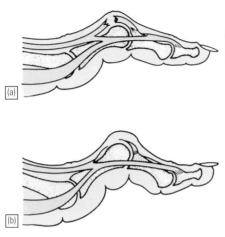

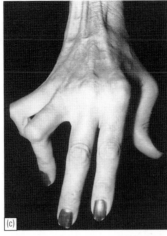

16.18 Boutonnière deformity
(a) When the middle slip of the extensor tendon ruptures it becomes difficult or impossible to extend the proximal interphalangeal joint. If it is not repaired (b), the lateral slips slide towards the volar surface, the knuckle pops through the 'buttonhole' in the extensor hood and the distal joint is drawn into hyperextension. (c) The same deformity is sometimes seen in rheumatoid arthritis.

16.9d). It is due to imbalance of extensor *versus* flexor action in the finger, and is often seen in rheumatoid arthritis. The deformity may be corrected by tendon rebalancing and joint stabilization.

'TRIGGER FINGER'

This common condition presents as an intermittent 'deformity', usually of the ring or middle finger, sometimes of the thumb. The patient complains that, when the hand is clenched and then opened, the finger (or thumb) gets stuck in flexion; with a little more effort, it suddenly snaps into full extension. The usual cause is thickening of the fibrous tendon sheath: the flexor tendon becomes temporarily trapped at the entrance to its sheath and then, on forced extension, it passes the constriction with a snap. A similar entrapment may occur due to a bulky tenosynovitis (e.g. in rheumatic disorders). A tender nodule or thickened tendon can usually be felt at the distal palmar crease.

Treatment

The condition often improves spontaneously, so there is no urgency about treatment. However, if it persists, or is particularly annoying, it can usually be cured by an injection of corticosteroid carefully placed at the entrance of the tendon sheath. Refractory cases need operation: the fibrous sheath is incised, allowing the tendon to move freely. In the case of the thumb, take particular care to avoid injuring the digital nerve, which runs close to the sheath.

Infantile trigger thumb

Parents sometimes seek help for a baby with a 'snapping thumb'. More often than not, the condition goes undiagnosed or is wrongly diagnosed as a 'dislocating thumb'; occasionally the child grows up with the thumb permanently bent or the distal phalanx underdeveloped. Feel for the tell-tale thickening on the palmar aspect at the base of the thumb – tenovaginitis of the tiny flexor sheath. Treatment (as above) can be deferred until the child is a year old, as spontaneous recovery is quite common.

BONE LESIONS

Malunited fractures may cause metacarpal or phalangeal deformity. Occasionally this needs correction by osteotomy and internal fixation.

CHAPTER 17

THE NECK

CLINICAL ASSESSMENT

HISTORY

The common symptoms of neck disorder are pain and stiffness.

Pain is felt in the neck itself, but it may also be referred to the shoulders or arms. It may start suddenly (as with an acute intervertebral disc prolapse) or gradually (as in chronic disc degeneration).

Stiffness may be either intermittent or continuous. Sometimes it is so severe that the patient can scarcely move the head.

Deformity usually appears as a wry neck; occasionally the neck is fixed in flexion.

Numbness, tingling and weakness in the upper limbs may be due to pressure on a nerve root; weakness in the lower limbs may result from cord compression in the neck.

Headache sometimes emanates from the neck, but if this is the only symptom, other causes should be suspected.

EXAMINATION

The entire upper trunk and both upper limbs should be exposed. Start the examination with the patient standing: neck posture and movements are most easily observed in this position. The shoulders also are examined while the patient is upright. The anterior structures (trachea, thyroid, oesophagus) are best felt with the patient seated and the examiner standing behind the chair. The third part of the examination is carried out with the patient lying down; it is easier (and more reliable) to feel for muscle spasm and point tenderness with the patient lying prone with his or her neck supported over a pillow. Neurological examination also is performed with the patient lying supine.

Look

Any deformity is noted. From the back, skin blemishes, scapular abnormalities or muscular asymmetry can be seen. One shoulder may be higher and there may be muscle wasting in the arm or hand.

Feel

The neck and shoulders should be carefully palpated for tender areas, lumps and muscle spasm.

Move

Flexion, extension, lateral flexion and rotation are tested and the range of movements noted. Shoulder movements, likewise, should be recorded.

Neurological examination

Neurological examination of the upper limbs is mandatory in all cases; in some, the lower limbs also should be examined. Muscle power, reflexes and sensation should be carefully tested; even small degrees of abnormality may be significant.

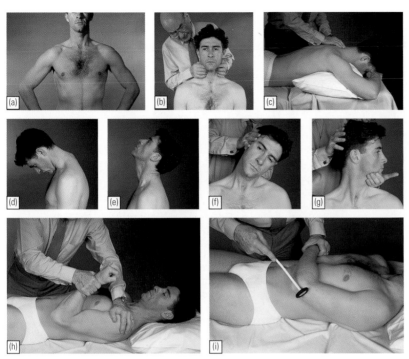

17.1 Examination (a) Look for any deformity or superficial blemish which might suggest a disorder affecting the cervical spine. (b) The front of the neck is felt with the patient seated and the examiner standing behind him. (c) The back of the neck is most easily and reliably felt with the patient lying prone over a pillow; this way muscle spasm is reduced and the neck is relaxed. (d–g) Movement: flexion ('chin on chest'); extension ('look up at the ceiling'); lateral flexion ('tilt your ear towards your shoulder'); and rotation ('look over your shoulder'). (h,i) Neurological examination is mandatory.

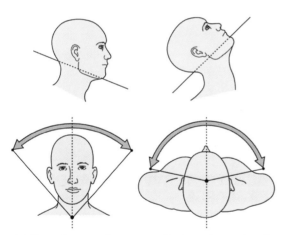

17.2 Normal range of movement Flexion and extension of the neck are best gauged by observing the angle of the occipitomental line – an imaginary line joining the tip of the chin and the occipital protuberance. In full flexion, the chin normally touches the chest; in full extension, the occipitomental line forms an angle of at least 45 degrees with the horizontal, and more than 60 degrees in young people. Lateral flexion is usually achieved up to 45 degrees and rotation to 80 degrees each way.

IMAGING

X-ray examination should include all levels from the base of the occiput to T1. The anteroposterior view should show the regular, undulating outline of the lateral masses; their symmetry may be disturbed by destructive lesions or fractures. A projection through the mouth is required to show the upper two vertebrae. In the lateral view, the disc spaces are inspected; disc-space narrowing and 'osteophyte' formation at the anterior and posterior edges of the vertebral bodies are features of intervertebral disc degeneration. Flexion and extension views are required to demonstrate instability.

CT and *MRI* are essential for defining the intervertebral discs, the neural structures and the outlines of the spinal canal and intervertebral foramina.

DEFORMITIES OF THE NECK

TORTICOLLIS ('WRY NECK', 'SKEW NECK')

In torticollis the chin is twisted upwards and towards one side. It may be either *congenital* or *secondary* to other local disorders.

Infantile (congenital) torticollis

Skew neck is sometimes seen in an infant or very young child. The sternomastoid muscle on one side is fibrous and fails to elongate as the child grows. In some cases, a well-defined lump is felt in the muscle during the first few weeks of life, but deformity may not become apparent until the

179

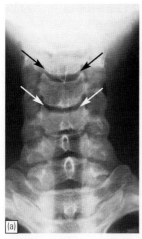

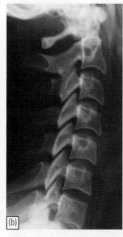

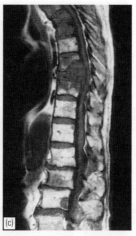

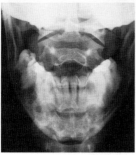

17.3 Imaging (a) Anteroposterior x-ray – note the smooth, symmetrical outlines and the clear, wide unco-vertebral joints (arrows). (b) Lateral view – showing all seven cervical vertebrae. (c) Open-mouth view – to show the odontoid process and atlantoaxial joints. (d) MRI of the lower cervical and upper thoracic spine, showing metastatic deposits (dark grey areas) in several vertebral bodies. The large tumour at T2/3 is encroaching perilously on the spinal canal.

child is 2 or 3 years old. As the neck grows, the contracted sternomastoid tethers the skull on one side, thus twisting the chin towards the opposite side. Secondary facial deformities may occur.

Treatment

If a child has a sternomastoid 'tumour', subsequent deformity may be prevented by gentle, daily manipulation of the neck. In established cases, the sternomastoid can be divided or elongated.

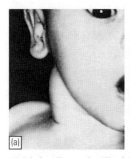

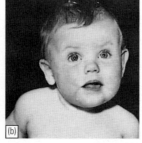

17.4 Infantile torticollis (a) A small lump or 'tumour' may be felt in the sternomastoid muscle. (b) The baby develops a wry-neck deformity, sometimes associated with facial hemi-atrophy.

Secondary torticollis

Wry neck, due to muscle spasm, may develop as a result of acute disc prolapse (the most common cause in adults), inflamed neck glands, vertebral infection, injuries of the cervical spine or ocular disorders.

ACUTE INTERVERTEBRAL DISC PROLAPSE

Cervical disc prolapse may be precipitated by local strain or injury, especially sudden unguarded flexion and rotation. In many cases (perhaps in all) there is a predisposing abnormality of the disc with increased nuclear tension.

The disc protrusion may press on: (1) the posterior longitudinal ligament, causing neck pain and stiffness; and (2) the nerve roots, causing pain and paraesthesia in one or both arms. Prolapse usually occurs immediately above or below the sixth cervical vertebra, so the commonly affected nerve root is C6 or C7.

Clinical features

The original attack may occasionally be related to a definite and severe strain. Subsequent attacks may be sudden or gradual in onset, and with trivial cause. The patient may complain of: (1) pain and stiffness of the neck, the pain often radiating to the scapular region and sometimes to the occiput; (2) pain and paraesthesia in one upper limb (rarely both), often radiating to the outer elbow, back of the wrist and to the index and middle fingers. Weakness is rare. Between attacks the patient feels well, although the neck may feel a bit stiff.

The neck may be tilted forwards and sideways. The muscles are tender and movements are restricted. The arms should be examined for neurological signs suggestive of nerve root irritation or compression.

Imaging

X-rays may show narrowing of the disc space. However, the diagnosis should be confirmed by MRI.

Differential diagnosis

Acute cervical disc prolapse should be differentiated from the following.

Acute soft-tissue strain

Acute strains of the neck can cause pain and stiffness which may last for weeks or months. The absence of neurological symptoms and signs is significant.

Neuralgic amyotrophy (acute brachial neuritis)

Pain is sudden and severe, and situated over the shoulder, or the back of the shoulder, rather than in the neck itself. Multiple neurological levels are affected. Look for signs of serratus anterior weakness (winging of the scapula).

Cervical spine infections

Pain is unrelenting and local spasm severe. X-rays show erosion of the vertebral end-plates.

Cervical tumours

Neurological signs are progressive and x-rays or MRI may show bone destruction.

Treatment

Heat and analgesics are soothing but, as with lumbar disc prolapse, there are only three satisfactory ways of treating the prolapse itself.

Rest

A collar will prevent unguarded movement; it may be made of felt, sponge-rubber or polythene.

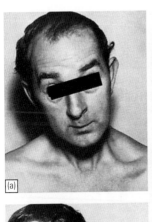
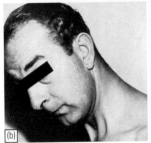
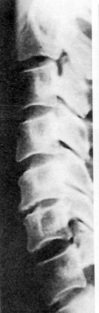
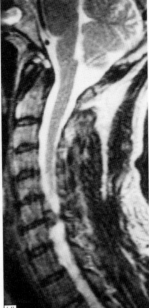
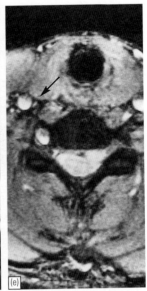

17.5 Acute disc prolapse (a,b) Acute wry neck due to a prolapsed disc. (c) The intervertebral disc space at C5/6 is reduced. (d,e) MRI in another case showing a large disc prolapse at C6/7.

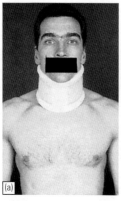
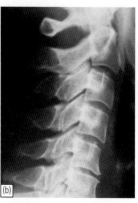

17.6 Cervical disc prolapse – treatment (a) For acute symptoms, rest in a polythene collar is often helpful. (b) Operative treatment usually consists of anterior discectomy and fusion of the affected segment.

Reduce

Traction may enlarge the disc space, permitting the prolapse to subside. The head of the couch is raised and weights (up to 8 kg) are tied to a harness fitting under the chin and occiput. Traction is applied intermittently for no more than 30 minutes at a time.

Remove

If symptoms are refractory and severe enough, the disc may be removed through an anterior approach; bone-grafts are inserted to fuse the affected area and to restore the normal intervertebral height. Nowadays the operation can also be performed using endoscopic techniques.

CHRONIC DISC DEGENERATION (CERVICAL SPONDYLOSIS)

Intervertebral disc degeneration is common from middle age onwards, even in people who have not been aware of any acute episode in former years. With time, the discs collapse and flatten, and bony spurs appear at the anterior and posterior margins of the vertebral bodies on either side of the affected discs; those that develop posteriorly may encroach upon the intervertebral foramina, causing pressure on the nerve roots. Several levels may be affected and the condition is then usually referred to as *spondylosis*. The condition is not always symptomatic, and many people go throughout life without experiencing anything more than slight stiffness.

Clinical features

Troublesome symptoms come on gradually. The patient, usually aged over 40, complains of neck pain and stiffness. The pain may radiate widely: to the occiput, the scapular muscles and down one or both arms. Paraesthesia, weakness and clumsiness are occasional symptoms. Typically there are exacerbations of more acute discomfort, and long periods of relative quiescence.

The appearance is usually normal. There may be tenderness in the soft tissues at the back of the neck and above the scapulae; neck movements are limited and painful at the extremes.

Careful neurological examination may show abnormal signs in one or both upper limbs.

X-rays

Typical x-ray features are narrowing of several disc spaces, bony spur formation at the anterior and posterior edges of the vertebral bodies and (in the anteroposterior view) osteoarthritic changes in the tiny unco-vertebral joints. Oblique views may show bony encroachment on the intervertebral foramina.

Differential diagnosis

Other disorders associated with neck or arm pain and sensory symptoms must be excluded. Cervical vertebral spur formation is very common in older people and this can be misleading in patients with other disorders.

Rotator cuff lesions

Pain around the shoulder may resemble the referred pain of cervical spondylosis. However, features such as rotator cuff tenderness and restricted shoulder movements should suggest a local problem.

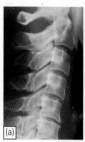
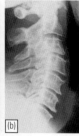
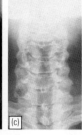

17.7 Cervical spondylosis – x-rays (a) Lateral x-ray showing disc narrowing and lipping of the anterior and posterior vertebral margins at C5/6. (b) A more advanced case. Spur formation is seen at several levels. (c) The anteroposterior view shows marked narrowing, and even obliteration, of the unco-vertebral joints (compare with Figure 17.3a).

Nerve entrapment syndromes

Median or ulnar nerve entrapment may give rise to intermittent symptoms of pain and paraesthesia in the hand. Characteristically, the symptoms are worse at night or are related to posture. In doubtful cases, nerve conduction studies and electromyography will help to establish the diagnosis. Remember, though, that the patient may have symptoms from both a peripheral and a central abnormality.

Cervical tumours

With tumours of the vertebrae, spinal cord, nerve roots or lymph nodes, the symptoms are unremitting. Imaging studies should reveal the diagnosis.

Treatment

During painful episodes, heat and massage are soothing; some patients benefit from a period in a restraining collar. Physiotherapy is the mainstay of treatment, patients usually being maintained in relative comfort by various measures including exercises, gentle passive manipulation and intermittent traction.

Operation is seldom indicated, but if severe symptoms are relieved only by a rigid and irksome support, anterior disc removal and fusion of the most painful level may be considered.

INFECTIONS

Pyogenic infection (usually staphylococcal) is uncommon and tuberculous infection rare. In both, destructive changes usually involve the intervertebral disc spaces and the neighbouring vertebrae. Later, pus may spread to form a retropharyngeal abscess, or into the spinal canal where it may compress the cord. Rest and

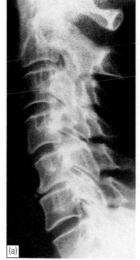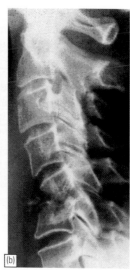

17.8 Pyogenic infection (a) The first x-ray, taken soon after the onset of symptoms, shows narrowing of the C5/6 disc space. (b) Three weeks later there is dramatic destruction and collapse of the adjacent vertebral bodies.

appropriate antibiotics are essential. Abscesses may need drainage and the spinal cord may need to be decompressed; this may be combined with fusion, though with pyogenic infection spontaneous fusion is usual.

RHEUMATOID ARTHRITIS

The cervical spine is severely affected in 30 per cent of patients with rheumatoid arthritis. Three types of lesion are common: (1) erosion of the atlantoaxial joints and the transverse ligament, with resulting instability; (2) erosion of the atlanto-occipital articulations, allowing the odontoid peg to ride up into the foramen

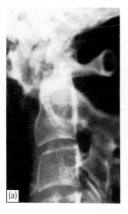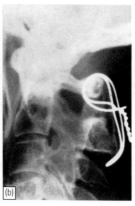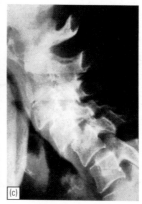

17.9 Rheumatoid arthritis
(a) Atlantoaxial subluxation is common; erosion of the joints and the transverse ligament has allowed the atlas to slip forward about 2 cm. (b) Reduction and posterior fusion with wire fixation. (c) In this case there is subluxation both at the atlantoaxial joint and in the mid-cervical region.

magnum; and (3) erosion of the facet joints in the mid-cervical region, sometimes ending in fusion but more often leading to subluxation.

The patient is usually a woman with advanced rheumatoid arthritis. She has neck pain, and movements are markedly restricted. Symptoms and signs of root compression may be present in the upper limbs; less often, there is lower limb weakness and upper motor neuron signs due to cord compression.

X-rays show an erosive arthritis, usually at several levels. Flexion and extension views may reveal subluxation at the atlantoaxial joint or in the mid-cervical region.

Treatment

Despite the startling x-ray appearances, serious complications are uncommon. Pain can usually be relieved by wearing a collar. Only if it is persistent and severe, or associated with increasing neurological deficit, is posterior spinal fusion advised.

CHAPTER 18

THE BACK

CLINICAL ASSESSMENT

HISTORY

The usual symptoms of back disorders are pain, stiffness and deformity in the back, and pain, paraesthesia or weakness in the legs. The mode of onset is very important: did it start suddenly (perhaps after lifting) or gradually? Are the symptoms constant, or are there periods of remission? Are they related to any particular posture?

Pain may be felt in the back, usually low down and on either side of the midline, or extending into the buttock and down the limb. Pain felt in the thigh and calf, though called sciatica, is rarely due to sciatic nerve disorder. It is referred pain, either from the dural sleeve of a lumbar or sacral nerve root or from an abnormal vertebral joint; pain referred from the root dura is characteristically more intense and often accompanied by numbness or paraesthesia, whilst pain referred from a joint or ligament is more inconstant and is not accompanied by neurological symptoms – but both are distributed more or less along the path of the sciatic nerve.

 'Sciatica' alone is non-specific. Sciatica plus neurological symptoms suggests nerve root compression.

Stiffness may be sudden and almost complete (after a disc prolapse) or continuous and predictably worse in the mornings (suggesting arthritis or ankylosing spondylitis).

Deformity is usually noticed by others, but the patient may become aware of shoulder asymmetry or of clothes not fitting well. In disc prolapse, arthritis and ankylosing spondylitis, deformity is usually secondary to, and overshadowed by, pain and stiffness. In structural disorders, such as scoliosis, it may be the only complaint.

Numbness or *paraesthesia* is felt anywhere in the lower limb, but can usually be mapped fairly accurately over one of the dermatomes. It is important to ask if it is aggravated by standing upright or walking and relieved by bending forward or sitting down – a classic feature of spinal stenosis.

Other symptoms important in back disorders are *urethral discharge, diarrhoea* and *sore eyes;* these are features of Reiter's disease, one of the causes of 'reactive' spondylitis.

SIGNS WITH THE PATIENT STANDING

Adequate exposure is essential; patients must strip to their underclothes.

Look

Begin by standing face to face with the patient and note his or her general physique and posture. Then move round and stand behind the patient. Does he or she stand upright or lean over to one side? Is the pelvis level, or is one leg shorter than the other? Does the spine look straight or curved *(scoliosis)*?

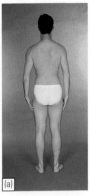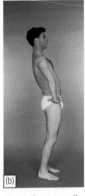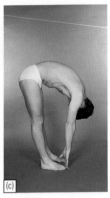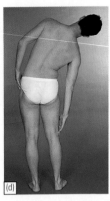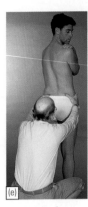

(a) (b) (c) (d) (e)

18.1 Examination With the patient standing upright (a), look at his general posture and note particularly the presence of any asymmetry or frank deformity of the spine. Then ask him to lean backwards (extension) (b), forwards to touch his toes (flexion) (c) and then sideways as far as possible (d), comparing his level of reach on the two sides. Finally, hold the pelvis stable and ask the patient to twist first to one side and then to the other (rotation). Note that rotation occurs almost entirely in the thoracic spine (e) and not in the lumbar spine.

Are there scars or other skin markings that may suggest a spinal disorder?

Seen from the side, the thoracic spine normally has a gentle forward curve or *kyphosis*. An unduly obvious kyphosis is sometimes called *hyperkyphosis;* if it is sharply angulated, the prominence is called a *kyphos.*

By contrast, the lumbar spine is normally bent slightly backwards *(lordosis).* In some conditions it may be unusually flat or excessively lordosed.

Feel

The spinous processes and the interspinous ligaments are palpated, noting any prominence or a 'step'.

Move

Flexion

Ask the patient to bend forward and try to touch the floor. Even with a stiff back, he or she may be able to do this by flexing the hips, so watch the lumbar spine to see if it really moves or, better still, measure the spinal excursion (see Fig. 18.2). The mode of flexion is also important: hesitant movements, especially on regaining the upright position, may signify pain or segmental instability.

Extension

Ask the patient to lean backwards; with a stiff spine, he or she may cheat by bending the knees. The 'wall test' will unmask a disguised loss of extension: standing with the back flush against a wall, the heels, buttocks, shoulders and occiput normally all make contact with the surface.

Lateral flexion

Ask the patient to bend first to one side and then to the other; compare the range of movement to right and left.

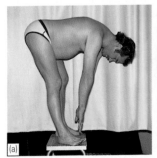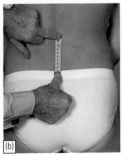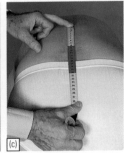

(a) (b) (c)

18.2 Measuring the range of flexion Bending down and touching the toes may look like lumbar flexion but this is not always the case. The patient in (a) has ankylosing spondylitis and a rigid lumbar spine, but he is able to reach his toes because he has good flexibility at the hips. Compare his flat back with the rounded back of the model in Figure 18.1c. You can measure the lumbar excursion. With the patient upright, select two bony points 10 cm apart and mark the skin (b); as the patient bends forward, the two points should separate by at least a further 5 cm (c).

Rotation

Ask the patient to twist the trunk to each side in turn while the pelvis is anchored by the examiner's hands; this is essentially a thoracic movement and should not be limited in lumbosacral disease.

Chest expansion

Rib excursion is assessed by measuring the chest circumference in full expiration and then full inspiration; the normal excursion is about 7 cm.

Muscle power

Distal muscle power is conveniently tested and compared by asking the patient to stand up on tiptoes (plantar flexion) and then to rock back on the heels (dorsiflexion); small differences between the two sides are easily spotted.

SIGNS WITH THE PATIENT PRONE

Bony outlines and small lumps can be felt more easily with the patient lying face down.

Deep tenderness is easy to localize, but difficult to ascribe to a particular structure.

Some neurological features are ideally elicited with the patient lying prone. *Hamstring power* is tested by having the patient flex the knee against resistance. The *femoral stretch test* is performed by bending the patient's knee with his or her hip flat against the couch; a positive sign is pain felt in the front of the thigh and the back, suggesting lumbar root tension.

Popliteal and posterior tibial pulses are conveniently felt in this position.

SIGNS WITH THE PATIENT SUPINE

The patient is observed for pain and stiffness while turning over. Hip and knee mobility are examined before testing for cord or nerve root involvement. Also check the femoral and pedal pulses.

The straight-leg raising test

This is the classic test for lumbosacral root tension. With the knee held absolutely straight, the leg is lifted from the couch until the patient experiences pain – not merely in the thigh (which is common and not significant), but in the buttock and back. The angle at which this occurs is noted; normally it should be possible to raise the leg to 90 degrees without causing undue discomfort. At this point, an additional stretch is imposed by passively dorsiflexing the foot. This may cause an additional stab of pain. If the knee is then slightly flexed, buttock pain is suddenly relieved; pain may then be re-induced by simply pressing on the common peroneal nerve behind the knee, to tighten it like a bowstring. Sometimes straight-leg raising on the unaffected side produces pain on the affected side. This 'crossed sciatic tension' is indicative of severe root tension, usually due to a prolapsed disc.

Neurological examination

A full neurological examination of the lower limbs is essential in every patient with a back problem.

General examination

While the patient is lying undressed, a rapid examination is carried out to detect the presence of any suspicious lumps in the breasts, abdomen or genitalia.

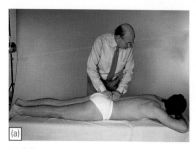 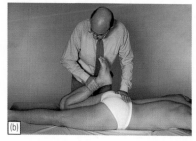 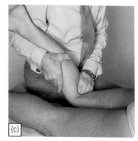

18.3 Examination with the patient prone (a) Feel for tenderness, watching the patient's face for any reaction. (b) Performing the femoral stretch test. You can test for lumbar root sensitivity either by hyperextending the hip or by acutely flexing the knee with the patient lying prone. Note the point at which the patient feels pain and compare the two sides. (c) While the patient is lying prone, take the opportunity to feel the pulses. The popliteal pulse is easily felt if the tissues at the back of the knee are relaxed by slightly flexing the knee.

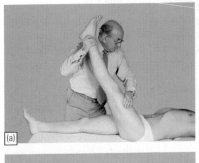
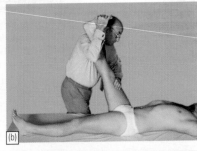
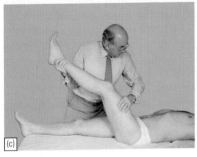
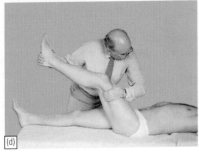

18.4 Sciatic stretch tests
(a) Straight-leg raising. The knee is kept absolutely straight while the leg is slowly lifted; note where the patient complains of tightness and pain in the buttock – normally around 80 or 90 degrees – and compare the two sides. (b) At that point, passive dorsiflexion of the foot causes an added stab of pain. (c) Sciatic tension can also be shown by the bow-string sign. At the point where the patient experiences pain during straight-leg raising, relax the tension by bending the knee slightly; the pain should disappear. Then apply firm pressure behind the lateral hamstrings (d); this tightens the common peroneal nerve and the pain recurs with renewed intensity.

IMAGING

X-rays

In the anteroposterior view, the spine should look perfectly straight. Individual vertebrae may show alterations in structure and the intervertebral spaces may be edged by bony spurs. The sacroiliac joints may show erosion or ankylosis.

In the lateral view, the normal thoracic kyphosis and lumbar lordosis should be regular and uninterrupted. There may be anterior shift of an upper segment upon a lower (spondylolisthesis). Individual vertebrae, which should be rectangular, may be wedged or biconcave. Compare the intervertebral disc spaces: there may be undue narrowing (flattening) of the disc at one or more levels.

Special techniques

CT, MRI and (occasionally) contrast myelography are useful for outlining the discs and the spinal canal.

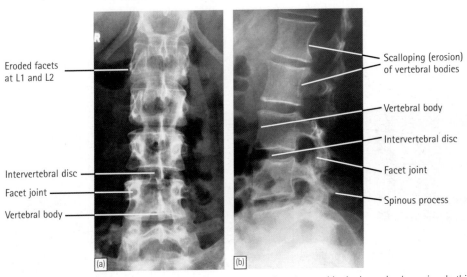

Eroded facets at L1 and L2

Intervertebral disc

Facet joint

Vertebral body

Scalloping (erosion) of vertebral bodies

Vertebral body

Intervertebral disc

Facet joint

Spinous process

18.5 Lumbar spine x-rays (a,b) The most important normal features are demonstrated in the lower lumbar spine. In this particular case there are also signs of marked posterior vertebral body and facet joint erosions at L1 and L2, features which are strongly suggestive of an expanding neurofibroma.

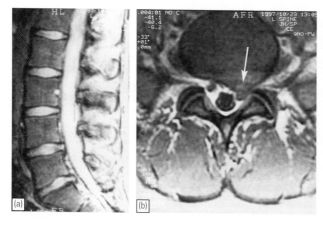

18.6 MRI (a) The lateral MRI shows a small posterior disc bulge at L4/5 and a larger protrusion at L5/S1. (b) Axial MRI demonstrated a disc prolapse encroaching on the intervertebral canal and the nerve root on the left side.

SCOLIOSIS

Seen from behind, the normal back is straight; in scoliosis it is curved to the side, and sometimes twisted. The deformity may be *postural* and correctable, or *structural* and fixed.

Postural scoliosis

In postural scoliosis the deformity is secondary or compensatory to some condition outside the spine, such as a short leg or pelvic tilt due to contracture of the hip; when the patient sits (thereby cancelling leg asymmetry), the curve disappears. Local muscle spasm associated with a prolapsed lumbar disc may cause a skew back: although sometimes called 'sciatic scoliosis', this, too, is a spurious deformity.

Structural scoliosis

Structural scoliosis is always accompanied by bony abnormality or vertebral rotation. The deformity is fixed and does not disappear with changes in posture. Secondary curves nearly always develop to counterbalance the primary deformity; they, too, may later become fixed. Once established, the deformity is liable to increase throughout the growth period (and sometimes even afterwards).

Several types of structural scoliosis are recognized.

Adolescent idiopathic scoliosis is far and away the most common, and this will be described in detail.

Infantile idiopathic scoliosis is seen in young children; some cases resolve spontaneously but others progress to severe deformity.

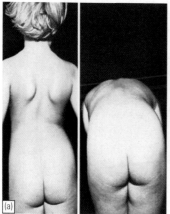
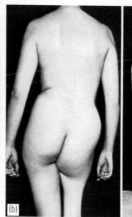
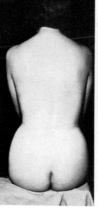
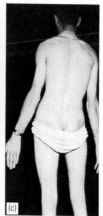

18.7 Postural scoliosis (a) This young girl presented with thoracolumbar 'curvature'. When she bends forward, the deformity disappears; this is typical of a postural or mobile scoliosis. (b) Short-leg scoliosis disappears when the patient sits. (c) Sciatic scoliosis disappears when the prolapsed disc settles down or is removed.

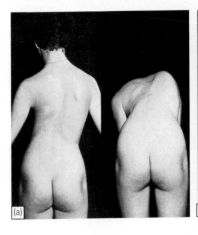
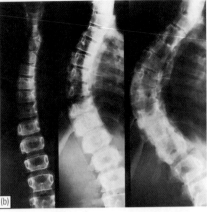

18.8 Structural scoliosis (a) A fixed (structural) curve becomes more obvious on flexion. In thoracic scoliosis this is largely because of prominence of the ribs on the convex side of the curve. (b) Over a period of 4 years this curve increased, most rapidly during the prepubertal growth spurt.

Osteopathic scoliosis is due to congenital vertebral anomalies. Although rare, curves may be severe and dangerously progressive.

Neuropathic scoliosis is due to asymmetrical muscle weakness (e.g. in poliomyelitis or cerebral palsy).

Myopathic scoliosis is sometimes seen in the rare muscular dystrophies.

Neurofibromatosis may be associated with a short, and often severe, deformity; why this occurs is not known.

ADOLESCENT IDIOPATHIC SCOLIOSIS

Idiopathic scoliosis usually presents before puberty and progresses until skeletal growth ceases; thereafter further deterioration is slight. The cause is unknown, but it has been suggested that localised extension (straightening out) of the normal dorsal kyphosis would inevitably force the spine to swivel round, thus producing the appearance of a lateral curvature.

Pathology

The curvature may occur anywhere in the thoracic or lumbar spine. The vertebrae that make up the curve are always rotated around the vertical axis, so the bodies point to the convexity and the spinous processes to the concavity of the curve. In thoracic curves the ribs on the convex side are also carried around posteriorly and stand out as a prominent hump.

Clinical features

Patients usually present between the ages of 10 and 15. Deformity is the only symptom and the severity depends largely on which part of the spine is involved: high curves are noticed early, whereas lumbar curves may pass virtually unnoticed. Whatever the deformity when the patient stands

upright, it always looks worse on flexion; this is in sharp contrast to a postural curve, which disappears on flexion. The shoulder is elevated on the side of the convexity and the hip sticks out on the side of the concavity. With thoracic scoliosis the breasts are asymmetrical and the rib angles protrude.

X-ray

This should include full-length views of the spine. The angle of curvature *(Cobb's angle)* is measured. X-ray of the pelvis shows when the iliac apophysis has ossified and fused *(Risser's sign)*, a sign of skeletal maturity after which progression of the curve is minimal.

Treatment

Prognosis is the key to treatment: the aim is to prevent the curve becoming severe. Generally speaking, the younger the child and the higher the curve, the worse the prognosis. A period of preliminary observation may be needed before deciding between conservative and operative treatment. At 4-monthly intervals the patient is examined, photographed and x-rayed so that the

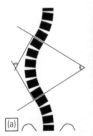
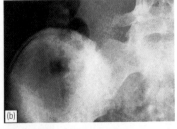

18.9 Scoliosis – Cobb's angle and Risser's sign (a) Cobb's method of measuring the primary curve. Lines projected from the uppermost and lowermost vertebral bodies in the curve show the angle of deformity. (b) When the iliac apophyses fuse, spinal maturity has been reached; there may be a further increase of curvature, but this will be slight.

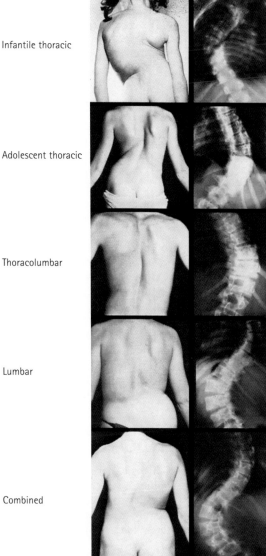

Infantile thoracic

60% male
90% convex to left.
Associated with ipsilateral plagiocephaly.
May be resolving or progressive.
Progressive variety becomes severe.

Adolescent thoracic

90% female
90% convex to right.
Rib rotation exaggerates the deformity.
50% develop curves of greater than 70°.

Thoracolumbar

Slightly more common in females.
Slightly more common to right.
Features mid-way between adolescent
thoracic and lumbar.

Lumbar

More common in females.
80% convex to left.
One hip prominent but no ribs to
accentuate deformity.
Therefore not noticed early, but backache
in adult life.

Combined

Two primary curves, one in each direction.
Even when radiologically severe, clinical
deformity relatively slight because always
well balanced.

18.10 Patterns of idiopathic scoliosis

curves can be measured and checked for progression. School screening should permit early diagnosis and regular assessment of the need for active treatment.

Conservative treatment

Exercises alone have no effect on the curve, but they help to maintain suppleness and are a useful adjunct to operative treatment.

Bracing is used: (1) for all progressive curves over 20 degrees but less than 40 degrees; (2) for well-balanced double curves; (3) with younger children needing operation, to hold the curve stationary until they reach adolescence, when fusion is more likely to succeed; and (4) to prevent recurrence after spinal fusion.

In the past, the *Milwaukee brace* was the one most commonly used. With an occipitocervical support proximally and a firm pelvic band distally, the spine is distracted; a mobile curve can thus be straightened to some extent. A lateral chest pad can also be used to apply pressure at the apex of the curve. The brace must be worn continuously, with a break of only 1 hour in 24. Needless to say, this injunction is often ignored by young patients;

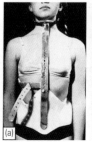
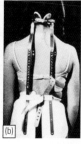
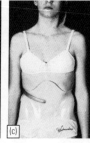

18.11 Structural scoliosis – conservative treatment
(a,b) The Milwaukee brace, which encouraged active postural correction, has lost some of its earlier popularity. (c) The Boston brace is much less cumbersome but is suitable only for curves below T9.

moreover, doubts have arisen as to the effectiveness of this uncomfortable treatment, and the shorter, less repugnant *Boston brace* has become more popular in recent years. This has the form of a thoracolumbar jacket, which is ideal for curves below T9.

Operative treatment

Operative correction is indicated for curves that progress to more than 40 degrees. The principle is to expose the entire length of the curve and, by applying a distraction rod to the concave side of the curve (anchored to the laminae of the proximal and distal vertebrae of the curve), to 'jack' the curved segment out as straight as possible without damaging the spine or injuring the cord. The entire length of the curve is then prepared for bone-grafting in the hope that it will fuse while the back is 'immobilized' in a plaster jacket.

Full correction is seldom, if ever, achieved; 50 per cent correction is regarded as satisfactory. In an attempt to improve on this, sublaminar wires have

been used to pull the apex of the curve closer to the metal rod on the concave side.

To correct severe curves, more robust forms of posterior or anterior instrumentation are employed; they carry a greater risk of neurological complications.

KYPHOSIS

Rather confusingly, the term 'kyphosis' is used to describe both the normal (the gentle rounding of the dorsal spine) and the abnormal (excessive dorsal curvature). In the latter sense it signifies a well-recognized deformity which may be progressive; some people prefer the term *hyperkyphosis*.

Postural kyphosis is common ('round back' or 'drooping shoulders') and may be associated with other postural defects such as flat-feet.

Structural kyphosis is fixed and associated with changes in the shape of the vertebrae. It may occur in osteoporosis of the spine (the common round back of elderly people), in ankylosing spondylitis and in Scheuermann's disease (adolescent kyphosis).

A *kyphos* (or *gibbus*) is a sharp posterior angulation due to localized collapse or wedging of one or more vertebrae. This may be the result of a congenital defect, a fracture (sometimes pathological) or spinal tuberculosis.

SCHEUERMANN'S DISEASE (ADOLESCENT KYPHOSIS)

This is a 'developmental' disorder of the growing spine in which there is irregular ossification, and possibly some fragmentation, of the vertebral body epiphyses – somewhat akin to other types of *'osteochondrosis'* in young adolescents (see page 51).

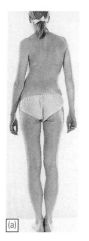
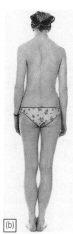
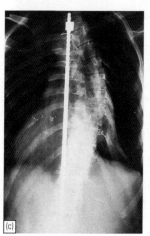
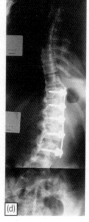

18.12 Structural scoliosis – operative treatment
(a,b) Clinical appearance before and after Harrington rod instrumentation and fusion. (c) X-ray of the same patient a year later, showing the Harrington distraction rod still in place. (d) Similar correction can be obtained by the anterior approach and compression on the convex side of the curve.

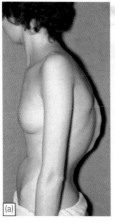
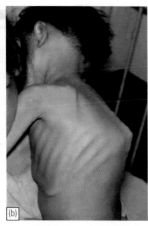

18.13 Kyphosis and kyphos (a) *Kyphosis*: a generalized exaggeration of the normal thoracic 'rounding' of the back, in this case due to Scheuermann's disease. (b) *Kyphos*: a localized spinal angulation, or gibbus, due to collapse of one or two spinal segments (here following tuberculous spondylitis).

This results in irregularity of the mature vertebral end-plates, sometimes associated with small central herniations of disc material into the vertebral body (*Schmorl's nodes*). With increasing growth and muscular activity, affected vertebrae in the thoracic spine (which is normally mildly kyphotic) may give way slightly and become wedge shaped. If this happens, the normal *kyphosis* is exaggerated. In the lumbar spine, the compressive forces are more evenly distributed and deformity does not occur.

Clinical features

Thoracic Scheuermann's disease

The usual form of Scheuermann's disease appears in the mid-thoracic vertebrae. The condition starts at or shortly after puberty and is more common in boys than in girls. The parents notice that the child, an otherwise fit teenager, is becoming increasingly 'round shouldered'. He may complain of backache and fatigue. Examination reveals a smooth but well-marked thoracic kyphosis (or 'hyperkyphosis') which does not improve with changes in posture (see Fig. 18.13a).

X-ray features are typical: in the lateral views one can see patchiness or irregularity of the vertebral end-plates and, in some cases, Schmorl's nodes at several intervertebral levels. Later, the vertebral bodies become noticeably wedge shaped.

Treatment depends on the severity of the clinical and x-ray changes. In some cases, the early features are so mild that they go unremarked, and it is only when, as an adult, the person is x-rayed for some unrelated reason that the features of an 'old Scheuermann's are recognized. If there is concern about back pain and/or deformity, an extension brace worn for a year or 18 months will often allow a return to normal vertebral growth. If this fails, or if the deformity is already marked when the patient is first seen, operative correction and fusion may be needed.

Thoracolumbar Scheuermann's disease

Thoracolumbar changes may appear together with thoracic kyphosis or may occur on their own. Compared to thoracic Scheuermann's, this condition is less common, tends to occur in late adolescence or early adulthood, does not give rise to local deformity and usually presents as low back pain. X-ray changes are similar to those seen in the thoracic spine, but with little or no vertebral wedging. Patients with low back pain may respond to back strengthening exercises. Operative treatment is not indicated unless there are associated features of discogenic disease.

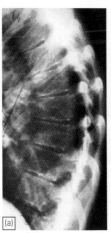
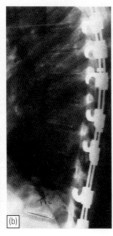
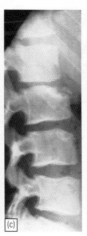
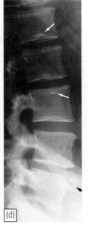

18.14 Scheuermann's disease – x-rays (a,b) X-rays before and after operative correction and fusion. (c,d) In lumbar Scheuermann's there is less wedging than in the thoracic region. End-plate fragmentation can be mistaken for a fracture of the vertebral body. Arrows show typical Schmorl's nodes.

TUBERCULOSIS

The spine is the most common site of skeletal tuberculosis, and the most dangerous.

Pathology

Blood-borne infection settles in a vertebral body adjacent to the intervertebral disc. Bone destruction and caseation follow, with infection spreading to the disc space and to the next vertebra. As the vertebral bodies collapse into each other, a sharp angulation (or kyphos) develops. Caseation and cold abscess formation may extend to neighbouring vertebrae or escape into the paravertebral soft tissues. There is a major risk of cord damage due to pressure by the abscess or displaced bone.

Clinical features

There is usually a long history of ill-health and backache. In some cases deformity is the dominant feature. Occasionally the patient presents with a cold abscess pointing in the groin, or with paraesthesia and weakness of the legs.

On examination, the characteristic finding in the thoracic spine is an angular kyphos (see Fig.18.13b); in the lumbar spine this is scarcely visible. There is local tenderness and muscle spasm. All movements are restricted.

The groins and lumbar regions should be examined for abscess formation, and the lower limbs must be examined for neurological changes.

X-rays

Early on there may be no more than disc space narrowing. With bone destruction there is collapse of adjacent vertebrae and obliteration of the disc space. A paravertebral abscess may be present. In long-standing cases there may be marked deformity involving a considerable length of the spine.

Investigations

The Mantoux test is positive and the erythrocyte sedimentation rate (ESR) may be raised. If there is an abscess, pus should be sent for bacteriological examination and culture.

Diagnosis

It is often difficult to distinguish tuberculosis from other types of infection or (in older patients) from metastatic disease. If there is doubt, a needle biopsy may provide the answer.

Treatment

Except for the more advanced cases with progressive bone destruction, conservative treatment is usually sufficient and curative. Anti-tuberculous chemotherapy should be rigidly supervised and continued for 6–12 months. If

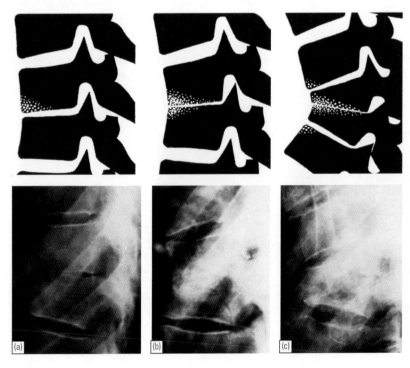

(a) (b) (c)

18.15 Spinal tuberculosis
(a–c) The diagrams and x-rays show progressively increasing destruction of the front of the vertebral bodies leading to vertebral collapse and kyphosis.

pain and spasm are marked, a period in hospital (sometimes on a frame) may be advisable; otherwise, a well-fitting brace is all that is needed.

The indications for operation are: (1) abscess formation (this must be drained); (2) marked bone destruction and progressive deformity (this requires spinal fusion); (3) threatened paraplegia that does not respond to conservative treatment.

POTT'S PARAPLEGIA

The spinal cord may be compressed by soft inflammatory material (an abscess, a caseous mass or granulation tissue) or by hard solid material (a bony sequestrum, a sequestrated disc or the ridge of bone at the kyphos). Occasionally fibrous tissue is the compressing agent.

Clinically the patient presents with signs of paraplegia added to those of spine tuberculosis. Clumsiness and weakness are early symptoms; later, muscle tone is increased and the tendon reflexes are brisk; clonus and extensor plantar responses may be found. Paraesthesia, or numbness, and disturbance of bladder control are common.

Early-onset paresis is due to pressure by an abscess or bony sequestrum. The diagnosis is confirmed by MRI or myelography. It is treated by early anterior decompression and debridement followed by spinal fusion. About 80 per cent recover, usually within a few weeks.

Late-onset paresis is due to increasing deformity, or reactivation of disease, or vascular insufficiency of the cord. Investigations should be carried out to establish the precise diagnosis. If MRI or myelography shows a block, operative removal of necrotic tissue is still worthwhile, even in late cases. If there is no block, operation is unlikely to be of use.

PYOGENIC INFECTION

Pyogenic organisms – usually staphylococci – may infect the vertebral body *(pyogenic spondylitis)* or the intervertebral disc *(discitis)*.

Clinical features

Pain is the chief complaint. It may be associated with acute muscle spasm; spinal movements are markedly restricted.

X-rays

Typical changes are narrowing of the disc space and destruction of the adjacent bone. Even before these signs appear, radioscintigraphy will almost always show increased activity. In late cases, new-bone formation is common – a point of distinction from tuberculous spondylitis. With healing, there may be fusion of adjacent vertebrae.

Investigations

The ESR is usually raised. A positive blood culture is unusual. Anti-staphylococcal antibodies may be present in high titres. Agglutination tests for salmonella and brucella should always be performed. A needle biopsy may be required to discover the offending organism.

Treatment

Treatment consists of bed-rest and intravenous antibiotics for 4–6 weeks; with a positive blood culture or biopsy sample, the most suitable drug can be selected. Once the acute infection has subsided, the patient is allowed up in a spinal brace, which is worn until x-rays and blood tests show that healing has occurred.

ANKYLOSING SPONDYLITIS (SPONDYLOARTHROPATHY)

This group of disorders is dealt with in Chapter 3.

INTERVERTEBRAL DISC LESIONS

Lumbar backache is one of the most common causes of chronic disability in Western societies, and in the majority of cases the backache is associated with some abnormality of the intervertebral discs at the lowest two levels of the spine (L4/5 and L5/S1).

PROLAPSED INTERVERTEBRAL DISC

In acute disc herniation, the gelatinous nucleus pulposus squeezes through the fibres of the annulus fibrosus and bulges posteriorly or posterolaterally beneath the posterior longitudinal ligament. Local oedema may add to the swelling, causing pressure on one of the nerve roots. With a complete rupture, part of the nucleus may sequestrate and lie free in the spinal canal.

Symptoms depend on the structure involved and the degree of compression. Pressure on the ligament probably accounts for backache; pressure on the dural envelope of the nerve root causes severe pain referred to the lower limb (sciatica); and compression of the nerve itself causes numbness, paraesthesia and muscle weakness.

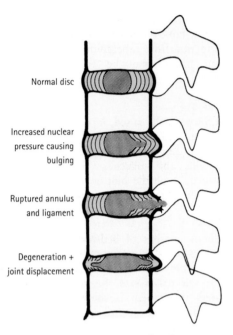

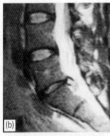

Normal disc

Increased nuclear
pressure causing
bulging

Ruptured annulus
and ligament

Degeneration +
joint displacement

18.16 Intervertebral disc rupture and prolapse
Diagrammatic representation of progressive stages in the
development of disc prolapse. At first there is only bulging of
the posterior part of the disc; the annulus fibrosus may go on
to rupture and the nucleus pulposus is extruded posteriorly to
one or other side. In disc degeneration, the disc may collapse
without actually rupturing.

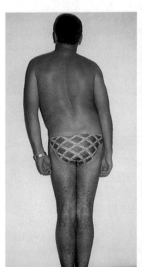

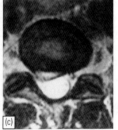

18.17 Prolapsed disc – clinical and MRI (a) This patient
presented with acute low back pain and sciatica. He has the
characteristic sideways list or tilt due to paravertebral muscle
spasm. (b,c) MRI showing the disc prolapse at L5/S1. In the
axial view (c), one can see that the disc protrusion encroaches
on the intervertebral foramen and nerve root at that level.

Clinical features

The patient is usually a fit young adult, although
children and old people can be affected. Typically,
while lifting or stooping (or perhaps merely
coughing), the patient is seized with back pain and
is unable to straighten up. Either then or a day or
two later, pain is felt in the buttock and lower limb
(sciatica). Both backache and sciatica are made
worse by coughing or straining. Later there may be
paraesthesia or numbness in the leg or foot, and
occasionally muscle weakness. *Cauda equina
compression* is rare but may cause urinary retention.

The patient usually stands with a slight list to
one side ('sciatic scoliosis'). All back movements
are severely limited, and during forward flexion
the list may increase.

There is often tenderness in the midline of the low
back, and paravertebral muscle spasm. Straight-leg
raising is limited and painful on the affected side;
dorsiflexion of the foot and bowstringing of the
lateral popliteal nerve may accentuate the pain.
Sometimes raising the unaffected leg causes acute
sciatic tension on the painful side ('crossed sciatic
tension'). With a prolapse at L3/4, the femoral
stretch test may be positive.

Neurological examination may show muscle
weakness (and, later, wasting), diminished reflexes
and sensory loss corresponding to the affected
level. L5 impairment causes weakness of big toe
extension and knee flexion, with sensory loss on
the outer side of the leg and the dorsum of the
foot. S1 impairment causes weak plantarflexion
and eversion of the foot, a depressed ankle jerk and
sensory loss along the lateral border of the foot.
Cauda equina compression causes urinary
retention and sensory loss over the sacrum.

> ⚠ Acute sciatica: always check for urinary retention –
> patients don't always tell you. Cauda equina damage
> may be irreversible.

Imaging

X-rays are essential, not to show an abnormal disc
space, but to exclude bone disease. After several
attacks the disc space may be narrowed. A
myelogram or radiculogram outlines the disc well,
but side-effects are unpleasant. *CT* and *MRI* are
the best ways of identifying the disc and localizing
the lesion.

Differential diagnosis

The full-blown syndrome is unlikely to be
misdiagnosed, but with repeated attacks and with
lumbar spondylosis gradually supervening, the

features often become atypical. Three groups of disorders must be excluded.

1. *Inflammatory disorders,* such as ankylosing spondylitis, cause severe and more generalized stiffness and typical x-ray changes.
2. *Vertebral tumours* cause constant pain; x-rays show bone destruction or a pathological fracture.
3. *Nerve tumours* may cause sciatica but pain is continuous; CT or MRI may delineate the lesions.

Treatment

Heat and analgesics soothe, and exercises strengthen muscles; but there are only three ways of treating the prolapse itself – *rest, reduction* and *removal;* equally important is the *rehabilitation* afterwards.

Rest

With an acute attack the patient should be kept in bed, with hips and knees slightly flexed and 10 kg traction to the pelvis. An anti-inflammatory drug such as indomethacin is useful. For mild attacks a spinal corset and reduced activity may suffice.

Reduction

Continuous bed-rest and traction for 2 weeks will reduce the herniation in more than 90 per cent of cases. If the symptoms and signs have not improved significantly by then, an *epidural injection* of corticosteroid and local anaesthetic may help. If conservative measures fail, discectomy is the treatment of choice.

Removal

The indications for operative removal of a disc are: (1) a cauda equina compression syndrome which does not clear up within 6 hours of starting bed-rest and traction – this is an emergency; (2) persistent pain and severely limited straight-leg raising after 2 weeks of conservative treatment; (3) neurological deterioration while under conservative treatment; and (4) frequently recurring attacks.

Through a posterior approach between adjacent vertebral laminae, the dural sac is retracted to one side and the bulging disc is exposed. The friable, partially shredded material is removed. This can be done by open operation or by endoscopic surgery (microdiscectomy).

Rehabilitation

After recovery from an acute disc rupture, or disc removal, the patient is taught isometric exercises and how to lie, sit, bend and lift with the least strain. Light work is resumed after a month and heavy work after 3 months. At that stage, if recovery is anything but total, the patient should be advised to avoid heavy lifting tasks altogether.

 Recurrent pain after discectomy: check for infection, recurrent disc, wrong level.

LUMBAR SEGMENTAL INSTABILITY AND OSTEOARTHRITIS

With disc degeneration, and especially after recurrent disc prolapse, there may be gradual flattening of the disc and displacement of the posterior facet joints. The disturbed movement in flexion and extension constitutes a type of segmental instability; symptoms are due to mechanical derangement and secondary osteoarthritis of the facet joints.

Clinical features

The patient may give a history of acute disc rupture followed by recurrent attacks of pain over several years. Backache is intermittent and related to spells of hard physical work, standing or walking a lot, or sitting in one position during a long journey; it is relieved by lying down. Pain is often referred to the buttock and sometimes it extends down the leg like sciatica. There may be acute incidents of 'locking' or 'giving way'.

The patient is usually over 40 and otherwise fit. Often, tender areas are felt in the back and buttocks. Lumbar movements are limited and may be painful at their extremes. A typical feature is difficulty in straightening up from the forward bend position. Neurological examination may show residual signs of an old disc prolapse (e.g. an absent ankle jerk).

X-rays

The classic features are narrowing of the disc space and marginal bony spurs ('osteophytes'). Osteoarthritis of the facet joints is often seen.

Treatment

Because the disability is seldom severe, and may even decrease with time (as the spine stabilizes itself), conservative measures are encouraged for as long as possible. These consist of instruction in modified activities, isometric exercises, manipulation during acute episodes, the wearing of a lumbar corset and small doses of anti-inflammatory drugs. If these measures, conscientiously applied, cannot control pain, spinal fusion may be indicated.

Chronic back pain can be psychologically debilitating; counselling and support are often welcomed by the patient.

SPONDYLOLISTHESIS

Spondylolisthesis means vertebral displacement. Normal laminae and facets constitute a locking mechanism which prevents each vertebra from moving forwards on the one below. Forward shift (or slip) occurs only when this mechanism fails. Listhesis is nearly always between L4 and L5, or between L5 and the sacrum. This usually happens for one of the following reasons:

- Dysplasia of the lumbosacral facet joints (20 per cent of cases).
- Separation or stress fracture (lysis) through the neural arch, allowing the anterior part of the vertebra to slip forward (50 per cent of cases).

- Osteoarthritic degeneration of the facet joints, causing them to lose their normal stability. This usually occurs at L4/5 (25 per cent of cases).
- Destructive conditions such as fracture, tuberculosis and neoplasia (5 per cent of cases).

Clinical features

Dysplastic spondylolisthesis is seen in children. It is usually painless, but the mother may notice the unduly protruding abdomen. There may be an associated scoliosis.

Lytic spondylolisthesis is the commonest variety. It occurs in adults, and intermittent backache is the usual presenting symptom. Pain may be initiated or exacerbated by exercise or strain. On examination, the buttocks look curiously flat, the sacrum appears to extend to the waist and transverse loin creases may be prominent. A 'step' can often be felt when the fingers are run down the spine. Movements are usually normal in younger

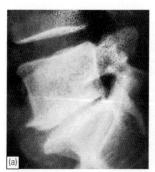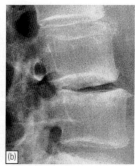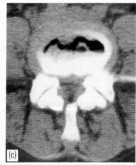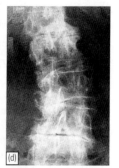

18.18 Spondylosis and osteoarthritis Typical x-ray features are (a) narrowing of the intervertebral disc space and anterior traction spurs, and (b) retrolisthesis and a vacant area in the disc space – the 'vacuum sign'. (c) CT showing the vacuum sign in the disc area and hypertrophic osteoarthritis of the facet joints. (d) In advanced cases, several levels are involved and there may be deformity of the spine.

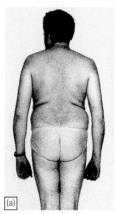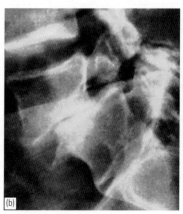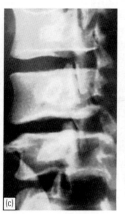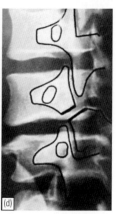

18.19 Spondylolisthesis (a) The transverse loin creases, short lumbar spine and long sacrum are characteristic. In the lateral x-ray (b), the slip may be obvious, but the defect in the pars interarticularis is better seen in the oblique view (c,d) where it is likened to a 'collar' around the 'neck' of an illusory 'dog'.

patients but may be restricted in older people.

Degenerative spondylolisthesis usually occurs in women over 40 years with long-standing backache due to facet joint arthritis. Sometimes the presenting symptom is spinal 'claudication' due to narrowing of the spinal canal (see under *Spinal stenosis* below).

Imaging

X-rays show the forward shift of the upper part of the spinal column on the stable vertebra below; elongation of the arch or defective facets may be seen. The gap in the pars interarticularis is more easily seen in oblique x-ray views, and best of all in CT scans.

Treatment

Conservative treatment is indicated (1) if the patient is no longer young and symptoms are not disabling, or (2) if there is doubt as to whether the symptoms arise from the slip or from an associated disc prolapse. It consists of bed-rest during an acute attack and a supporting corset between attacks.

Operative treatment is indicated (1) at any age if the symptoms are disabling, or (2) in the young adult with even moderate symptoms, and (3) if neurological compression is marked. Spinal fusion is carried out to fix the unstable segment.

SPINAL STENOSIS

One of the long-term consequences of disc degeneration and osteoarthritis is narrowing of the spinal canal due to hypertrophy at the posterior disc margin and the facet joints. This is more likely if the canal was always small, or if a spondylolisthesis decreases its anteroposterior diameter.

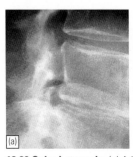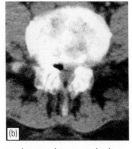

18.20 Spinal stenosis (a) A lateral x-ray shows marked narrowing of the spinal canal, but the CT scan (b) provides even more convincing evidence.

Clinical features

Typically, a patient with backache complains of aching and/or numbness and paraesthesia in the thighs, legs or feet. The symptoms come on after standing upright or walking for 5–10 minutes and are consistently relieved by sitting or squatting with the spine somewhat flexed (hence the term 'spinal claudication'). Symptoms may be unilateral, suggesting an asymmetrical stenosis or intervertebral canal stenosis.

Examination, especially after getting the patient to reproduce the symptoms by walking, may show neurological defects in the lower limbs. Always check the upper limbs for signs of polyneuropathy and the lower limbs for evidence of peripheral vascular disease.

Nerve conduction studies and electromyography are helpful in establishing the diagnosis and the severity of neurological change.

Imaging

Lateral view x-rays may show degenerative spondylolisthesis or advanced disc degeneration and osteoarthritis. Measurement of the spinal canal may be carried out on plain films, but more reliable information is obtained from CT. If operation is planned, myelography or MRI is essential to show the extent of spinal canal narrowing.

Treatment

Conservative measures, including instruction in spinal posture, may suffice. If they fail to provide sufficient relief, operative decompression may reduce the neurological symptoms. However, patients must be warned that the operation will not improve their backache. If there are clear-cut signs of spinal instability, segmental fusion may also be needed.

THE BACKACHE PROBLEM

Backache is such a frequent cause of disability that it has become almost a disease in itself. Careful history taking and examination will uncover one of five patterns.

Transient backache following muscular activity

This suggests a simple back strain, which will respond to a period of rest followed by gradually increasing exercise.

Sudden, acute pain and sciatica

In young people (those under 20) it is important to exclude infection and spondylolisthesis. Patients aged 20–40 years are more likely to have an acute disc prolapse. Elderly patients may have osteoporotic compression fractures.

Chronic low back pain, with or without 'sciatica'

If the patient is over 40 and has had recurrent episodes of pain, the most likely diagnosis is facet joint dysfunction, segmental instability or osteoarthritis. However, disorders such as ankylosing spondylitis, chronic infection or other bone disease must be excluded by appropriate imaging and blood investigations. Treatment is almost always conservative. *NB. 'Sciatica' does not necessarily connote sciatic nerve irritation. More* *often it as a manifestation of referred pain from other vertebral structures.*

Back pain plus pseudoclaudication

These patients are usually aged over 50 and give a history of long-standing back trouble. The diagnosis of spinal stenosis should be confirmed by suitable imaging studies.

Severe and constant pain

This suggests local bone pathology such as infection, a fracture, Paget's disease, a tumour or metastatic disease. Imaging studies should clinch the diagnosis.

CHAPTER 19

THE HIP

CLINICAL ASSESSMENT

HISTORY

Pain arising in the hip joint is felt in the groin, down the front of the thigh and, sometimes, in the knee; occasionally knee pain is the only symptom! Pain at the back of the hip is seldom from the joint: it usually derives from the lumbar spine.

Stiffness may cause difficulty with putting on socks or sitting in a low chair.

Limp is common, and sometimes the patient complains that the leg is 'getting shorter'.

Walking distance may be curtailed or, reluctantly, the patient starts using a walking stick.

SIGNS WITH THE PATIENT UPRIGHT

The *gait* is noted, and also whether the patient uses any form of support. If there is a limp, it may be due to pain *(antalgic gait)*, to shortening *(short-leg limp)* or to abductor weakness *(Trendelenburg lurch)*.

The *Trendelenburg test* is used to assess stability. The patient is asked to stand, unassisted, on each leg in turn; while standing on one leg, he or she has to lift the other leg by bending the knee (but not the hip). Normally the weight-bearing hip is held stable by the abductors and the pelvis rises on the unsupported side; if the hip is unstable, or very painful, the pelvis drops on the unsupported side.

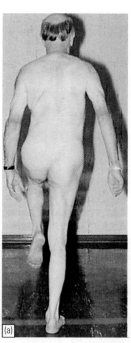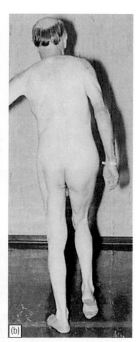

19.1 Examination – Trendelenburg's sign (a) This man has osteoarthritis of the left hip. Standing on his right leg he is well supported by his right hip, the pelvis is level or, if anything, tilted towards the right and the left buttock fold is higher than the right. (b) Standing on his left leg is more difficult. His left hip cannot support him properly; the pelvis tilts towards the right and the right buttock fold drops below the left. The Trendelenburg test is positive for the left side (i.e. abnormal).

A positive Trendelenburg test is found in (1) dislocation or subluxation of the hip; (2) weakness of the abductors; (3) shortening of the femoral neck; or (4) any painful disorder of the hip.

SIGNS WITH THE PATIENT LYING SUPINE

Look

Make sure that the patient is lying comfortably with the pelvis horizontal (both anterior superior iliac spines at the same level) and the legs placed symmetrically. Now check to see if the medial malleoli are at the same level, or if one leg seems to be shorter than the other. Look for scars or sinuses, swelling or wasting and any obvious deformity or malposition of one of the limbs. In babies, asymmetry of skin creases may be important.

Limb length

Provided the pelvis is truly at right angles to the trunk and lower limbs, any visible discrepancy in limb length is real. This can be confirmed by placing the two lower limbs in comparable positions in relation to the pelvis and then measuring the distance from the anterior superior iliac spine to the medial malleolus on each side.

If shortening is present, it is usually possible to establish where the fault lies. With the knees flexed and the heels together, it can be seen whether the discrepancy is below or above the knee. If it is above, the next question is whether the abnormality lies above the greater trochanter. The thumbs are pressed firmly against the anterior superior iliac spines and the middle fingers feel for the tops of the greater trochanters; any elevation of the trochanter on one side is readily felt.

Apparent shortening or lengthening

Measurement may show that the discrepancy in limb length is only *apparent* and not real. This occurs when the pelvis is tilted and one limb is hitched upwards. Almost invariably this is due to an uncorrectable deformity in the hip: with fixed adduction on one side, the limbs would tend to be crossed; when the legs are placed side by side, the pelvis has to tilt upwards on the affected side, giving the impression of a shortened limb. The

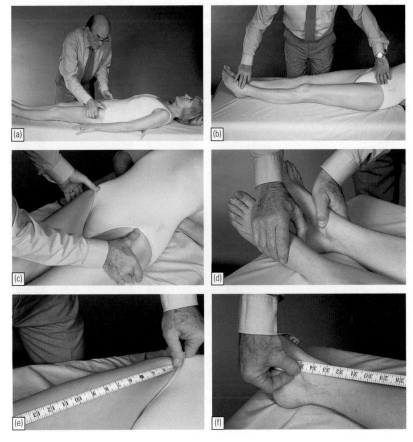

19.2 Measurement (a,b) Make sure the patient is lying straight on the examination couch and that the pelvis is absolutely level – the anterior superior iliac spines at the same level in relation to the longitudinal axis of the body (c). Then check the medial malleoli (d); discrepancy in leg length will usually be obvious. (e,f) Leg length is most accurately assessed by measuring from the anterior superior iliac spine to the tip of the medial malleolus on each side.

exact opposite occurs when there is fixed abduction, and the limb seems to be longer on the affected side.

Feel

Bone contours are felt when levelling the pelvis and judging the height of the greater trochanters. Tenderness may be elicited in and around the joint. The surface marking of the femoral head is halfway between the anterior superior iliac spine and the pubic tubercle.

Move

The assessment of hip movements is difficult because any limitation can easily be obscured by movement of the pelvis. Thus, even a gross limitation of extension, causing a *fixed flexion deformity,* can be completely masked simply by arching the back into excessive lordosis. Fortunately, it can be just as easily unmasked by performing

Thomas' test: both hips are flexed simultaneously to their limit, thus completely obliterating the lumbar lordosis; holding the 'sound' hip firmly in this position (and thus keeping the pelvis still), the other limb is lowered gently; with any flexion deformity, the knee will not rest on the couch. Meanwhile the full range of *flexion* will also have been noted; the normal range is about 130 degrees.

Similarly, when testing *abduction,* the pelvis must be prevented from tilting sideways. This is achieved by placing the 'sound' hip (the hip opposite to the one being examined) in full abduction and keeping it there, thus fixing the pelvis in the coronal plane. A hand is placed on one iliac crest to detect the slightest movement of the pelvis. Then, after checking that the anterior superior iliac spines are level, the affected joint is moved gently into abduction. The normal range is about 45 degrees. Adduction is tested by crossing one limb over the other; the pelvis must be watched and felt to

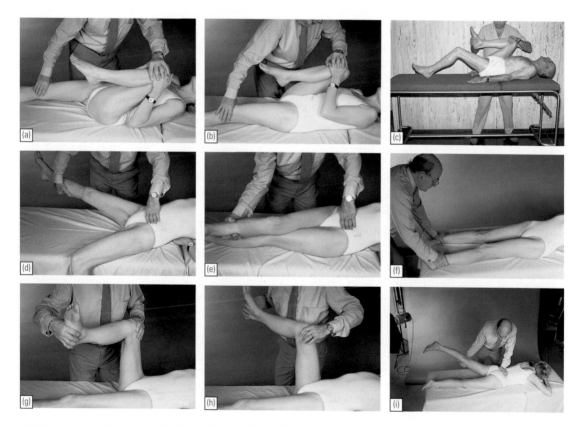

19.3 Movement (a) Forcing one hip into full flexion will straighten out the lumbar spine; the other hip should still be capable of full extension in this position. (b) Now the position is reversed; the right hip is held in full flexion. (c) If the hip cannot straighten out completely, this is referred to as a *fixed flexion deformity.* (d) Testing for abduction. The pelvis is kept level by placing the opposite leg over the edge of the examination couch with that hip also in abduction (the examiner's left hand checks the position of the anterior spines) before abducting the target hip. (e) Testing for adduction. (f–h) External and internal rotation are assessed (f) first with the hips in full extension and then (g,h) in 90 degrees of flexion. (i) Testing for extension.

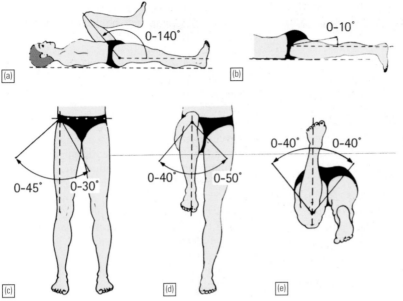

19.4 Normal range of movements

determine the point at which it starts to tilt. The normal range of adduction is about 30 degrees.

To test *rotation,* both legs, lifted by the ankles, are rotated first internally then externally; the patellae are watched to estimate the amount of rotation. Rotation in flexion is tested with the hip and knee each flexed 90 degrees.

Abnormal movement, i.e. movement greatly in excess of the norm, or the ability to elicit 'telescoping' by alternately pulling and pushing the limb in its long axis, suggests either instability or an established pseudarthrosis of the hip.

SIGNS WITH THE PATIENT LYING PRONE

Scars, sinuses or wasting are noted. Extension of the two hips is most accurately compared with the patient lying prone. Rotation also can be assessed by flexing both knees and then moving the legs (like two handles), first away from each other and then crossing each other.

IMAGING

The minimum required is an anteroposterior x-ray view of the pelvis showing both hips and a lateral view of each hip separately. The two sides can be compared: any difference in the size, shape or position of the femoral heads is important. With a normal hip, Shenton's line, which continues from the inferior border of the femoral neck to the inferior border of the pubic ramus, looks continuous; any interruption in the line suggests an abnormal position of the femoral head. Narrowing of the joint 'space' is a sign of articular cartilage loss, a feature of both inflammatory and non-inflammatory arthritis. Increased radiographic density in the femoral head is associated with avascular necrosis; however, the early changes of femoral head necrosis can be detected only on MRI.

Ultrasonography is the ideal method for demonstrating neonatal hip dysplasia; x-rays are unable to display an image of the cartilaginous femoral head and acetabulum.

THE DIAGNOSTIC CALENDAR

Hip disorders are characteristically seen in certain well-defined age groups. Whilst there are exceptions to this rule, it is sufficiently true to allow the age of onset to serve as a guide to the probable diagnosis (Table 19.1).

Table 19.1 The diagnostic calendar: age of onset can be a guide to probable diagnosis

Age of onset (years)	Probable diagnosis
0 (birth)	Developmental dysplasia
0–5	Infections
5–10	Perthes' disease
10–20	Slipped epiphysis
Adults	Arthritis

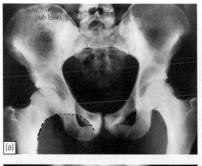
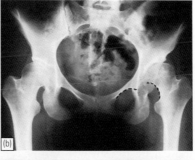
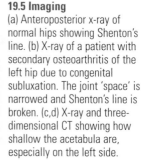
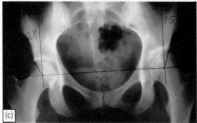
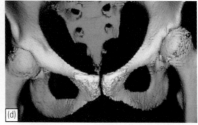

19.5 Imaging
(a) Anteroposterior x-ray of normal hips showing Shenton's line. (b) X-ray of a patient with secondary osteoarthritis of the left hip due to congenital subluxation. The joint 'space' is narrowed and Shenton's line is broken. (c,d) X-ray and three-dimensional CT showing how shallow the acetabula are, especially on the left side.

DEVELOPMENTAL DYSPLASIA OF THE HIP

The condition formerly known as congenital dislocation of the hip and now called developmental dysplasia of the hip (DDH) comprises a spectrum of disorders: frank dislocation during the neonatal period; subluxation or partial displacement; and an unusually shallow acetabulum (acetabular dysplasia) without actual displacement. Whether the instability comes first and then affects acetabular development because of imperfect seating of the femoral head, or is the result of a primary acetabular dysplasia, is still not known for certain. Both mechanisms might be important.

The reported incidence of neonatal hip instability is 5–20 per 1000 live births; however, most of these hips stabilize spontaneously, and on re-examination 3 weeks after birth the incidence of instability is only 1 or 2 per 1000 infants. Girls are much more commonly affected than boys, the ratio being about 7:1. The left hip is more often affected than the right; in 1 in 5 cases the condition is bilateral.

Aetiology and pathogenesis

Genetic factors must be important, for DDH tends to run in families and even in entire populations (e.g. along the northern and eastern Mediterranean seaboard). Two heritable features which could predispose to hip instability are generalized joint laxity and shallow acetabula.

Hormonal changes in late pregnancy may aggravate ligamentous laxity in the infant.

Intrauterine malposition, especially a breech position with extended legs, would favour dislocation.

Postnatal factors play a part in maintaining any tendency to instability. This may account for the unusually high incidence of DDH in Lapps (Sami), North American Indians and Eskimos (Inuit), who swaddle their babies and carry them with hips and knees fully extended; compare the rarity of DDH in African peoples, who carry their babies astride their backs with hips abducted.

Pathology

The acetabulum is unusually shallow (shaped like a saucer instead of a cup) and its roof slopes too steeply; the femoral head slides out posteriorly and then rides upwards. The joint capsule, though stretched, remains intact and, by folding inwards, may impede reduction. The fibrocartilaginous labrum is often turned into the acetabulum and this acts as a further obstacle to reduction. Maturation of the acetabulum and femoral epiphysis is retarded and the femoral neck is unduly anteverted.

Clinical features

The ideal, still unrealized, is to diagnose every case at birth. For this reason, every newborn child should be examined for signs of hip instability. Where there is a family history of congenital dislocation, and with breech presentations, extra care is taken and the infant may have to be examined more than once.

Neonatal diagnosis

There are several ways of testing for instability. In *Ortolani's test*, the baby's thighs are held with the thumbs medially and the fingers resting on the greater trochanters; the hips are flexed to 90 degrees and gently abducted. Normally there is smooth abduction to almost 90 degrees. In congenital dislocation the movement is usually impeded, but if pressure is applied to the greater trochanter there is a soft 'clunk' as the dislocation reduces, and then the hip abducts fully (the 'jerk of entry'). If abduction stops halfway and there is no jerk of entry, there may be an irreducible dislocation.

Barlow's test is performed in a similar manner, but here the examiner's thumb is placed in the groin and, by grasping the upper thigh, an attempt is made to lever the femoral head in and out of the acetabulum during abduction and adduction. If the femoral head is normally in the reduced position, but can be made to slip out of the socket and back in again, the hip is classed as 'dislocatable' (i.e. unstable).

Every hip with signs of instability – however slight – should be examined by *ultrasonography.* This provides a dynamic assessment of the shape of the cartilaginous socket and the position of the femoral head.

Late features

Ideally, all children should be examined again at 6 months, 12 months and 18 months of age, so as to be sure that late-appearing signs of DDH are not missed. Occasionally dislocation does not occur until several months after birth.

Parents may notice that walking is delayed; in the most obvious cases the child walks with a limp. With unilateral dislocation, the skin creases

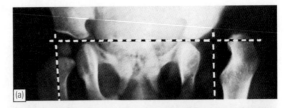
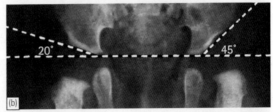
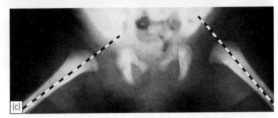
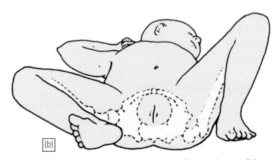

19.7 DDH – x-rays (a) The left hip is dislocated, the femoral head is underdeveloped and the acetabular roof slopes upwards much more steeply than on the right side. In this case the features are very obvious, but lesser changes can be gauged by geometrical tests. The epiphysis should lie medial to a vertical line which defines the outer edge of the acetabulum (Perkins' line) and below a horizontal line which passes through the triradiate cartilages (Hilgenreiner's line). (b) The acetabular roof angle should not exceed 30 degrees. (c) Von Rosen's lines: with the hips abducted 45 degrees, the femoral shafts should point into the acetabula. In each case the left side is shown to be abnormal.

are asymmetrical, the hip does not abduct fully and the leg is slightly short and rotated internally.

Bilateral dislocation is more difficult to detect because there is no asymmetry and the characteristic waddling gait may be mistaken for

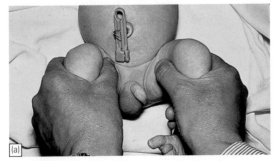

19.6 Developmental dysplasia of the hip (DDH) – early signs (a) Position of the hands for performing Ortolani's test. (b) Showing why abduction is limited.

normal toddling. However, the perineal gap is abnormally wide and abduction is limited.

X-ray examination is helpful in older children. The bony part of the acetabular roof slopes upwards abnormally and the socket is unusually shallow. The ossific centre of the femoral head is underdeveloped, and from its position it may be apparent that the head is displaced upwards and outwards.

Prognosis

Children in whom treatment is started only after the first year of life probably have no more than a 50 per cent chance of remaining free of trouble in later life.

Untreated, congenital dislocation leads to progressive deformity and disability, although with bilateral involvement, because the changes are symmetrical, disability is for some years less marked.

The earlier treatment is begun, the more likely is it that the child will develop a normal (or near-normal) hip. A good, modern health service should ensure that treatment is started within a week or two of birth; even then, careful follow-up is necessary to be certain that redislocation has not occurred and that the acetabulum is developing normally.

Treatment under 6 months of age

The simplest and safest policy is to regard all infants with a positive Ortolani or Barlow test as probably unstable and to nurse them in double napkins or with an abduction pillow between the legs for the first 6 weeks. At that stage they are re-examined: those with stable hips are left free but kept under observation for at least 6 months; those with persistent instability are treated by more formal abduction splintage (see below) until the hip is stable and x-ray shows that the acetabular roof is developing satisfactorily (usually 3–6 months).

Where facilities for ultrasound scanning are available, newborn infants with a high-risk background (a family history or extended breech delivery) or a suggestion of hip instability are examined by ultrasonography. If this shows that the hip is reduced and has a normal cartilaginous outline, no treatment is required, but the child is kept under observation for 3–6 months. If the anatomy is less than perfect, the hip is splinted in abduction and at 6 weeks ultrasound scanning is repeated. Some hips will now appear normal and these need no further treatment, apart from routine observation for 3–6 months. A few will show persistent abnormality, and for these, splintage is continued until a further scan at 3 months or an x-ray at 6 months shows a well-formed acetabular roof.

Splintage

It is crucial to ensure that the hip is properly reduced before it is splinted; this can be checked by ultrasound. The object is to hold the hips about 100 degrees flexed and somewhat abducted. Extreme positions are avoided and the joints should be allowed some movement in the splint. For the newborn, double napkins or a soft abduction pillow may suffice. For larger infants, the Pavlik harness is better.

Treatment of persistent dislocation: 6 months to 6 years

If, after early treatment, the hip is still incompletely reduced, or if the child presents late with a 'missed' dislocation, the hip must be reduced and held reduced until acetabular development is satisfactory.

Closed reduction

Manipulation under anaesthesia carries a high risk of femoral head necrosis. To minimize this risk, reduction must be gradual; traction is applied to both legs, preferably on a vertical frame, and abduction is gradually increased until, by 3 weeks, the legs are widely separated. This manoeuvre alone (aided if necessary by adductor tenotomy)

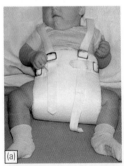
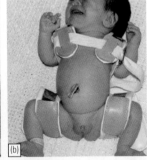
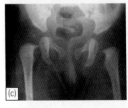
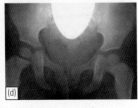

19.8 DDH – early treatment (a,b) Various types of abduction splint. (c,d) X-rays showing result of splintage for DDH of the right hip at 3 months and 18 months.

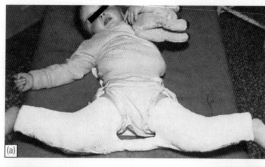

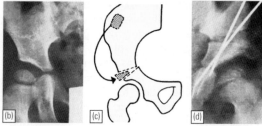

19.9 DDH – later treatment (a) Reduced open but stable only in medial rotation. If the femoral head remains poorly covered (b), this can be treated by innominate osteotomy (c,d).

may achieve stable, concentric reduction. Arthrography at this stage will show whether the femoral head is fully seated in the acetabulum.

Splintage

If concentrically reduced, the hips (both) are held in a plaster spica at 60 degrees of flexion, 40 degrees of abduction and 20 degrees of internal rotation. After 6 weeks, the plaster is replaced by a splint that prevents adduction but allows movement. Within a few months, x-rays may show a concentric femoral

head with a normal acetabular roof; if so, splintage is gradually discarded.

Open reduction

If, at any stage, concentric reduction has not been achieved, open operation is needed. Any obstruction is dealt with and the hip is reduced and held in a spica for 3 months. If reduction can be achieved only by markedly internally rotating the hip, a corrective osteotomy of the femur is carried out either at the time of open reduction or 6 weeks later. If the head, though reduced, is poorly covered, it should be provided with a bony roof – usually by repositioning the innominate bone and acetabulum (innominate osteotomy).

Treatment after the age of 6 years

For unilateral dislocation, operative reduction is still feasible, at least up to the age of 10; as in the former group, it may be necessary to combine this with corrective osteotomy of the femur or innominate osteotomy of the pelvis. In older children, the force needed for reduction may damage the hip and cause avascular necrosis, so it may be better to leave well alone and wait until pain and abnormal function call for further reconstructive surgery.

With bilateral dislocation, the deformity is symmetrical and therefore less noticeable; the risk of operative intervention is also greater because failure on one or other side results in asymmetrical deformity. Therefore, most surgeons avoid operation unless pain or deformity is unusually severe. The untreated patient waddles through life and may be surprisingly uncomplaining. However,

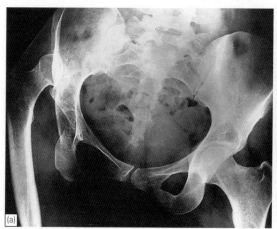

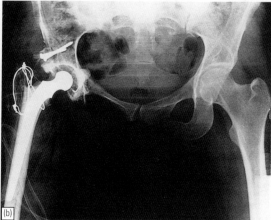

19.10 Untreated DDH (a) This patient, aged 35 years, had a short leg, a severe limp and back pain. (b) Hip replacement restored her to near normality.

if disability becomes severe, hip replacement may be justified.

ACETABULAR DYSPLASIA AND SUBLUXATION OF THE HIP

Acetabular dysplasia may be genetically determined or may follow incomplete reduction of a congenital dislocation, damage to the lateral acetabular epiphysis or maldevelopment of the femoral head. The socket is unusually shallow, the roof is sloping and there is deficient coverage of the femoral head; in some cases the hip subluxates. Faulty load transmission in the lateral part of the joint may lead to secondary osteoarthritis in later life.

Clinical features

During infancy, limited abduction of the hip is suspicious and ultrasonography may reveal a deficient acetabulum.

In children the condition is usually asymptomatic and discovered only when the pelvis is x-rayed for some other reason. Sometimes, however, the hip is painful – especially after strenuous activity – and the child may develop a limp. If there is subluxation, the Trendelenburg sign is positive, leg length may be asymmetrical and movement – particularly abduction in flexion – is restricted.

Adolescents and young adults may complain of pain over the lateral side of the hip, probably due to muscle fatigue and/or increased bone stress in the lateral part of the acetabulum. Some experience episodes of sharp pain in the groin, possibly the result of a labral tear or detachment. However, the majority go through life without experiencing really intrusive symptoms.

Older adults (those in their forties) may present with features of secondary osteoarthritis. Indeed, in Southern Europe dysplasia of the hip is the commonest cause of symptomatic osteoarthritis.

Imaging

X-rays should be taken lying and standing (the latter may show minor degrees of incongruity). The acetabulum looks shallow, the roof is sloping and the femoral head is uncovered. Lesser degrees of dysplasia are revealed by measuring the depth of the socket and the relationship between the centre of the femoral head and the edge of the acetabulum – Wiberg's centre-edge (CE) angle, which should be no less than 30 degrees. If the femoral head is displaced, Shenton's line will be broken.

CT and *MRI* are helpful when operative treatment is being considered. Three-dimensional CT reconstruction is particularly useful in providing an accurate picture of the anatomy.

Treatment

Infants with subluxation are treated as for dislocation: the hip is splinted in abduction until the acetabular roof looks normal.

Children and adolescents, provided the hip is reducible and congruent, often manage with no more than muscle strengthening exercises. If symptoms persist, they may need an operation to augment the acetabular roof, either a lateral shelf procedure or a pelvic osteotomy, both of which may be combined with a varus osteotomy of the proximal femur.

Adults with pain, weakness, instability and subluxation of the hip are candidates for one of the newer types of periacetabular osteotomy and three-dimensional reorientation of the entire hip. This involves cutting through the innominate bone, the ischium and the lateral part of the superior pubic ramus, so that the entire segment containing the acetabulum can be repositioned to cover the load-bearing part of the femoral head.

Patients with secondary osteoarthritis may need intertrochanteric osteotomy or total hip replacement.

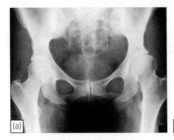 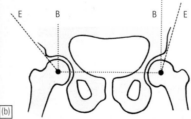 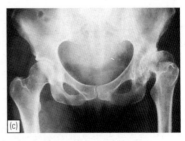

19.11 Acetabular dysplasia (a) X-ray showing a dysplastic left acetabulum. The socket is shallow and the roof sloping, leaving much of the femoral head uncovered. (b) Method of measuring Wiberg's centre-edge (CE) angle. (c) Left untreated, this sometimes progresses to severe osteoarthritis.

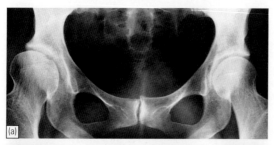

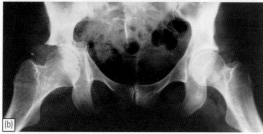

19.12 Acetabular reconstruction (a) Acetabular dysplasia of the right hip. (b) X-ray after innominate osteotomy.

ACQUIRED DISLOCATION OF THE HIP

Dislocation occurring after the first year of life is usually due to one of three causes: *pyogenic arthritis, muscle imbalance* or *trauma*.

Dislocation following sepsis

Pyogenic infection of the joint, whether primary or secondary to osteomyelitis of the femoral neck, carries a serious risk of enzymatic 'digestion' of the articular cartilage. In years gone by, septic arthritis in early childhood (when the epiphysis is still mainly cartilaginous) often resulted in partial or complete dissolution of the femoral head and dislocation of the hip – a so-called Tom Smith dislocation. On x-ray, the femoral head appears to be completely absent; however, part of it often survives, although it is too osteoporotic to be seen.

The dislocation should be treated by traction, followed, if necessary, by open reduction. In the absence of a femoral head, the greater trochanter can be placed in the acetabulum; varus osteotomy of the upper femur helps to achieve stability. Further reconstructive surgery may be needed in later life.

Dislocation due to muscle imbalance

Unbalanced paralysis in childhood may result in the hip abductors being weaker than the adductors. This is seen in cerebral palsy, in myelomeningocele and after poliomyelitis (see

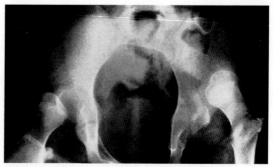

19.13 Acquired dislocation of the hip Muscle imbalance in a child with spina bifida has led to bilateral hip dislocation.

Chapter 10). The greater trochanter fails to develop properly, the femoral neck becomes valgus and the hip may subluxate or dislocate. Treatment is similar to that of very late congenital dislocation, but in addition some muscle rebalancing operation is essential.

Traumatic dislocation

Occasionally, dislocation of the hip is missed while attention is focused on some more distal (and more obvious) injury. Reduction is essential, if necessary by open operation; even if avascular necrosis or hip stiffness supervenes, a hip in the anatomical position presents an easier prospect for reconstructive surgery than one that remains persistently dislocated.

PROTRUSIO ACETABULI

In this condition the socket is too deep and bulges into the cavity of the pelvis. The 'primary' form shows a slight familial tendency. It affects females much more often than males and develops soon after puberty; at this stage there are usually no symptoms, although movements are limited. X-rays

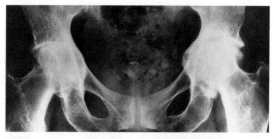

19.14 Protrusio acetabuli X-ray examination of the pelvis shows the typical bulging of the inner wall of the acetabulum on each side. The condition has been present since adolescence and has resulted in osteoarthritis.

show the sunken acetabulum, with the inner wall bulging beyond the iliopectineal line. Secondary osteoarthritis may develop in later life, but until then the condition does not require treatment.

Protrusio may occur in later life secondary to bone 'softening' disorders, such as osteomalacia or Paget's disease, and in long-standing cases of rheumatoid arthritis. If pain is severe, or movements are markedly restricted, joint replacement is indicated.

COXA VARA

The normal femoral neck-shaft angle is 160 degrees at birth, decreasing to 125 degrees in adult life. An angle of less than 120 degrees is called coxa vara. The deformity may be either congenital or acquired.

Congenital coxa vara

This is a rare disorder of infancy and early childhood. It is due to a defect of endochondral ossification in the medial part of the femoral neck. When the child starts to crawl or stand, the femoral neck bends or develops a stress fracture; with continued weight-bearing, it collapses increasingly into varus. Sometimes there is also shortening or bowing of the femoral shaft.

The condition is usually diagnosed when the child starts to walk. The leg is short and the thigh may be bowed. X-ray shows that the physeal line is too vertical; typically, in the infant, there is a separate triangular fragment of bone in the inferior portion of the metaphysis (Fairbank's triangle).

With bilateral coxa vara the patient may not be seen until he or she presents as a young adult with osteoarthritis.

If shortening is progressive, the deformity should be corrected by a subtrochanteric valgus osteotomy. Varus does not recur, but there may be some permanent shortening.

Acquired coxa vara

Coxa vara can develop at any age if the bone at the femoral neck gives way. This is seen in certain of the osteochondral dystrophies, in rickets, following severe grades of slipped femoral epiphysis and in adult osteomalacia. Malunited or ununited femoral neck fractures also may result in varus deformity of the femoral neck.

Often no treatment is required, but if the condition is troublesome, it can be improved by corrective intertochanteric or subtrochanteric osteotomy.

FEMORAL ANTEVERSION (IN-TOE GAIT)

The commonest cause of in-toe gait is excessive anteversion of the femoral neck, so that internal rotation of the hip is increased and external rotation diminished. The gait may look clumsy, but is no bar to athletic prowess and usually improves with growth. These children often sit on the floor in the 'television position' (with the knees facing each other), but should be encouraged to adopt the 'Buddha position'. Correction by osteotomy is feasible, but rarely indicated, and certainly not before the age of 8.

PERTHES' DISEASE (COXA PLANA)

Perthes' disease is a disorder of childhood characterized by necrosis of the femoral head. Although the incidence is only 1 in 10 000, it should always be considered in the differential diagnosis of hip pain in young children. Patients are usually 4–8 years old and often show delayed skeletal maturity; boys are affected four times as often as girls.

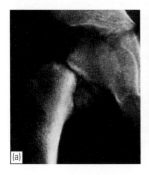 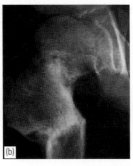 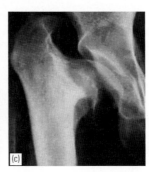

19.15 Infantile coxa vara (a) Typical x-ray features before displacement of the femoral neck. The physis is too vertical and there is a large triangular fragment of bone on the undersurface of the femoral neck. (b) Abduction osteotomy in a young patient with established coxa vara. (c) Untreated coxa vara.

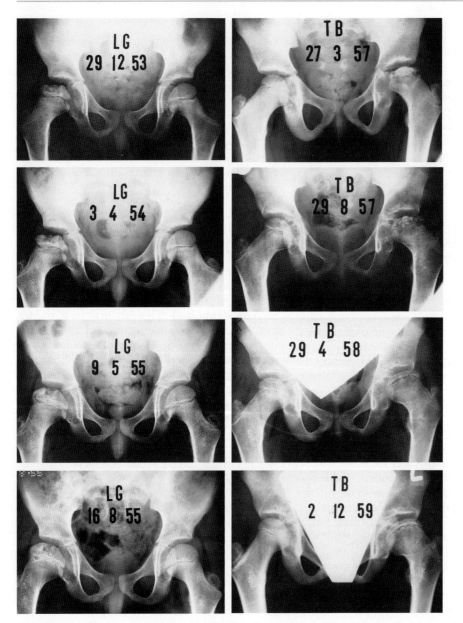

19.16 Perthes' disease – prognostic classification The Herring classification is based on the severity of structural disintegration of the lateral pillar of the femoral epiphysis. Column 1 shows the changes in a boy with moderately severe Perthes' disease of the right hip. Although the central part of the epiphyseal ossific centre seems to be 'fragmented', the lateral part of the epiphysis is intact throughout the natural progress of the disease. This is a favourable feature and serial x-rays show how the femoral head has gradually re-formed. Column 2 shows progressive changes in another young boy with severe Perthes' disease of the left hip. The epiphysis is widely involved from the outset, 'fragmentation' extends to the most lateral portion of the epiphysis and there is progressive flattening of the epiphysis resulting in permanent distortion of the femoral head.

Pathogenesis

Up to the age of 4 months, the femoral head is supplied by: (1) metaphyseal vessels which penetrate the growth disc; (2) lateral epiphyseal vessels running in the retinacula; and (3) scanty vessels in the ligamentum teres. The metaphyseal supply gradually declines until, by the age of 4 years, it has virtually disappeared; by the age of 7, however, the vessels in the ligamentum teres have developed. Between 4 and 7 years of age, the femoral head may depend for its blood supply almost entirely on the lateral epiphyseal vessels, whose situation in the retinacula makes them susceptible to stretching and to pressure from an effusion. The precipitating cause is probably an effusion into the hip joint following either trauma, of which there is a history in more than half the cases, or a non-specific synovitis.

Pathology

The pathological process takes 2–4 years to complete, passing through three stages.

Stage 1: bone death

Following one or more episodes of ischaemia, part of the bony femoral head dies; it still looks normal on plain x-ray but it stops enlarging.

Stage 2: revascularization and repair

New blood vessels enter the necrotic area and new bone is laid down on the dead trabeculae, producing the appearances of increased density on the x-ray. If only part of the epiphysis is involved and the repair process is rapid, the bony architecture may be completely restored.

Stage 3: distortion and remodelling

If a large part of the bony epiphysis is damaged, or the repair process is slow, the epiphysis may collapse and subsequent growth at the head and neck will be distorted. Sometimes the epiphysis ends up flattened ('coxa plana') but enlarged ('coxa magna') and the femoral head is incompletely covered by the acetabulum.

Clinical features

The patient – usually a boy of 4–8 years – complains of pain and starts to limp. The hip looks deceptively normal, although there may be a little wasting. Early on, the joint is irritable, so all movements are diminished and their extremes painful. Often the child is not seen till later, when most movements are full; but abduction is nearly always limited and usually internal rotation also.

X-rays

Even before x-ray changes appear, the ischaemic area can sometimes be demonstrated as a 'void' on radioisotope scanning. The earliest changes are increased density of the bony epiphysis and apparent widening of the joint space. Flattening, fragmentation and lateral displacement of the epiphysis follow, with rarefaction and broadening of the metaphysis. The picture varies with the age of the child, the extent of ischaemia and the stage of the disease.

Various prognostic grading systems are employed, based mainly on x-ray appearances. The one described by Herring is recommended (Herring JA: *Journal of Bone and Joint Surgery* 76A, 448–58, 1994) (see Fig. 19.16).

Differential diagnosis

The commonest cause of hip pain in children is a non-specific transient synovitis – the so-called *irritable hip*. Ultrasound may show a joint effusion, but the x-rays are always normal. Symptoms last for a week or two and clear up completely. The child should be kept in bed until pain disappears and the effusion resolves.

Treatment

As long as the hip is painful, the child should be in bed with skin traction applied to the affected leg. Once pain has subsided, which usually takes about 3 weeks, further treatment is dictated by an assessment of prognosis in each case.

Favourable prognostic signs are: (1) onset under the age of 6; (2) only partial involvement of the femoral head; (3) absence of metaphyseal rarefaction; and (4) normal femoral head shape.

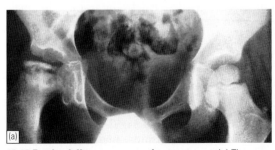 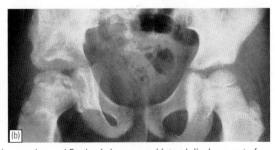

19.17 Perthes' disease – operative treatment (a) The x-ray shows advanced Perthes' changes and lateral displacement of the right femoral head. (b) Following an innominate osteotomy, the femoral head is much better 'contained' and, although not normal, is developing reasonably well.

Children in this category need no active treatment, though they should be followed up; 'supervised neglect' is an apt description.

Unfavourable signs are: (1) onset over the age of 6; (2) involvement of the whole femoral head; (3) severe metaphyseal rarefaction; and (4) lateral displacement of the femoral head. Children in this category need treatment by containment of the femoral head.

'Containment'

This means keeping the femoral head well seated within the acetabulum. Surrounded by its socket, it is more likely to retain its normal shape during the period of healing and remodelling. Containment can be achieved by holding the hips widely abducted in plaster or in a removable splint until the bone changes have run their course (at least a year). This is so encumbering that most orthopaedic surgeons nowadays prefer to achieve the same effect by performing a varus osteotomy of the femur or an innominate osteotomy of the pelvis (Fig. 19.17).

In those with the very worst x-ray changes, the outcome is dubious whatever the treatment, so some surgeons prefer not to subject such children to unrewarding splintage or operation.

SLIPPED UPPER FEMORAL EPIPHYSIS

Displacement of the proximal femoral epiphysis – also known as *epiphysiolysis* – is uncommon and virtually confined to children going through the pubertal growth spurt. Boys are affected more often than girls.

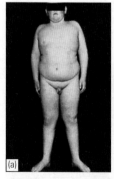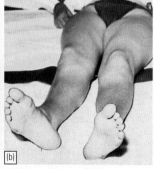

19.18 Slipped epiphysis – clinical features (a) This boy complained only of pain in his right knee. His build is unmistakable and the resting posture of his right lower limb tends towards external rotation (b). On examination, abduction and internal rotation were restricted.

Cause and pathology

A slipped epiphysis is, to all intents and purposes, an insufficiency fracture through the hypertrophic zone of the cartilaginous growth plate. Trauma may be the precipitating cause, but often an underlying abnormality predisposes to slipping. The disorder occurs around puberty, and often in very tall children or very fat children with delayed gonadal development. Perhaps this means that these children have an imbalance between pituitary growth hormone (which stimulates bone growth) and gonadal hormone (which promotes physeal fusion). Thus, during the pubertal growth spurt, the relatively immature physis might be too weak to resist the stress imposed by the increased body weight.

Clinical features

The patient – usually a boy of 14 or 15 years – presents with pain in the groin, the anterior part of the thigh or the knee (referred pain); he may also limp. The onset may be sudden and in 30 per cent there is a history of trauma ('acute slip'). However, in the majority, symptoms are protracted ('chronic slip'), or else a long period of pain may culminate in a sudden climax following minor trauma ('acute-on-chronic slip'). Two-thirds of the patients are fat and sexually underdeveloped, or unusually tall and thin.

On examination, the leg is externally rotated and is 1 or 2 cm short. Characteristically there is limitation of abduction and medial (internal) rotation. Following an acute slip, the hip is irritable and all movements are accompanied by pain.

X-rays

Even when slipping is trivial, changes can be seen. In the anteroposterior view the epiphyseal plate seems to be too wide and too 'woolly'. A line drawn along the superior surface of the neck remains superior to the head instead of passing through it *(Trethowan's sign)*. In the lateral view the femoral epiphysis is tilted backwards; small degrees of tilt can be detected by measuring the angle between the epiphyseal base and the femoral neck (see Fig. 19.19).

Complications

Avascular necrosis is the most serious complication. It is seen only after a slip has been reduced or pinned, and is presumably due to the remaining leash of vessels being damaged.

Coxa vara deformity may result if the displacement is not reduced and the epiphysis fuses in its deformed position. The patient limps but the condition is usually painless. Osteotomy

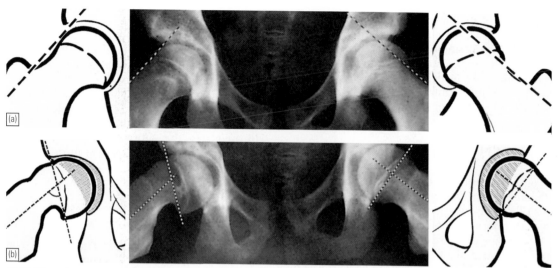

19.19 Slipped epiphysis – x-rays Careful x-ray examination is the key to diagnosis: even minute differences between the two sides may be important. In the anteroposterior view (a) Trethowan's line passes just above the femoral head on the right but cuts through the superior part of the femoral head on the left (normal) sign. The lateral view (b) is diagnostically more reliable; even minor degrees of slip can be shown by drawing lines through the base of the epiphysis and up the middle of the femoral neck – if the angle indicated is less than 90 degrees, the epiphysis has slipped posteriorly.

may be needed to correct the deformity and in the hope of preventing secondary osteoarthritis.

Slipping at the opposite hip occurs in a third of cases – sometimes while the patient is in bed. Forewarned is forearmed: at the least suspicion of symptoms, the epiphysis should be pinned.

Secondary osteoarthritis is a likely sequel if displacement has not been reduced, and inevitable if there has been avascular necrosis.

Treatment

Manipulation is dangerous and should be avoided.

Minor displacement

Displacement of less than one-third the width of the epiphysis is treated by accepting the position and

fixing the epiphysis with two thin threaded pins or screws. This is always done under x-ray control.

Moderate displacement

Displacements of one-third to one-half the epiphyseal width can often be treated by pinning alone. With further growth, the proximal femur may be remodelled to an acceptable degree; if this does not happen, the residual deformity can be corrected later by an osteotomy lower down.

Severe displacement

If the displacement is more than half the epiphyseal width, corrective surgery will be needed. In skilled hands this can be achieved by exposing the slip, removing a small piece of the femoral neck in order

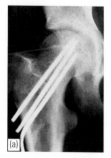
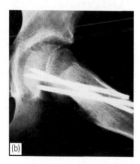
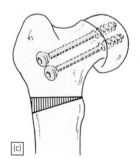
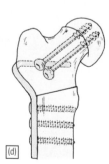

19.20 Slipped epiphysis – treatment (a,b) In this case slipping was minimal so no reduction was attempted, but further slipping was prevented by pinning the epiphysis in that position. (c,d) In more severe degrees of slip, the epiphysis should be fixed without attempting reduction and then, at a later stage, a complex compensatory osteotomy (d) can be performed to restore the normal position of the limb.

to permit replacement of the epiphysis, and pinning. A safer method is to fix the epiphysis in the displaced position and follow this some time later with a compensatory osteotomy lower down. The femur is divided just below the greater trochanter; the distal fragment is repositioned and fixed in valgus, flexion and medial rotation.

PYOGENIC ARTHRITIS

Pyogenic arthritis of the hip is usually seen in children under the age of 2 years. The organism (usually a staphylococcus) reaches the joint either directly from a distant focus or by local spread from osteomyelitis of the femur. Unless the infection is rapidly aborted, the femoral head, which is largely cartilaginous at this age, is liable to be destroyed by the proteolytic enzymes of bacteria and pus.

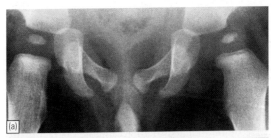
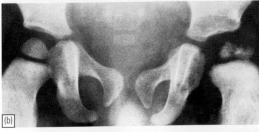
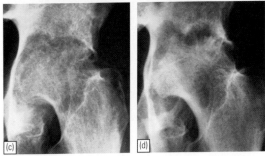

19.21 Pyogenic arthritis (a,b) *In an infant:* the left hip is distended and the head is drifting out of the socket. Six months later the epiphysis appears to be necrotic. (c,d) *In an adult:* rapid bone destruction over a period of 3 weeks!

Clinical features

The child is ill and in pain, but it is often difficult to tell exactly where the pain is! The affected limb may be held absolutely still and all attempts at moving the hip are resisted. With care and patience, it may be possible to localize a point of maximum tenderness over the hip; the diagnosis is confirmed by aspirating pus from the joint.

In neonates the most common presenting feature is a total lack of movement in the affected limb (pseudoparalysis). Local signs of inflammation are usually absent and blood tests are often normal.

X-rays

During the acute stage of bone infection, x-rays may show slight lateral displacement of the femoral head, suggesting the presence of a joint effusion. Ultrasound scans also will help to reveal a joint effusion. In children the epiphysis may become necrotic and later appear unusually dense or 'fragmented' on x-ray. In adults the defining feature is rapidly progressive erosion of the articular surfaces.

Treatment

Antibiotics should be given as soon as the diagnosis is reasonably certain, but not before obtaining a sample of joint fluid (or pus) for microbiological investigation and testing for antibiotic sensitivity. The joint is aspirated under general anaesthesia and, if pus is withdrawn, arthrotomy is advisable; antibiotics are instilled locally and the wound is closed without drainage. The hip is kept on traction or splinted in abduction until all evidence of disease activity has disappeared.

TUBERCULOSIS

The disease may start as a synovitis, or as an osteomyelitis in one of the adjacent bones. Once arthritis develops, destruction is rapid and may result in pathological dislocation. Healing usually leaves a fibrous ankylosis with considerable limb shortening and deformity.

Clinical features

Pain in the hip is the usual presenting symptom, though in late, neglected cases a cold abscess may point in the thigh or buttock. The patient walks with a limp; muscle wasting may be obvious and joint movements are limited and painful.

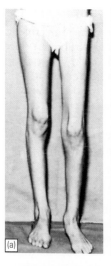

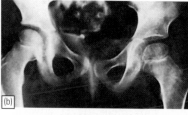

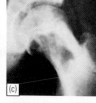

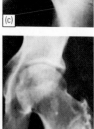

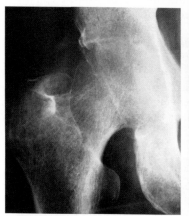

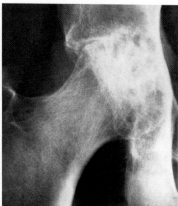

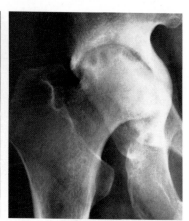

19.22 Tuberculous arthritis
(a) This patient presented with pain in the left hip. (b) The x-ray shows rarefaction of the bones on either side of the hip joint, a typical feature of an inflammatory disorder of the joint. (c) Localized abscess in the femoral neck. (d) Advanced tuberculosis causing joint destruction and marked cystic erosion of the bones on both sides of the joint.
(e) Trochanteric infection, which rarely extends to the joint.

19.23 Hip tuberculosis – drug treatment In this patient, anti-tuberculous drugs alone resulted in healing – though hip movements were still restricted.

X-rays

The first x-ray change is general rarefaction of bone around the hip, a sign of inflammatory joint disease. In a child, the femoral epiphysis may be enlarged, again suggestive of chronic synovitis. Later changes are erosion and eventually destruction of the articular surfaces on both sides of the joint. The resemblance to rheumatoid arthritis is liable to lead to misdiagnosis in areas where tuberculosis is uncommon. A more unusual radiographic feature is the appearance of a bone abscess in the femoral neck or the greater trochanter.

Complications

Early disease may heal leaving a normal or almost normal hip. However, if the joint is destroyed, the usual result is an unsound fibrous ankylosis. The leg is scarred and thin, and shortening is likely to be severe.

Treatment

If the disease is caught early, anti-tuberculous chemotherapy should result in healing. During the acute phase, the joint may need to be splinted in abduction or held in traction until the symptoms subside. An abscess in the femoral neck is best evacuated. After the disease subsides the patient is got up, but chemotherapy should be continued for several months (see Chapter 2).

If the joint has been destroyed, arthrodesis may become necessary, but usually not before the age of 14. In adults joint replacement is feasible.

RHEUMATOID ARTHRITIS

The hip joint is frequently affected in rheumatoid arthritis. The hallmark of the disease is progressive bone destruction on both sides of the joint without any reactive osteophyte formation.

Clinical features

Usually the patient already has rheumatoid disease affecting many joints. Pain in the groin comes on insidiously; limp, though common, may be ascribed to pre-existing arthritis of the foot or knee. With advancing disease the patient has difficulty getting into or out of a chair, and even movement in bed may be painful.

Wasting of the buttock and thigh is often marked, and the limb is usually held in external rotation and fixed flexion. All movements are restricted and painful.

X-rays

During the early stages there is osteoporosis and diminution of the joint space; later, the acetabulum and femoral head are eroded. In the worst cases (and especially in patients on corticosteroids) there is gross bone destruction and the floor of the acetabulum may be perforated.

Treatment

If the disease can be arrested by general treatment, hip deterioration may be slowed down. But once cartilage and bone are eroded, no treatment will influence the progression to joint destruction. Total joint replacement is then the best answer. It relieves pain and restores a useful range of movement. It is advocated even in younger patients, because the polyarthritis so limits activity that the implants are not unduly stressed.

OSTEOARTHRITIS

Osteoarthritis is the commonest non-traumatic disorder of the hip in middle and late age. Usually no specific 'cause' is identified, but in younger patients (those under the age of 40) osteoarthritis may appear as a sequel to acetabular dysplasia, coxa vara, Perthes' disease or slipped epiphysis. Secondary osteoarthritis is also seen in older patients after rheumatoid arthritis, avascular necrosis or Paget's disease.

Pathology

The articular cartilage becomes soft and fibrillated whilst the underlying bone shows cyst formation and sclerosis. These changes are most marked in the

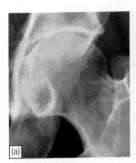
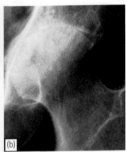
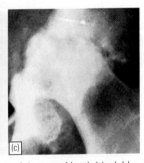

19.24 Rheumatoid arthritis Three stages in the development of rheumatoid arthritis: (a) loss of joint space; (b) erosion of the bone after cartilage has disappeared; (c) perforation of the acetabular floor – such marked destruction is more likely to occur if the patient is being treated with corticosteroids. Note how similar these changes are to those of tuberculous arthritis (Figure 19.23).

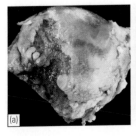
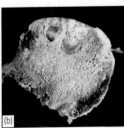
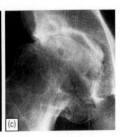

19.25 Osteoarthritis (a,b) Pathology – loss of articular cartilage over the dome of the femoral head and osteophyte formation around the periphery. Subarticular cysts are seen in the coronal section (b). These features are well demonstrated in the x-ray (c).

area of maximal loading (chiefly the top of the joint); at the margins of the joint there are the characteristic osteophytes. Synovial hypertrophy and capsular fibrosis may account for joint stiffness.

Clinical features

Pain is felt in the groin but may radiate to the knee. Typically it occurs after periods of activity, but later it is more constant and sometimes disturbs sleep. Stiffness at first is noticed chiefly after rest; later it increases progressively until putting on socks and shoes becomes difficult. Limp is often noticed early and, if the hip is adducted, the patient may think the leg is getting shorter.

The patient is usually fit and over 50, but secondary osteoarthritis can occur at 30 or even 20. There may be an obvious limp and, except in early cases, a positive Trendelenburg sign. The affected leg usually lies in external rotation and adduction, so it appears short; there is nearly always some fixed flexion, although this may only be revealed by Thomas' test. Muscle wasting is detectable but rarely severe. Deep pressure may elicit tenderness, and the greater trochanter is somewhat high and posterior. Movements, though often painless within a limited range, are restricted.

X-rays

The earliest sign is a decreased joint space (loss of articular cartilage), usually maximal in the superior weight-bearing region but sometimes affecting the entire joint. Later signs are subarticular sclerosis, cyst formation and osteophytes at the edges of the joint. There may also be tell-tale signs of previous abnormalities dating back to childhood or adolescence.

Treatment

Analgesics and anti-inflammatory drugs are helpful, and warmth is soothing. The patient is encouraged to use a walking stick (held in the opposite hand) and to try to preserve movement and stability by performing exercises within the range of comfort. Joint manipulation sometimes relieves pain for long periods.

Patients should be advised on ways of changing their lifestyle so as reduce impact loading on the affected hip: e.g. cutting down on uphill walking, climbing up and down stairs, carrying heavy weights or even sitting in one position for very

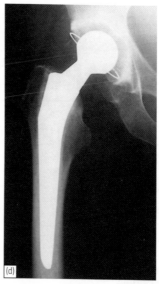

19.26 Osteoarthritis – treatment X-ray appearance after total hip replacement.

long periods. Functional aids will help with daily activities such as bathing and dressing. Of course none of these measures will restore damaged cartilage, but they will lessen the patient's symptoms.

Operative treatment

Details of operative treatment can be found in Chapter 12. The indications for surgery are relentlessly intrusive pain, a progressive decrease in joint movements, increasing difficulty with activities of daily living and x-ray signs of progressive joint deterioration. The procedure of choice will usually be *total joint replacement*, especially if the patient is over 50 years of age and unlikely to stress the hip excessively during his or her remaining lifetime. In experienced hands the results are likely to be good over a period of 15–20 years, but the patient should be warned that failures do occur and may necessitate revision of the arthroplasty. For younger patients, who will probably need at least one revision during their remaining lifetime, other procedures are worth considering. If the hip is dysplastic and a significant area of articular cartilage still preserved, a repositioning osteotomy may buy 5–10 years of satisfactory function, by which time a total hip replacement may be more suitable.

CHAPTER 20

THE KNEE

CLINICAL ASSESSMENT

HISTORY

Pain is the most common knee symptom, so much so that in young patients the term 'anterior knee pain' has become a virtual diagnosis in itself. With inflammatory or degenerative disorders it is usually diffuse, but with mechanical disorders (and especially after injury) it is often localized – the patient can, and should, point to the painful spot. If he or she can remember the mechanism of the injury, this is extremely useful.

Swelling may be localized or diffuse. If there was an injury, it is important to ask whether the swelling appeared immediately (suggesting a haemarthrosis) or only after some hours (typical of a torn meniscus). Chronic swelling is usually due to synovitis or arthritis.

Stiffness also is common. Ask whether it fluctuates and when it feels worse or better. Early morning stiffness suggests an inflammatory disorder; stiffness after periods of inactivity is typical of osteoarthritis.

Locking is an ambiguous term. The joint is not really 'locked' in the sense that it cannot move at all. One minute it moves perfectly well and the next it can still flex as before but it cannot extend fully; something has got jammed between the articular surfaces (usually a torn meniscus or loose body). *Unlocking* is even more suggestive: the obstructing object has moved and the joint can now move freely again.

Three causes of:
Giving way
Torn meniscus
Torn ligaments
Unstable patella
Acute swelling
Synovitis
Haemarthrosis
Septic arthritis
Chronic swelling
Rheumatoid arthritis
Osteoarthritis
Tuberculosis

Deformity, especially if it is of recent onset, is quickly noticed. It may be unilateral or bilateral: *valgus* or *varus, fixed flexion* or *hyperextension.* Knock-knees and bandy-legs are common in children and usually correct spontaneously as the child grows.

Giving way can be due to muscle weakness, but more often it is caused by a mechanical disorder such as a torn meniscus or a faulty patellar extensor mechanism.

Loss of function manifests as a progressively diminishing walking distance, inability to run and difficulty going up and down steps.

Pain in the knee: check the hip as well – it could be referred pain.

SIGNS WITH THE PATIENT UPRIGHT

Valgus or *varus deformity* is best seen with the patient standing. Symmetrical knock-knee and bow-legs can, of course, be normal variations; unilateral deformities, especially if progressive, are much more significant. The patient should be observed walking, noting any instability or limp.

SIGNS WITH THE PATIENT LYING SUPINE

Look

The first thing that strikes you is the *position of the knee (or knees):* it may lie in valgus or varus, partially flexed or hyperextended. *Swelling* also may be obvious. Then look more closely for *old scars* or *sinuses,* and for small *lumps.*

Wasting of the quadriceps is a sure sign of joint disorder. The visual impression can be checked by *measuring* the girth of the thigh at the same level (e.g. a fixed distance above the joint line or a hand's breadth above the patella) in each limb.

Feel

Increased *warmth* is detected by comparing the two knees. The 'temperature gradient' can also be felt by running a hand down the length of the limb: normally there is a linear decrease in warmth from proximal to distal.

The *soft tissues* and *bony outlines* are then palpated systematically, feeling for abnormal outlines and localized tenderness. This is easier if the knee is bent and the examiner sits on the edge of the couch facing the knee. By placing both hands over the front of the knee, the anatomical outlines of the joint margins, the patellar ligament, the collateral ligaments, the iliotibial band and the pes anserinus are then easily traced with the fingers. The knee is then placed flat on the couch (extended) and the edges of the patellofemoral joint are palpated while pushing the patella first to one side and then to the other

Synovial thickening is best appreciated as follows: placing the knee in extension, the examiner grasps the edges of the patella in a pincer made of the thumb and middle finger, and tries to lift the patella forwards; normally the bone can be grasped quite firmly, but if the synovium is thickened, the fingers simply slip off the edges of the patella.

Move

Normally the knee flexes until the calf meets the ham, and extends completely with a snap; even slight loss of extension – or 'springiness' on attempting it – is important. While moving the knee, feel for crepitus – a sign of patellofemoral degeneration or wear.

Tests for intra-articular fluid

Cross-fluctuation

This test is applicable only if there is a large joint effusion. The left hand compresses and empties the suprapatellar pouch while the right hand straddles the front of the joint below the patella; by squeezing with each hand alternately, a fluid impulse is transmitted across the joint.

The patellar tap

The suprapatellar pouch is compressed with the left hand, while the index finger of the right hand pushes the patella sharply backwards; with a positive test, the patella can be felt striking the femur and bouncing off again.

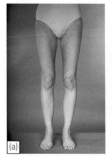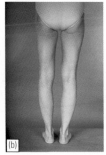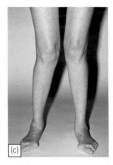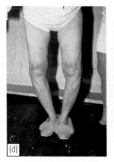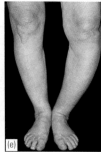

20.1 Examination standing (a,b) Look at the general shape and posture, first from in front and then from behind. Normally the knees are in slight valgus. Look for swelling of the joint or wasting of the thigh muscles; quadriceps wasting occurs very quickly. (c) This patient has rheumatoid arthritis and bilateral valgus deformities; in contrast, osteoarthritis is likely to lead to varus deformities (d); unilateral deformity is easier to notice and almost always pathological – this man has Paget's disease of the tibia (e).

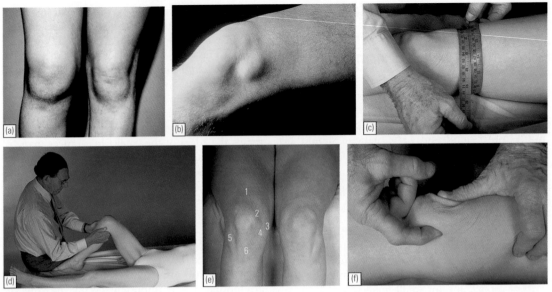

20.2 Examination with the patient supine Swelling may either involve the whole joint, as in this patient (a) with acute synovitis, or may be due to some localized lesion, as in patient (b) with a large loose body in the joint. (c) Muscle wasting can be diagnosed by measuring the thigh girth at a fixed distance above the joint line of the knee and comparing the two sides. (d) This is the best position for feeling for tenderness. Important points are marked in (e): (1) quadriceps tendon, (2) edge of patella, (3) medial collateral ligament, (4) joint line, (5) lateral collateral ligament, (6) patellar ligament. (f) By pushing the patella to one or other side of the mid-line, one can feel under its edge.

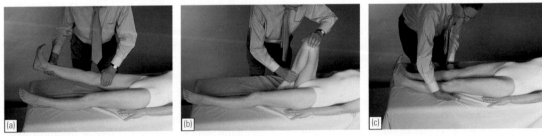

20.3 Movement The knee should move from full extension (a) through a range of 150 degrees to full flexion (b). Small degrees of flexion deformity (loss of full extension) can be detected by placing the hands under the knees while the patient forces the legs down on the couch (c); if your hand can be extracted more easily on one side than the other, this indicates loss of the final few degrees of complete extension.

The bulge test

This is useful when very little fluid is present. The medial compartment is emptied by pressing on that side of the joint whilst at the same time the suprapatellar pouch is kept closed by the other hand; the first hand is then lifted away from the medial side and moved to the lateral side, which is then sharply compressed; a distinct ripple is seen on the flattened medial surface.

The patellar hollow test

When the normal knee is flexed, a hollow appears lateral to the patellar ligament and disappears with further flexion; with excess fluid, the hollow fills and disappears at a lesser angle of flexion.

Patellar tests

The patellar friction test

Rubbing the patella against the femoral trochlea may be painful. Another way of testing for patellofemoral pain is to press against the patella and ask the patient to contract the quadriceps muscles.

The apprehension test

Pressing the patella laterally with the thumb while flexing the knee slightly may induce intense anxiety and resistance to further movement. This is diagnostic of recurrent patellar subluxation or dislocation.

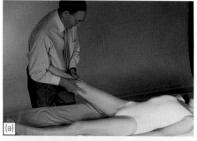
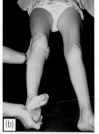
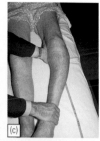
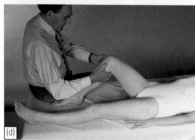
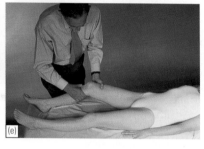

20.4 Testing for instability There are two ways of testing the collateral ligaments (side-to-side stability): (a) by gripping the foot close to your body and guiding the knee alternately towards valgus and varus; (b) by gripping the femoral condyles (provided your hand is big enough) and then forcing the leg alternately into valgus and varus. (c) In this case there was gross instability on the lateral side, allowing the knee to be pulled into marked varus. Cruciate ligament instability can be assessed by either the drawer test (d) or the Lachman test (e), as described in the text.

Tests for ligamentous stability

The *medial* and *lateral ligaments* are tested by stressing the knee into valgus and varus: this is best done by tucking the patient's foot under your arm and supporting the knee firmly with one hand on each side of the joint; the leg is then angulated alternately towards abduction and adduction. The test is performed at 30 degrees of flexion and again at full extension. There is normally some mediolateral movement at 30 degrees, but if this is excessive (compared to the normal side), it suggests a torn or stretched collateral ligament.

The *cruciate ligaments* are tested by examining for abnormal gliding movements in the anteroposterior plane. With both knees flexed 90 degrees and the feet resting on the couch, the upper tibia is inspected from the side; if its upper end has dropped back, or can be gently pushed back, this indicates a tear of the posterior cruciate ligament (the 'sag sign'). With the knee in the same position, the foot is anchored by the examiner sitting on it (provided this is not painful); then, using both hands, the upper end of the tibia is grasped firmly and rocked backwards and forwards to see if there is any anteroposterior glide (the *drawer test*). When doing this, make sure that the hamstrings are relaxed. Excessive anterior movement (a positive anterior drawer sign) denotes anterior cruciate laxity; excessive posterior movement (a positive posterior drawer sign) signifies posterior cruciate laxity. More sensitive is the *Lachman test:* the patient's knee is flexed 20 degrees; with one hand grasping the lower thigh and the other the upper part of the leg, the joint surfaces are shifted backwards and forwards upon each other. If the knee is stable, there should be no gliding.

SIGNS WITH THE PATIENT LYING PRONE

Scars or lumps in the popliteal fossa are noted. If there is a swelling, is it in the midline (most likely a bulging capsule) or to one side (possibly a bursa)? A semimembranosus bursa is usually just above the joint line, a Baker's cyst below it. (The joint line is located about a finger's breadth below the flexion crease.)

The soft tissues are carefully palpated. If there is a lump, where does it originate? Does it pulsate? Can it be emptied into the joint?

Apley's test

The knee is flexed to 90 degrees and rotated while a compression force is applied; this, the *grinding test,* reproduces symptoms if a meniscus is torn.

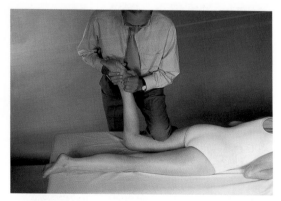

20.5 Apley's test The knee is flexed to 90 degrees and rotated while applying first a compression force and then a distraction force. Pain and/or clicking on compression is suggestive of a meniscal lesion.

Rotation is then repeated while the leg is pulled upwards with the surgeon's knee holding the thigh down; this, the *distraction test,* produces increased pain only if there is ligament damage.

Imaging

Anteroposterior and lateral views are standard, but sometimes patellofemoral (or skyline) and intercondylar (or tunnel) views are needed. MRI is useful in doubtful meniscal or ligament injuries.

Arthroscopy

Arthroscopy is useful: (1) to establish or refine the accuracy of diagnosis; (2) to help in deciding whether to operate, or to plan the operative approach with more precision; (3) to record the progress of a knee disorder; and (4) to perform certain operative procedures. Arthroscopy is not a substitute for clinical examination: a detailed history and meticulous assessment of the physical signs are indispensable preliminaries and remain the sheet anchor of diagnosis.

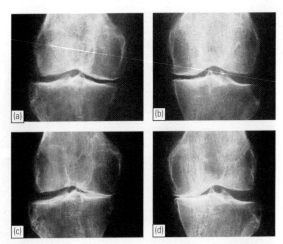

20.6 X-rays Anteroposterior views should always be taken with the patient standing. (a,b) X-rays with the patient lying down show only slight narrowing of the medial joint space on each side; but with weight-bearing (c,d) it is clear that these changes are much more marked.

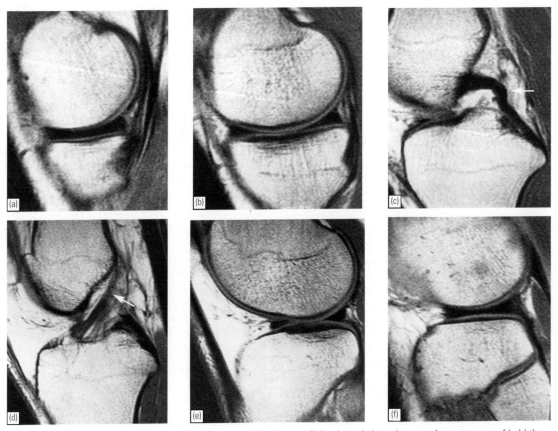

20.7 MRI A series of saggital T_1-weighted images proceeding from medial to lateral show the normal appearances of (a,b) the medial meniscus, (c) the posterior cruciate ligament, (d) the somewhat fan-shaped anterior cruciate ligament and (e,f) the lateral meniscus.

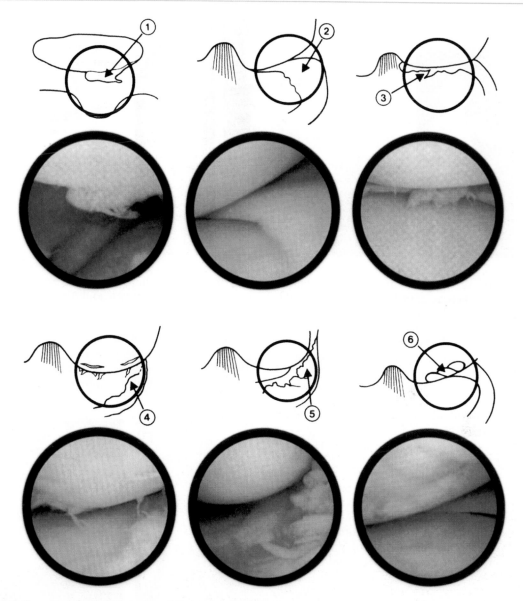

20.8 Arthroscopy Arthroscopic images of the interior of the right knee from the lateral side, showing (1) chrondomalacia patellae; (2) normal medial meniscus; (3) torn medial meniscus; (4) degenerate medial meniscus and osteoarthritic femoral condyle; (5) rheumatoid synovium; (6) osteochondritis dissecans of medial femoral condyle.

BOW-LEGS (GENU VARUM) AND KNOCK-KNEES (GENU VALGUM)

By the end of growth, the knees are normally in 5–7 degrees of valgus. Theoretically, anything more or less than that would be classed as deformity, though often it bothers nobody unless it is unilateral, of recent onset or progressive.

In practice, deformity is usually gauged from simple observation; this is best done with the patient standing and bearing weight. Bilateral *genu*

varum (bow-leg) can be recorded by measuring the distance between the knees with the legs straight and the medial malleoli just touching; it should be less than 6 cm. Similarly, *genu valgum* (knock-knee) can be estimated by measuring the distance between the medial malleoli when the knees are held touching with the patellae facing forwards; it is usually less than 8 cm.

In children these deformities are so common that they are considered to be normal stages of development; most correct spontaneously by the

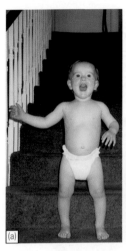
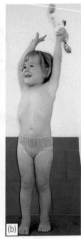
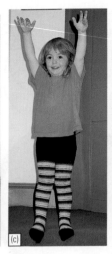
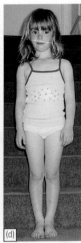

(a) (b) (c) (d)

20.9 Bow-legs and knock-knees in children Two sisters with natural self-correcting 'deformities' of the knees. (a,b) Tamzin at 1½ and 2½ years; (c,d) Jessy at 3 and 4½ years.

age of 10–12. Treatment is unnecessary, but the parents should be reassured and the child should be seen at intervals of 6 months to record progress. In the occasional case where, by the age of 10, the deformity is still marked, operative correction should be advised. This can be done by stapling one side of the physis to slow growth on that side (epiphyseodesis), or at a later stage by osteotomy.

Bone dysplasias and rickets are associated with more intractable deformities which are likely to need operative correction.

Blount's disease is particularly challenging. This is a progressive bow-leg deformity associated with abnormal growth of the posteromedial part of the proximal tibia. Children are often overweight and start walking early; deformity is usually bilateral and may include a rotational element. X-rays show characteristic features such as abnormal flattening or sloping of the medial half of the epiphysis. Spontaneous resolution is rare and operative correction is usually needed.

Valgus and varus deformities in adults – especially if they are unilateral or asymmetrical – are likely to be secondary to disorders such as joint injury, rheumatoid arthritis (usually valgus) or osteoarthritis (usually varus). Slight degrees of bow-leg and knock-knee are well tolerated, but if the deformity is marked or associated with instability, it can be corrected by joint reconstruction or osteotomy (supracondylar femoral for valgus deformity and proximal tibial for varus).

LESIONS OF THE MENISCI

MENISCAL TEARS

The menisci have an important role in (1) increasing the stability of the knee, (2) control-

ling the complex rolling and gliding actions of the joint and (3) distributing load during movement.

Tears are common in young adults. The meniscus is split in its length by a force grinding it between the femur and the tibia. In the young this usually occurs when weight is being taken on the flexed knee and there is a twisting strain; hence the frequency in footballers. In middle life, when

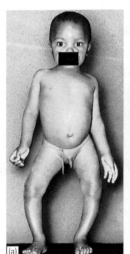
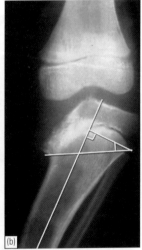

(a) (b)

20.10 Blount's disease In contrast to the children in Figure 20.9, this young boy developed progressive bow-legged deformities from the time he started walking. X-rays showed the typical features of Blount's disease: marked distortion of the tibial epiphysis, as if one half of the growth plate (physis) had fused and stopped growing. Changes can be accurately assessed by measuring the *metaphyseo-diaphyseal angle*: a line is drawn perpendicular to the long axis of the tibia and another across the metaphyseal flare, as shown on the x-ray; the acute angle formed by these two lines should normally not exceed 11 degrees.

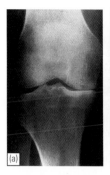
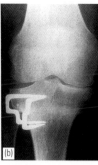
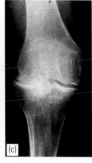
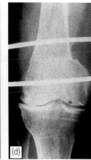

20.11 Osteotomy (a,b) For varus deformity, a high tibial osteotomy is the most effective. (c,d) For valgus deformity, the osteotomy should be on the femoral side of the joint.

fibrosis has restricted mobility of the meniscus, tears occur with relatively little force.

The medial meniscus is affected far more frequently than the lateral, partly because its attachments to the capsule make it less mobile. Different patterns of tears are recognized.

- *Bucket-handle tears* are when the split is vertical but runs along part of the circumference of the meniscus, creating a loose sliver still attached anteriorly and posteriorly. The torn sliver sometimes displaces towards the centre of the joint and becomes jammed between femur and tibia, causing a block to extension ('locking').
- *Horizontal tears* are usually 'degenerative' or due to repetitive minor trauma. Some are associated with meniscal cysts.

Most of the meniscus is avascular, and spontaneous repair does not occur unless the tear is in the outer third, which is vascularized from the capsule. The loose tag acts as a mechanical irritant, giving rise to recurrent synovial effusion and, in some cases, secondary osteoarthritis.

Clinical features

The patient is usually a young person who sustains a twisting injury to the knee on the sports field. Pain is often severe and further activity is avoided; occasionally the knee is 'locked' in partial flexion. Almost invariably, swelling appears some hours later, or perhaps the following day.

With rest, the initial symptoms subside, only to recur periodically after trivial twists or strains. Sometimes the knee gives way spontaneously and this is again followed by pain and swelling.

It is important to remember that in patients aged over 40 the initial injury may be unremarkable and the main complaint is of recurrent 'giving way' or 'locking'.

'Locking' – that is, the sudden inability to extend the knee fully – suggests a bucket-handle tear. The patient sometimes learns to 'unlock' the knee by bending it fully or by twisting it from side to side.

On examination, the joint may be held slightly flexed and there is often an effusion. In late presentations, the quadriceps will be wasted. Tenderness is localized to the joint line, in the vast majority of cases on the medial side. Flexion is usually full but extension is often slightly limited.

Between attacks of pain and effusion there is a disconcerting paucity of signs. The history is helpful, and Apley's grinding test may be positive.

Investigations

Imaging

Plain x-rays are normal but MRI is a reliable method for confirming the diagnosis, and may even reveal tears that are missed by arthroscopy.

Arthroscopy

Arthroscopy has the advantage that, if a lesion is identified, it can be treated at the same time. You have to be certain, though, that the lesion which you can see is the one causing the patient's symptoms!

Treatment

In the past, meniscal tears were treated by open operation. Nowadays arthroscopic surgery is preferable. For peripheral tears, operative repair is feasible. In other cases, the displaced portion should be cleanly excised. Postoperative physiotherapy is an important part of the treatment.

MENISCAL CYSTS

A meniscal cyst can be likened to a ganglion, inasmuch as it contains gelatinous fluid and is surrounded by fibrous tissue, but in reality it is distinct. It is probably traumatic in origin, arising from either a small horizontal tear or repeated squashing of the peripheral part of the meniscus.

The patient presents with pain, and a small lump can be seen and felt, usually on the lateral side of

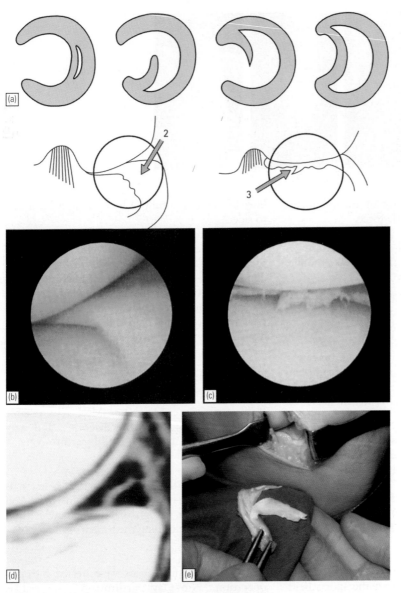

20.12 Meniscal tears The meniscus is torn by a twisting force with the knee bent. (a) The initial split may extend posteriorly and anteriorly, leaving either a 'bucket-handle' or a free-ended tag. Arthroscopy provides a means of confirming the diagnosis and treating the problem at the same time: (b) shows a normal meniscus with an intact and smooth edge and (c) a pathological meniscus with a ragged, torn edge. (d) MRI is now the standard method of diagnosing meniscal lesions. This image shows a horizontal tear of the posterior horn of the medial meniscus. (e) Most meniscal tears are excised, but some tears at the periphery can be repaired.

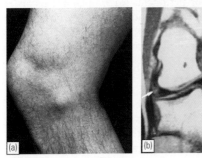

20.13 Meniscal cyst (a) A small, firm swelling at or just below the joint line on the lateral side is typical. (b) MRI showing the cyst arising from the edge of the lateral meniscus.

the joint; it may feel surprisingly firm (or tense), particularly when the knee is extended.

If the symptoms are sufficiently troublesome, the cyst can be decompressed or removed arthroscopically; any meniscal lesion can be dealt with at the same time.

OSTEOCHONDRITIS DISSECANS

A small, well-demarcated, avascular fragment of bone and overlying cartilage sometimes separates from one of the femoral condyles and appears as a loose body in the joint. The most likely cause is trauma, either a single impact with the edge of the

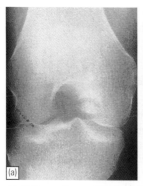
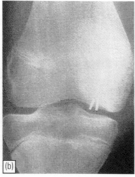
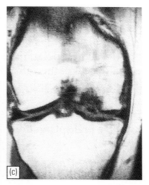

20.14 Osteochondritis dissecans The lesion is often missed in the standard anteroposterior x-ray and is better seen in the 'tunnel view', usually along the inner side of the medial femoral condyle (a). Here the osteochondral fragment has remained in place, but sometimes it appears as a separate body elsewhere in the joint. (b) An unstable fragment can be fixed with pins or screws. (c) MRI shows a much wider area of involvement than is apparent in the plain x-ray.

patella or repeated contact with an adjacent tibial ridge. More than 80 per cent of lesions occur on the lateral part of the medial femoral condyle and lesions are bilateral in 25 per cent of cases.

Clinical features

The patient, usually a male aged 15–20 years, presents with intermittent ache or swelling. Later, there are attacks of 'giving way' and the knee feels unreliable. From time to time the knee may 'lock'.

The quadriceps muscle is wasted and the joint may be slightly swollen; there is usually a small effusion. Two signs which are almost diagnostic are (a) tenderness localized to one femoral condyle, and (b) Wilson's sign: if the knee is flexed to 90 degrees, rotated medially and then gradually straightened, pain is felt; if the test is repeated with the knee rotated laterally, the patient feels no pain.

Imaging

Plain x-rays, especially intercondylar (tunnel) views, may show a line of demarcation around a lesion, usually in the lateral part of the medial femoral condyle. Once the fragment has become detached, the empty hollow may be seen – and possibly a loose body elsewhere in the joint. Radionuclide scans show increased activity around the lesion, and MRI consistently shows an area of low signal intensity in the T_1-weighted images.

Treatment

In the earliest stage, when the cartilage is intact and the lesion 'stable', no treatment is needed, but activities are curtailed for 6–12 months. Small lesions often heal spontaneously.

If the fragment is 'unstable' – i.e. surrounded by a clear boundary with sclerosis of the underlying

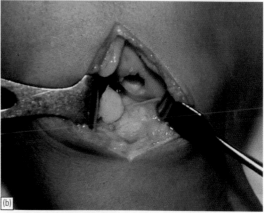

20.15 Osteochondritis dissecans Intraoperative pictures showing the articular lesion (a) and the defect left after removal of the osteochondral fragment (b).

bone, or showing MRI features of separation, or even detached – treatment will depend on the size of the lesion. A small or ill-fitting fragment should be removed by arthroscopy and the base drilled; the bed will eventually be covered by fibrocartilage. A large fragment (say more than 1 cm in diameter) or one that can be shaped to fill the crater should be fixed in situ with pins or Herbert screws. After any of the above operations, the knee is held in a cast for 6 weeks; thereafter movement is encouraged, but weight-bearing is deferred until x-rays show signs of healing.

In recent years attempts have been made to fill the condylar defect by cartilage transplantation. Long-term results are still awaited.

LOOSE BODIES

The knee – relatively capacious, with large synovial folds – is a haven for loose bodies. These may be produced by: (1) injury (a chip of bone or cartilage); (2) osteochondritis dissecans (which may produce one or two fragments); (3) osteoarthritis (pieces of cartilage or osteophyte); (4) Charcot's disease (large osteocartilaginous bodies are separated by repeated trauma in a joint that has lost protective sensation);

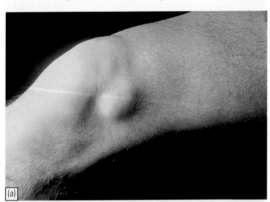

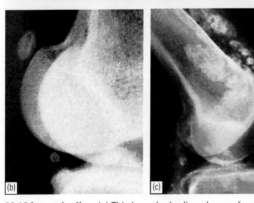

20.16 Loose bodies (a) This loose body slipped away from the fingers when touched; the term 'joint mouse' seems appropriate. (b) Which is the loose body here? Not the large one (which is a normal fabella), but the small lower one opposite the joint line. (c) Multiple loose bodies are seen in synovial chrondromatosis, a rare disorder of cartilage metaplasia in the synovium.

and (5) synovial chondromatosis (cartilage metaplasia in the synovium, sometimes producing hundreds of loose bodies).

Clinical features

The patient may be symptomless, or may complain of sudden 'locking' without injury. The joint gets stuck in a position which varies from one attack to another. Sometimes the 'locking' is only momentary and usually the patient can wriggle the knee until it suddenly unlocks. The patient may be aware of something 'popping in and out of the joint'. Sometimes, especially after the first attack, the knee swells up, due to synovitis. In some cases there is evidence of an underlying cause. A pedunculated loose body may be felt; one that is truly loose tends to slip away during palpation (aptly named 'joint mouse').

X-rays

Most loose bodies are radio-opaque. The films may also show an underlying joint abnormality.

Treatment

A loose body causing symptoms should be removed unless the joint is severely osteoarthritic. This can usually be done with the aid of arthroscopy.

TUBERCULOSIS

Tuberculosis of the knee may appear at any age, but it is more common in children than in adults.

Clinical features

Pain and limp are early symptoms, or the child may present with a swollen joint and a low-grade fever. The thigh muscles are wasted, thus accentuating the joint swelling. The knee feels warm and there is synovial thickening. Movements are restricted and often painful. The Mantoux test is positive and the erythrocyte sedimentation rate (ESR) may be increased.

X-rays

Common features are periarticular osteoporosis and, in children, enlargement of the bony epiphyses. Joint-space narrowing and progressive erosion are late signs.

Diagnosis

Monoarticular rheumatoid synovitis, or juvenile chronic arthritis, may closely resemble tuberculosis. A synovial biopsy may be necessary to establish the diagnosis.

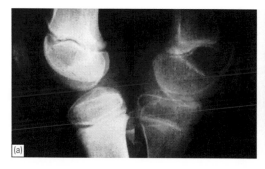
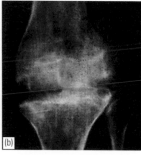

20.17 Tuberculosis (a) Lateral views of the two knees. On one side the bones are porotic and the epiphyses enlarged, features suggestive of a severe inflammatory synovitis. (b) Later the articular surfaces are eroded.

Treatment

Anti-tuberculous chemotherapy should be given for 3–6 months, while the knee is rested in a splint. At that stage, if the swelling has disappeared and x-rays show that the joint surfaces are intact, the knee is mobilized and the patient is allowed to start walking. However, if the joint surfaces are destroyed and the knee is stiff, arthrodesis is recommended; in adults this can be done as soon as the disease is inactive, but in children the operation is deferred until growth ceases.

RHEUMATOID ARTHRITIS

Occasionally, rheumatoid arthritis starts in the knee as a chronic monoarticular synovitis. Sooner or later, however, other joints become involved.

Clinical features

During stage 1 (synovitis) the patient complains of pain and chronic swelling. There is some wasting, there may be a large effusion and the thickened synovium is easily palpable.

In stage 2 (articular erosion) there is increasing instability of the joint, muscle wasting is marked and there is some loss of flexion and extension. X-rays may show loss of joint space and marginal erosions; the condition is easily distinguishable from osteoarthritis by the complete absence of osteophytes.

In stage 3 (deformity) pain and disability are usually severe. In some patients the joint has only a jog of painful movement; in others, it becomes increasingly unstable and deformed. X-rays reveal the bone destruction characteristic of advanced disease.

Treatment

In addition to general treatment, local splintage and injection of triamcinolone will usually reduce the synovitis. A more prolonged effect may be obtained by injecting radiocolloids such as yttrium-90 (^{90}Y).

Synovectomy is indicated if other measures fail to control the synovitis (which nowadays is rare) and can be done very effectively by arthroscopy.

If deformity is marked, a femoral or tibial osteotomy may improve function and relieve pain. However, once bone destruction is present and the joint is unstable, total joint replacement is advised.

OSTEOARTHRITIS

The knee is one of the commonest sites for osteoarthritis. Often there is a predisposing factor: injury to the articular surface, a torn meniscus and

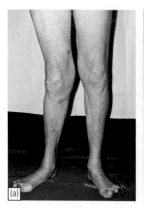
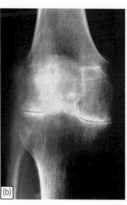
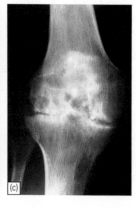

20.18 Rheumatoid arthritis (a) A patient with rheumatoid arthritis showing the typical valgus deformity of the right knee; the feet and toes also are affected. (b,c) X-rays showing progressive erosive arthritis resulting in joint destruction and deformity.

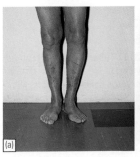
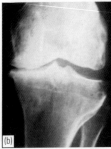
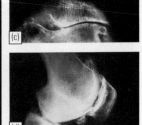

20.19 Osteoarthritis (a,b) Slight varus deformity of the left knee suggesting loss of cartilage thickness in the medial compartment. X-ray shows diminished joint space and peripheral osteophytes on the medial side of the knee. (c,d) Sometimes it is the patellofemoral joint that is mainly affected.

ligamentous instability or pre-existing deformity of the knee. However, in many cases no obvious cause can be found, and here the condition is often bilateral and has a strong association with Heberden's nodes.

Cartilage breakdown usually starts in an area of excessive loading. Thus, with long-standing varus the changes are most marked in the medial compartment. The characteristic features of cartilage fibrillation, sclerosis of the subchondral bone and peripheral osteophyte formation are usually present.

Clinical features

Patients are usually over 50 years old; they tend to be overweight and may have long-standing bow-leg deformity.

Pain is the leading symptom, worse after use or (if the patellofemoral joint is affected) on stairs. After rest, the joint feels stiff and it hurts to 'get going' after sitting for any length of time. Swelling is common, and giving way or locking may occur.

On examination, there may be an obvious deformity (usually varus) or the scar of a previous operation. The quadriceps muscle is usually wasted.

Except during an exacerbation, there is little fluid and no warmth; nor is the synovial membrane thickened. Movement is somewhat limited and is often accompanied by patellofemoral crepitus.

X-rays

A weight-bearing view is essential. The tibiofemoral joint space is diminished (often only in one compartment) and there is subchondral sclerosis. Osteophytes and subchondral cysts are usually present and sometimes there is soft-tissue calcification in the suprapatellar region or in the joint itself (chrondrocalcinosis).

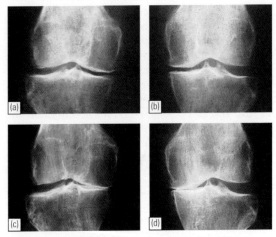

20.20 Osteoarthritis – x-rays Always obtain weight-bearing views of the knees. X-rays taken with the patient lying down (a,b) suggest only minor cartilage loss on the medial side of each knee. (c,d) Weight-bearing views show the true position: there is severe loss of articular cartilage.

Treatment

If symptoms are not severe, treatment is conservative. Analgesics can be prescribed for pain. Local measures include quadriceps exercises and the application of warmth (e.g. radiant heat or short-wave diathermy). Joint loading is lessened by using a walking stick.

Operative treatment

The indications for operative treatment are persistent pain unresponsive to conservative treatment, progressive deformity and instability. *Arthroscopic washouts,* with trimming of degenerate meniscal tissue and osteophytes, may give temporary relief; this is a useful measure when there are contraindications to reconstructive surgery.

Realignment osteotomy (typically an upper tibial valgus osteotomy for medial compartment disease in a young patient) is often successful in relieving symptoms and staving off the need for 'end-stage' surgery.

Replacement arthroplasty is indicated in older patients with progressive joint destruction. This is usually a 'resurfacing' knee replacement; with modern techniques and meticulous attention to anatomical alignment of the knee, the results are excellent.

PATELLOFEMORAL DISORDERS

RECURRENT DISLOCATION OF THE PATELLA

Dislocation of the patella usually results from an acute strain. In 15–20 per cent of cases the initial episode is followed by recurrent dislocation or subluxation after minimal stress. Sometimes, however, recurrent dislocation develops without any prior injury. Predisposing causes are: (1) generalized ligamentous laxity; (2) underdevelopment of the lateral femoral condyle and flattening of the intercondylar groove; (3) maldevelopment of the patella, which may be too high or too small; (4) valgus deformity of the knee; and (5) a primary muscle defect.

Repeated dislocation damages the contiguous surfaces of patella and femoral condyle; this may result in further flattening of the condyle, thus facilitating further dislocations. A late complication is secondary osteoarthritis.

Clinical features

Girls are affected more commonly than boys and the condition is often bilateral. There is acute pain, the knee is stuck in flexion and the patient may fall; although the patella always dislocates laterally, the patient may think it has displaced medially because the uncovered medial femoral condyle stands out prominently.

If the knee is seen while the patella is dislocated, the diagnosis is obvious. There is usually tenderness on the medial side of the joint. Later the joint becomes swollen, and aspiration may reveal a blood-stained effusion.

Between attacks, clinical signs are sparse; however, the *apprehension test* is positive (see Fig. 20.21c and page 222).

Treatment

If the patella is still dislocated, it is pushed back into place while the knee is gently extended. A plaster cylinder or splint is applied and retained for 2–3 weeks; isometric quadriceps-strengthening exercises are encouraged and the patient is allowed to walk with the aid of crutches. Exercises should be continued for at least 3 months, concentrating on strengthening the vastus medialis muscle.

If recurrences are few and far between, conservative treatment may suffice; as the child grows older, the patellar mechanism tends to stabilize. However, about 15 per cent of children with patellar instability suffer repeated and

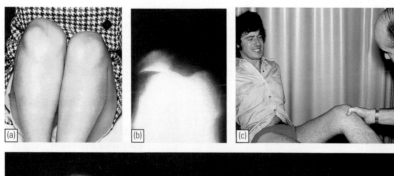

20.21 Patellofemoral instability (a,b) This young girl presented with recurrent subluxation of the right patella. The knee looks abnormal and the x-ray shows the patella riding on top of the lateral femoral condyle. (c) The apprehension test: watch the patient's face. (d) Tangential x-ray views showing both patellae slightly tilted. This is not necessarily symptomatic, but it is sometimes seen in patients with anterior knee pain and maltracking of the patella.

distressing episodes of dislocation and for these patients surgical reconstruction is indicated.

Operative treatment

The principles of operative treatment are (a) to repair or strengthen the medial patellofemoral ligaments and (b) to re-align the extensor mechanism so as to produce a mechanically more favourable angle of pull. Some methods are illustrated in Figure 20.22.

PATELLOFEMORAL OVERLOAD (PATELLAR PAIN SYNDROME; CHONDROMALACIA OF THE PATELLA)

Anterior knee pain is common among active adolescents and young adults. It is often associated with softening and fibrillation of the articular surface of the patella – *chondromalacia patellae.*

The basic disorder is probably repetitive mechanical overload of the patellofemoral joint due to either (1) malcongruence of the patellofemoral surfaces because of some abnormal shape of the patella or intercondylar groove, or (2) malalignment of the extensor mechanism, or relative weakness of the vastus medialis, which causes the patella to tilt, or subluxate, or bear more heavily on one facet than the other during flexion and extension.

Clinical features

The patient, often a teenage girl or an athletic young adult, complains of pain over the front of the knee or 'underneath the knee-cap'. Symptoms are aggravated by activity or climbing stairs, or when standing up after prolonged sitting. The quadriceps may be wasted and there may be a small effusion.

Patellofemoral pain is elicited by pressing the patella against the femur and asking the patient to

Common causes of anterior knee pain

1.	*Referred from hip*
2.	*Patellofemoral disorders*
	Patellar instability
	Patellofemoral overload
	Patellofemoral osteoarthritis
	Osteochondral injury
3.	*Joint disorders*
	Osteochondritis dissecans
	Loose body in the joint
	Synovial chondromatosis
4.	*Periarticular disorders*
	Patellar tendinitis
	Patellar ligament strain
	Bursitis
	Osgood–Schlatter's disease

contract the quadriceps – first with central pressure, then compressing the medial facet and then the lateral. If, in addition, the apprehension test is positive, this suggests previous subluxation or dislocation.

Imaging

X-ray examination should include skyline views of the patella, which may show abnormal tilting or subluxation, and a lateral view with the knee partly flexed to see if the patella is high or small.

The most accurate way of showing and measuring patellofemoral malposition is by CT or MRI with the knees in full extension and varying degrees of flexion.

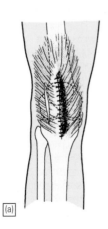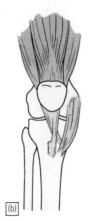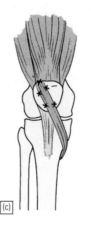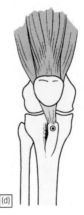

20.22 Patellar instability – operative treatment Several methods are employed.
(a) Lateral release and vastus medialis tethering.
(b) Transposition of lateral half of patellar ligament towards the medial side (Roux–Goldthwait).
(c) Medial tethering by using semitendinosus tendon.
(d) Medial transposition of patellar ligament insertion (Elmslie–Trillat).

Arthroscopy

Cartilage softening is common in asymptomatic knees, and painful knees may show no abnormality. However, arthroscopy is useful in excluding other causes of anterior knee pain.

Differential diagnosis

Other causes of anterior knee pain must be excluded before finally accepting the diagnosis of patellofemoral overload (see Box).

Treatment

In the vast majority of cases the patient will be helped by adjustment of stressful activities and physiotherapy, combined with reassurance that most patients recover. Exercises are directed specifically at strengthening the medial quadriceps so as to counterbalance the tendency to lateral tilting or subluxation of the patella.

If symptoms persist, surgery can be considered – lateral release, or lateral release combined with one of the realignment procedures illustrated in Figure 20.22 if there is any sign of patellar instability. Arthroscopic shaving of fibrillated cartilage is sometimes performed, but its efficacy is questionable. Exposed areas of subchondral bone can be drilled, in the hope that revacularization may encourage repair with fibrocartilage.

OSGOOD–SCHLATTER'S DISEASE

Painful swelling of the tibial tubercle is a fairly common complaint among adolescents, particularly those engaged in strenuous sports. Although often called *osteochondritis,* it is nothing more than a traction injury of the apophysis into which part of the patellar ligament is inserted.

On examination, the tibial tuberosity is unusually prominent and tender. Sometimes active extension of the knee against resistance is also painful.

X-rays show displacement or fragmentation of the tibial apophysis.

Treatment

Spontaneous recovery is usual, but takes time, and it is wise to restrict such activities as cycling and football.

SWELLINGS AROUND THE KNEE

A fairly common complaint is of swelling – either of the entire joint or asymmetrically on one or

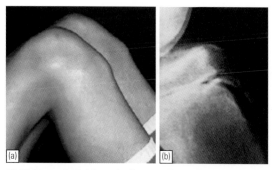

20.23 Osgood–Schlatter's disease This boy complained of a painful bump below the knee. X-ray shows the traction injury of the tibial apophysis.

other aspect of the joint. The following conditions should be considered.

ACUTE SWELLING OF THE ENTIRE JOINT

Post-traumatic haemarthrosis

Swelling immediately after injury means blood in the joint. The knee is very painful and it feels warm, tense and tender. Later there may be a 'doughy' feel. Movements are restricted. X-rays are essential to see if there is a fracture; if there is not, suspect a tear of the anterior cruciate ligament.

Non-traumatic haemarthrosis

In patients with clotting disorders, the knee is the most common site for acute bleeds. If the appropriate clotting factor is available, the joint should be aspirated and splinted.

Acute septic arthritis

The joint is swollen, painful and inflamed, the white cell count and ESR are elevated and aspiration reveals pus in the joint. Fluid should be sent for microbiological investigation, including anaerobic culture. *This should always be done before starting antibiotic treatment.* The organism is usually *Staphylococcus aureus,* but in adults gonococcal infection is almost as common. Treatment consists of intravenous antibiotics and drainage of the joint.

Traumatic synovitis

Injury stimulates a reactive synovitis; typically, the swelling appears only after some hours, unlike the almost immediate appearance of a haemarthrosis, and subsides spontaneously over a period of days. There is inhibition of quadriceps action and the thigh wastes. If the amount of fluid is considerable, its aspiration hastens muscle recovery.

Aseptic non-traumatic synovitis

Acute swelling, without a history of trauma or signs of infection, suggests gout or pseudogout. Aspiration will provide fluid which may look turbid, resembling pus, but it is sterile and microscopy (using polarized light) reveals the crystals. Treatment with anti-inflammatory drugs is usually effective.

CHRONIC SWELLING OF THE ENTIRE JOINT

Arthritis

The commonest causes of chronic swelling are osteoarthritis and rheumatoid arthritis. Other signs, such as deformity, loss of movement or instability, may be present and x-ray examination will usually show characteristic features.

Synovial disorders

The most important condition to exclude is *tuberculosis*. There has been a resurgence of cases during the past 10 years and the condition should be seriously considered whenever there is no obvious alternative diagnosis. Investigations should include Mantoux testing, synovial biopsy and microbiological investigations. The ideal is to

start anti-tuberculous chemotherapy before joint destruction occurs.

SWELLINGS IN FRONT OF THE JOINT

Prepatellar bursitis ('housemaid's knee')

This fluctuant swelling is confined to the front of the patella, and the joint itself is normal. It is an uninfected bursitis due to constant friction between skin and bone. As such, it is seen mainly in carpet layers, paving workers, floor cleaners and miners who do not use protective knee pads. Treatment consists of firm bandaging, and kneeling is avoided; occasionally aspiration is needed. In chronic cases the lump is best excised.

Infrapatellar bursitis ('clergyman's knee')

The swelling is below the patella and superficial to the patellar ligament, being more distally placed than prepatellar bursitis. Treatment is similar to that for prepatellar bursitis.

SWELLINGS AT THE BACK OF THE KNEE

Semimembranosus bursa

The bursa between the semimembranosus and the medial head of gastrocnemius may become enlarged in children or adults. It presents usually as a painless lump behind the knee, slightly to the

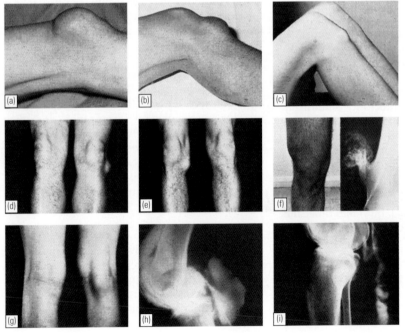

20.24 Lumps around the knee
In front: (a) prepatellar bursa; (b) infrapatellar bursa; (c) Osgood–Schlatter's disease.

On either side: (d) cyst of lateral meniscus; (e) cyst of medial meniscus; (f) cartilage-capped exostosis.

Behind: (g) semi-membranosus bursa; (h) arthrogram of Baker's cyst; (i) leaking cyst.

medial side of the midline, and is most conspicuous with the knee straight. The lump is fluctuant and transilluminates. The knee joint is normal. A waiting policy is wise, even if the lump causes an ache, as it usually disappears with time.

Popliteal 'cyst'

Bulging of the posterior capsule and synovial herniation may produce a swelling in the popliteal fossa. It is most likely to be caused by rheumatoid arthritis or osteoarthritis, but it is still often called a 'Baker's cyst' (even though the original description by William Morrant Baker in 1877 probably referred to an association with tuberculous arthritis). Occasionally the 'cyst' ruptures and the synovial contents spill into the muscle planes, causing pain and swelling in the calf – a combination which can easily be mistaken for deep vein thrombosis.

The swelling may diminish following aspiration and injection of hydrocortisone; excision is not advised, because recurrence is common unless the underlying condition is treated.

SWELLINGS AT THE SIDE OF THE JOINT

Meniscal cyst

This presents as a small, tense swelling, usually on the lateral side at or just below the joint line. Sometimes it is so tense that it can easily be mistaken for a bony lump. It is usually tender on pressure (see also page 227).

Calcification of the collateral ligament

An acutely painful swelling may suddenly appear, usually on the medial side of the joint. It is rubbery in consistency and acutely tender. Operative decompression will confirm the diagnosis (the calcific material is extruded like toothpaste) and provide immediate relief.

Bony swellings

Bony lumps arising in the long-bone metaphyses may cause visible and palpable swellings in the vicinity of a joint. Large, non-discrete and painful bone swellings should suggest a tumour. The diagnosis is usually revealed by x-ray examination but may need to be confirmed by biopsy.

CHAPTER 21

THE ANKLE AND FOOT

CLINICAL ASSESSMENT

HISTORY

The most common presenting symptoms are pain, deformity, swelling and 'giving way'. It is important to know whether standing or walking provokes the symptoms and whether shoe pressure is a factor.

Pain over a bony prominence or a joint is probably due to a local disorder. Pain across the entire forefoot *(metatarsalgia)* is less specific and is often associated with uneven loading and muscle fatigue.

Deformity may be in the ankle, the foot or the toes. Parents often worry about their children who are 'flat-footed' or 'pigeon-toed'. Elderly patients may complain chiefly of having difficulty fitting shoes.

Swelling can be diffuse and bilateral, or localized. Swelling over the medial side of the first metatarsal head (a bunion) is common in older women.

'Giving way' may be due to pain or instability at the ankle or subtalar joint.

Corns and callosities are a frequent cause for complaints. These hardened, often tender, patches of skin on the toes and soles of the feet are produced by localized pressure and friction, usually from ill-fitting shoes.

Numbness and paraesthesia may be felt in all the toes or in a circumscribed field served by a single nerve.

SIGNS WITH THE PATIENT STANDING AND WALKING

The patient, whose lower limbs should be exposed from the knees down, stands first facing the surgeon, then with his or her back to the surgeon. Normally the heels are in slight valgus while standing and inverted when on tiptoes; the degree of inversion should be equal on the two sides, showing that the subtalar joints are mobile and the tibialis posterior muscles functioning.

Deformities such as flat-foot, cavus (high-arched) foot, hallux valgus and crooked toes are noted. Corns over the proximal toe joints and callosities on the soles are common in older people.

Ask the patient to walk. Note whether the gait is smooth or halting and whether the feet are well balanced. Foot problems may cause a limp, usually from stiffness, muscle weakness, deformity or pain. The position and mobility of the ankle are important. A fixed equinus deformity results in the heel failing to strike the ground at the beginning of the walking cycle; sometimes the patient forces heel contact by hyperextending the knee. If the ankle dorsiflexors are weak, the forefoot may strike the ground prematurely, causing a 'slap'; this is referred to as foot-drop (or drop-foot). During swing-through, the leg is lifted higher than usual

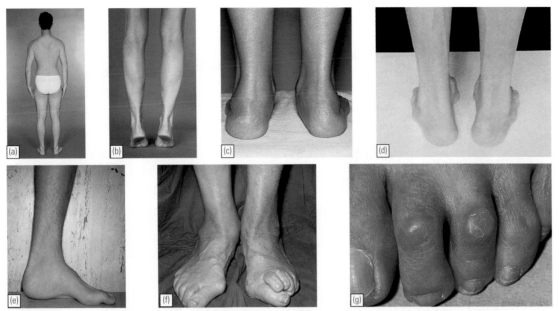

21.1 Examination with patient standing Look at the patient as a whole, first from in front and from behind. (a,b) The heels are normally in slight valgus and should invert equally when a patient stands on his/her toes. (c) This patient has flat-feet (pes planus), while the patient in (d) has the opposite deformity, varus heels and an abnormally high longitudinal arch – pes cavus (e). From the front you can again notice (f) the dropped longitudinal arch in the patient with pes planus, as well as the typical deformities of bilateral hallux valgus and overriding toes. (g) Corns on the top of the toes are common.

so that the foot can clear the ground; this is known as a high-stepping gait.

Don't forget to examine the shoes for uneven wear and distortion of the uppers; they provide valuable information about faulty stance and gait.

SIGNS WITH THE PATIENT SITTING OR LYING

The patient is next examined lying on a couch, or it may be more convenient if he or she sits opposite the examiner and places each foot in turn on the examiner's lap.

Look

The heel is held square so that the shape of the foot can be properly assessed. The toes are now examined more closely for deformities and the soles are examined for callosities.

Feel

The skin temperature is assessed and the pulses are felt. If there is tenderness in the foot, it must be precisely localized, for its site is often diagnostic. Any swelling, oedema or lumps must be examined. Sensation may be abnormal.

Move

The foot is constructed as a series of joints, each of which should be examined methodically, noting the ranges of both passive and active movements. Muscle power can be tested at the same time.

Ankle joint

With the heel grasped in the left hand and the midfoot in the right, plantarflexion and dorsiflexion are tested.

Subtalar joint

When assessing inversion and eversion, make sure that the ankle is fully plantigrade (at a right angle to the leg); this prevents the ankle tilting to one or other side.

Mid-tarsal joint

The heel is held still with one hand while the other moves the tarsus up and down and from side to side.

Toes

The metatarsophalangeal and interphalangeal joints are tested.

Tests for stability

Ankle stability should be tested in both coronal and sagittal planes, always comparing the two sides. The ankle is held in 10 degrees of

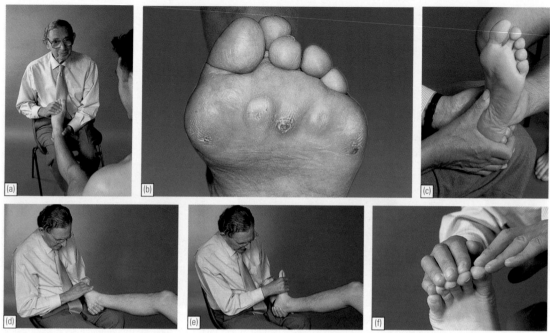

21.2 Examination with patient sitting (a) The patient is seated with his foot on the examiner's lap. Keep your eye on the patient's face as well as on the foot. (b) Look for superficial scars and deformities, especially of the toes; don't forget the sole of the foot, where callosities go together with toe deformities. (c) Feel for tenderness over every joint from the ankle to the toes and along the major ligaments of the foot. (d–f) Then test for movements in the ankle and the toes.

plantarflexion and the joint stressed into valgus and then varus. Anteroposterior stability is assessed by performing an anterior 'drawer test': with the ankle held in 10 degrees of plantarflexion, the distal tibia is gripped with one hand while the other grasps the heel and tries to shift the hindfoot forwards and backwards. Patients with recent ligament injury may have to be examined under anaesthesia. The same tests can be performed under x-ray and the positions of the two ankles measured and compared (see page 380).

General examination

If there are any symptoms or signs of vascular or neurological impairment, or if multiple joints are affected, a more general examination is essential.

Imaging

Anteroposterior and lateral *x-rays* of the ankle and foot are routine. Standing films, stress films and special views are sometimes needed. *CT* is useful for displaying the anatomy of complex fractures and looking for abnormal bridges between the tarsal bones (coalitions). *Radioisotope scanning,* though non-specific, is excellent for localizing areas of abnormal blood flow or bone remodelling activity; it is useful in the diagnosis of covert infection. *MRI*

and *ultrasound* are used to demonstrate soft-tissue problems, such as tendon and ligament injuries.

DEFORMITIES OF THE FOOT

The normal position of the foot is *plantigrade* – i.e. when the patient stands, the sole is at right angles to the leg. *Equinus* (like a horse's foot) means that the hindfoot is fixed in plantarflexion (pointing downwards). *Plantaris* looks similar, but the ankle is neutral and only the forefoot is plantarflexed. *Calcaneus* is fixed dorsiflexion at the ankle. A dorsiflexion deformity in the mid-foot produces a *rocker-bottom foot.*

Normally the medial border of the foot, even when weight-bearing, forms a *longitudinal arch.* The arrangement of the metatarsals also produces an *anterior* or *transverse arch* in the forefoot. Flattening of the longitudinal arch is referred to as a *planus deformity* or *flat-foot;* and a dropped metatarsal arch as *anterior flat-foot.* An excessively high arch produces a *cavus deformity.*

Common deformities of the toes are lateral deviation of the big toe *(hallux valgus),* proximal interphalangeal flexion of one of the lesser toes *(hammer-toe)* and flexion of both interphalangeal joints of several toes *(claw-toes).*

CONGENITAL TALIPES EQUINOVARUS (IDIOPATHIC CLUB-FOOT)

In this deformity the heel is in equinus (pointing downwards), the entire hindfoot in varus (tilted towards the midline) and the mid-foot and forefoot adducted and supinated (twisted medially and the sole turned upwards). It is relatively common; the incidence is 1 or 2 per 1000 births and boys are affected twice as often as girls. The condition is bilateral in one-third of cases. Similar deformities are seen in neurological disorders, e.g. myelomeningocele, and in arthrogryposis.

The skin and soft tissues of the calf and the medial side of the foot are short and underdeveloped. If the condition is not corrected early, secondary growth changes occur in the bones and these are permanent. Even with treatment, the foot is liable to be short and the calf may remain thin.

Clinical features

The deformity is usually obvious at birth; the foot is both turned and twisted inwards so that the sole faces posteromedially. The heel is usually small and high, and deep creases appear posteriorly and medially. In a normal baby the foot can be dorsiflexed and everted until the toes almost touch the front of the leg. In club-foot this manoeuvre meets with varying degrees of resistance and in severe cases the deformity is fixed.

The infant must always be examined for associated disorders such as congenital hip dislocation and spina bifida.

X-rays

The tarsal bones are incompletely ossified at this age and the anatomy is therefore difficult to define. However, the shape and position of the tarsal ossific centres are helpful in assessing progress after treatment.

Treatment

The aim of treatment is to produce and maintain a plantigrade, supple foot that will function well. There are several methods of treatment, but relapse is common, especially in babies with associated neuromuscular disorders.

Conservative treatment

Treatment should begin early, preferably within a day or two of birth. This consists of repeated manipulation and adhesive strapping or application of plaster-of-Paris casts, which will maintain the correction. If adhesive strapping is used, parents are

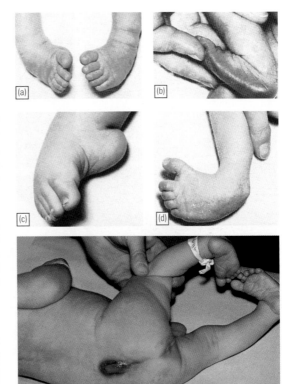

21.3 Talipes equinovarus (club-foot) (a) True club-foot is a fixed deformity, unlike (b) postural talipes, which is easily correctable by gentle passive movement. (c,d) With true club-foot, the poorly developed heel is higher than the forefoot, which points downwards and inwards (varus). (e) Always examine the hips for congenital dislocation and the back for spina bifida (as in the case illustrated here).

taught how to do the manipulation and they can then carry out gentle stretches on a regular basis with the strapping still in place. Treatment is supervised by a physiotherapist, who alters the strapping as correction is gradually obtained. Plaster-of-Paris casting requires serial changes and manipulations in a clinic setting. Sometimes surgical release of the Achilles tendon is needed to complete the correction.

Operative treatment

Resistant cases will need surgery. The objectives are (a) the complete release of joint tethers (capsular and ligamentous contractures and fibrotic bands) and (b) lengthening of tendons so that the foot can be positioned normally without undue tension. A detailed knowledge of the pathological anatomy is a sine qua non. After operative correction, the foot is immobilized in its corrected position in a plaster

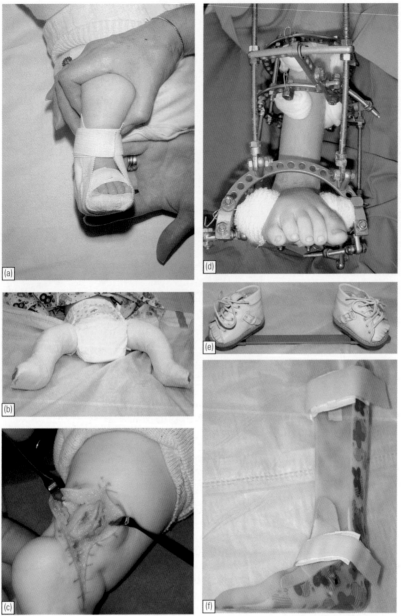

21.4 Congenital talipes equinovarus – treatment
First-line treatment is non-operative. This may be by manipulation and strapping (a) or serial casting (b). If insufficient correction is achieved, a formal open release may be needed (c). Severe relapses need more radical forms of treatment such as the Ilizarov fixator (d). After successful correction of deformity, relapses may be prevented by using Dennis Browne boots in infants (e) or moulded ankle–foot orthoses (f) in older children.

cast. Kirschner wires are sometimes inserted across the intertarsal and ankle joints to augment the hold. The wires and cast are removed at 6–8 weeks, after which hobble boots (Dennis Browne) or a customized orthosis are used to maintain the correction.

LATE OR RELAPSED CLUB-FOOT

Late presenters often have severe deformities with secondary bony changes, and the relapsed club-foot is complicated by scarring from previous surgery. A revision of the soft-tissue releases may be considered;

this can be combined with shortening of the lateral side of the foot by calcaneocuboid fusion or cuboid enucleation (Dilwyn Evans). Alternatively, gradual correction by means of a circular external fixator (the Ilizarov method) has proved effective in treating difficult relapsed cases and severe deformities; the early results are encouraging.

Despite initially successful surgery, deformities do still recur. A deformed, stiff and painful foot in an adolescent is best salvaged by corrective osteotomies and fusions.

FLAT-FOOT

The problems associated with flat-foot deformities differ significantly between infants, children and adults.

INFANTILE FLAT-FOOT (CONGENITAL VERTICAL TALUS)

This rare neonatal condition usually affects both feet. In appearance it is the very opposite of a club-foot. The foot is turned outwards (valgus) and the medial arch is not only flat, it actually curves the opposite way from the normal, producing the appearance of a 'rocker-bottom' foot. X-ray features are characteristic: the calcaneum is in equinus and the talus points into the sole of the foot, with the navicular dislocated dorsally onto the neck of the talus. Passive correction is impossible; by the time the child is seen, the tendons and ligaments on the dorsolateral side of the foot are usually shortened. The only effective treatment is by operation, ideally before the age of 2 years.

FLAT-FOOT IN CHILDREN AND ADOLESCENTS

Flat-foot is a common complaint among children and teenagers, or rather their parents – the children themselves usually don't seem to mind! When weight-bearing, the foot is turned outwards and the medial border of the foot is in contact (or nearly in contact) with the ground; the heel becomes valgus (hence the medical terms *pes planus* and *pes valgus*). Two forms of the condition are recognized: flexible and rigid.

Flexible flat-foot appears in toddlers as a normal stage in development, and it usually disappears after a few years when medial arch development is complete; sometimes, though, it persists into adult life. The arch can often be restored by simply dorsiflexing the great toe (the jack, or great-toe extension, test) and during this manoeuvre the tibia rotates externally. Many of these children have ligamentous laxity and there may be a family history of both flat-feet and joint hypermobility.

Stiff (or 'rigid') *flat-foot* which cannot be corrected passively should alert the examiner to an underlying abnormality. In older children and adolescents, conditions to be considered are tarsal coalition (often a bar of bone connecting the calcaneum to the talus or the navicular), an inflammatory joint condition or a neurological disorder.

Clinical assessment

In the common *flexible flat-foot* there are no symptoms, but the parents notice that the feet are flat or that the shoes wear badly. The deformity becomes noticeable when the youngster stands.

The first test is to ask the patient to go up on tiptoes: if the heels invert, it is a flexible (or mobile) deformity. Next, examine the foot with the child sitting or lying. Feel for localized tenderness and test the range of movement in the ankle, the subtalar and midtarsal joints. A tight Achilles tendon may induce a *compensatory flat-foot* deformity.

Teenagers and young adults sometimes present with a *painful, rigid flat-foot*. On examination, the peroneal and extensor tendons appear to be in spasm (the condition is sometimes called *spasmodic flat-foot*). In some cases a definite cause may be found (e.g. a tarsal coalition or inflammatory arthritis), but in many no specific cause is identified.

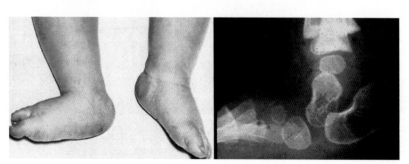

21.5 Congenital vertical talus
The infant's foot is in marked valgus and has a rocker-bottom shape. The deformity is rigid and cannot be corrected. X-ray shows the vertical talus pointing downwards towards the sole and the other tarsal bones rotated around the head of the talus.

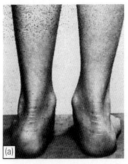
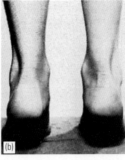

21.6 Mobile flat-feet (a) Standing with the feet flat on the floor, the medial arches appear to have dropped and the heels are in valgus. (b) When the patient goes up on his toes, the medial arches are restored, indicating that these are 'mobile' flat-feet. If this does not occur, look carefully for a tarsal coalition.

The spine, hips and knees should always be examined. The clinical assessment is completed by a swift general examination for joint hypermobility and signs of neuromuscular abnormalities.

Imaging

X-rays are unnecessary for asymptomatic, flexible flat-feet. For pathological flat-feet (which are usually painful or stiff), standing anteroposterior, lateral and oblique views may help to identify underlying disorders. CT scanning is the most reliable way of demonstrating tarsal coalitions.

Treatment

Young children with flexible flat-feet require no treatment. Parents need to be reassured and told that the 'deformity' will probably correct itself in time; even if it does not fully correct, function is unlikely to be impaired.

Where the condition is obviously due to an underlying disorder such as poliomyelitis, splintage or operative correction and muscle rebalancing may be needed.

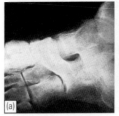
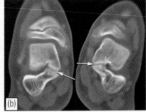

21.7 Tarsal coalition (a) X-ray appearance of a calcaneonavicular bar. (b) CT image showing incompletely ossified talocalcaneal bars bilaterally (arrows).

Spasmodic flat-foot is relieved by rest in a cast or a splint. If there is an abnormal tarsal bar or other bony irregularity, this may have to be removed; in late cases, if pain is intolerable, a triple arthrodesis may be necessary.

FLAT-FOOT IN ADULTS

When adults present with symptomatic flat-feet, the first thing to ask is whether they always had flat-feet or whether it is of recent onset. Constitutional flat-feet which have been more or less asymptomatic for many years may start causing nagging pain after a change in daily activities (e.g. taking on work which requires a lot of standing and walking). More recent deformities may be due to an underlying disorder such as rheumatoid arthritis or generalized muscular weakness; and unilateral flat-foot should make one think of tibialis posterior synovitis or rupture.

Where there is no underlying abnormality, little can be done apart from giving advice about sensible footwear and arch supports. Patients with painful, rigid flat-feet may require more robust splintage (and, of course, treatment for any generalized condition such a rheumatoid arthritis). Those with tibialis posterior rupture can be helped by operative repair or replacement of the defective tendon.

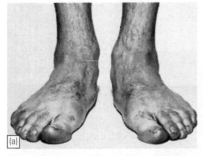
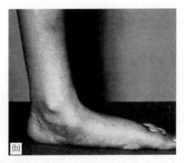
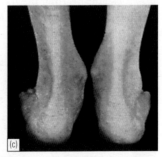

21.8 Flat-foot in adults – clinical features (a) The medial arches have dropped and the feet appear to be pronated. (b) The medial border of the foot is flat and the tuberosity of the navicular looks prominent. (c) The heels are in valgus and the toes are visible lateral to the outer edge of the heel on the left side (the 'too-many-toes' sign).

PES CAVUS

In pes cavus the arch is higher than normal, and often there is also clawing of the toes. The close resemblance to deformities seen in neurological disorders where the intrinsic muscles are weak or paralysed suggests that all forms of pes cavus are due to some type of muscle imbalance.

Clinical features

The foot is highly arched and the toes are drawn up into a 'clawed' position, forcing the metatarsal heads down into the sole. Often the heel is inverted and the soft tissues in the sole are tight. The metatarsal heads are prominent and the overlying skin may be calloused.

The deformity may be noticed by the parents or the school doctor before there are any symptoms. At first the deformities are mobile and can be corrected passively by pressure under the metatarsal heads: as the forefoot lifts, the toes flatten out automatically. Later the deformities become fixed. Pain may then be felt under the metatarsal heads or over the toes where shoe pressure is most marked. Callosities appear at the same sites and walking tolerance is reduced.

Spinal disorders and neuromuscular abnormalities rank high as causes and must be looked for.

Treatment

Often no treatment is required; apart from the difficulty of fitting shoes, the patient has no complaints. However, if the patient has significant discomfort, custom-made shoes with moulded supports may provide relief. If this is unsuccessful and the deformities are still passively correctable, a tendon rebalancing operation may be worthwhile: the long toe flexors are released and transplanted into the extensor expansions to pull the toes straight.

A painful foot with fixed deformities presents a much more difficult problem. The toes can be straightened by a combination of soft-tissue releases, tendon transfers and arthrodesis of the interphalangeal joints. More complex operations on the arch itself should be deferred until the age of 16. Severe deformities may require triple arthrodesis of the hindfoot.

HALLUX VALGUS

Hallux valgus is the commonest of the foot deformities (and probably of all musculoskeletal deformities). In people who have never worn shoes the big toe is in line with the first metatarsal, retaining the slightly fan-shaped appearance of the forefoot. In people who habitually wear shoes the hallux assumes a valgus position; but only if the angulation is excessive is it referred to as 'hallux valgus'.

Splaying of the forefoot, with varus angulation of the first metatarsal, predisposes to lateral angulation of the big toe in people who wear shoes. This *metatarsus primus varus* may be congenital, or it may result from loss of muscle tone in the forefoot in elderly people. Hallux valgus is also common in rheumatoid arthritis.

The elements of the deformity are lateral deviation and rotation of the hallux, together with hypertrophy ('exostosis') of the medial part of the metatarsal head and an overlying bursa which together form a prominent bump (or *bunion*) on the medial side. Lateral deviation of the hallux may lead to overcrowding of the lateral toes and sometimes overriding.

Clinical features

Hallux valgus is most common in women between 50 and 70 years, and is usually bilateral. An

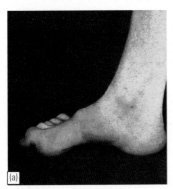
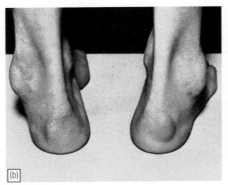
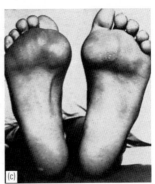

21.9 Pes cavus and claw-toes (a) Typical appearance of 'idiopathic' pes cavus. Note the high arch and claw-toes. (b) This is associated with varus heels. (c) Look for callosities under the metatarsal heads.

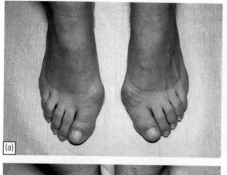

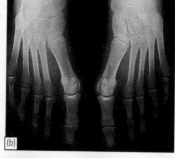

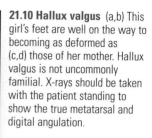

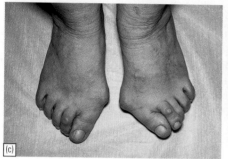

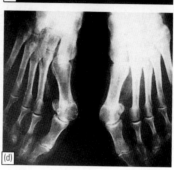

21.10 Hallux valgus (a,b) This girl's feet are well on the way to becoming as deformed as (c,d) those of her mother. Hallux valgus is not uncommonly familial. X-rays should be taken with the patient standing to show the true metatarsal and digital angulation.

important sub-group, with a strong familial tendency, appears during late adolescence.

Often there are no symptoms apart from the deformity. Pain, if present, may be due to (1) shoe pressure on a large or an inflamed bunion, (2) splaying of the forefoot and muscle strain (metatarsalgia), (3) associated deformities of the lesser toes, or (4) secondary osteoarthritis of the first metatarsophalangeal joint.

X-rays

X-rays should be taken with the patient standing, to show the degree of metatarsal and hallux angulation. The first metatarsophalangeal joint may be subluxated, or it may look osteoarthritic.

Treatment

Adolescents

Deformity is usually the only 'symptom', but the mother is anxious to prevent it becoming as severe as her own. Conservative treatment is justified as a first measure (operative correction carries a 20–40 per cent recurrence rate in this age group). The patient is encouraged to wear shoes with deep toe-boxes, soft uppers and low heels. If the deformity progresses, a corrective osteotomy of the first metatarsal and soft-tissue rebalancing around the metatarsophalangeal joint may produce a satisfactory correction.

Adults

Surgical treatment is more readily offered to older patients. This usually takes the form of excision of the bunion, metatarsal osteotomy and soft-tissue rebalancing. However, if the metatarsophalangeal joint is frankly osteoarthritic, arthrodesis of the joint may be a better option.

HALLUX RIGIDUS

'Rigidity' of the first metatarsophalangeal joint may be due to local trauma or osteochondritis dissecans of the first metatarsal head, but in older people it is usually caused by long-standing joint disorders such as gout, pseudogout or osteoarthritis. In contrast to hallux valgus, men and women are affected with equal frequency. Clinical problems are due to the fact that, because the big toe cannot extend (dorsiflex), push-off at the end of the stance phase of gait becomes painful and clumsy.

Clinical features

Pain on walking, especially on slopes or rough ground, is the predominant symptom. The hallux is straight and the metatarsophalangeal joint feels knobbly; a tender dorsal 'bunion' (actually a large osteophyte) is characteristic. Dorsiflexion is restricted and painful; plantarflexion is also limited, but less so.

X-ray

The changes are those of osteoarthritis: the joint space is narrowed, there is bone sclerosis and, often, large osteophytes at the joint margins.

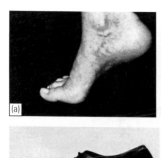
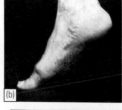
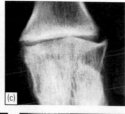
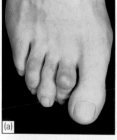
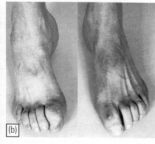
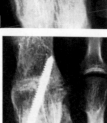

21.11 Hallux rigidus (a) In normal walking, the big toe dorsiflexes (extends) considerably. With rigidus (b), dorsiflexion is limited. (c) The usual cause is osteoarthritis of the first metatarsophalangeal joint. (d) A rocker sole may be all that is needed to relieve symptoms. Operations include joint replacement (e) and arthrodesis (f).

Treatment

A rocker-soled shoe may abolish pain by allowing the foot to 'roll' without the necessity for dorsiflexion at the metatarsophalangeal joint.

If walking is painful despite this type of shoe adjustment, an operation is advised. For young patients, the best procedure is a simple extension osteotomy of the proximal phalanx, to mimic dorsiflexion at the interphalangeal joint. In older patients, cheilectomy is the procedure of choice: the dorsal osteophytes and the dorsal edge of the metatarsal head are removed in an attempt to restore extension (dorsiflexion) at the metatarsophalangeal joint. Arthrodesis of the metatarsophalangeal joint is a good solution for the badly arthritic joint.

DEFORMITIES OF THE LESSER TOES

Common deformities of the lesser digits are hammer-toe, claw-toe and overlapping toe.

HAMMER-TOE

Hammer-toe is an isolated flexion deformity of the proximal interphalangeal joint of one of the lesser toes – usually the second or third. The distal interphalangeal joint remains straight or is pulled into hyperextension. Shoe pressure may then produce a painful corn on the dorsally projecting proximal interphalangeal 'knuckle', and the metatarsophalangeal joint is forced into hyperextension.

Treatment

Operative correction is indicated for pain or for difficulty with shoes. The toe is shortened and straightened by excising the joint; often this ends in fusion of the proximal and middle phalanges, but some surgeons prefer to fix the toe in the straight position with a Kirschner wire.

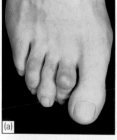
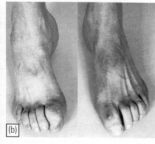
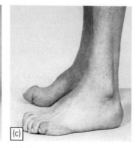
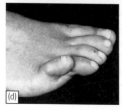

21.12 Disorders of the lesser toes (a) Hammer-toe deformity. (b,c) Claw-toes. This patient suffered from peroneal muscular atrophy, a neurological disorder causing weakness of the intrinsic muscles and cavus feet. (d) Overlapping fifth toe.

CLAW-TOES

In this deformity, all the toes are affected to a greater or lesser degree. The metatarsophalangeal joints are hyperextended and the interphalangeal joints are flexed. This suggests that the intrinsic muscles are relatively weak, and it is not surprising that the deformity is seen in neurological disorders (e.g. peroneal muscular atrophy, poliomyelitis and peripheral neuropathies) and in rheumatoid arthritis. Often, however, no cause is found. The condition may also be associated with pes cavus.

Clinical features

The patient complains of pain in the forefoot and under the metatarsal heads. Usually the condition is bilateral, and walking may be severely restricted.

At first the joints are mobile and can be passively corrected; later, the deformities become fixed and the metatarsophalangeal joints subluxed or dislocated. Painful corns and callosities develop and in the most severe cases the skin ulcerates at the pressure sites.

Treatment

As long as the toes can be passively straightened, the patient may obtain relief by wearing a metatarsal support (pressure under the metatarsal heads will straighten the mobile joints). If this fails to relieve discomfort, 'dynamic' correction is achieved by transferring the long toe flexors to the extensors. When the deformity is fixed, it may either be accepted and accommodated by special footwear, or treated by interphalangeal arthrodesis combined with tendon transfers.

OVERLAPPING TOES

This is often seen when a markedly valgus big toe forces the adjacent second toe to find room for itself by riding up on top of the hallux. The overlapping toe may fall back into position once the hallux valgus is corrected, but sometimes surgical correction is needed.

Overlapping fifth toe is a congenital anomaly. If it is sufficiently bothersome, the toe may be straightened by performing a dorsal V/Y-plasty together with transfer of the flexor to the extensor tendon. The toe has to be held in the corrected position with tape or a Kirschner wire for 6 weeks while the soft tissues heal.

RHEUMATOID ARTHRITIS

The ankle and foot are affected almost as often as the wrist and hand. During stage 1, there is synovitis of the metatarsophalangeal, intertarsal and ankle joints, as well as of the sheathed tendons (usually the peronei and tibialis posterior). In stage 2, joint erosion and tendon dysfunction prepare the ground for the progressive deformities of stage 3.

THE ANKLE AND HINDFOOT

The earliest symptoms are pain and swelling around the ankle. Walking becomes increasingly difficult and, later, deformities appear. On examination, swelling and tenderness are usually localized to the back of the medial malleolus (tenosynovitis of tibialis posterior) or the lateral malleolus (tenosynovitis of the peronei). Less often, the ankle swells (joint synovitis) and its movements are restricted. Inversion and eversion may be painful and limited. In the late stages the tibialis posterior may rupture (all too often this is missed), or become ineffectual with progressive erosion of the tarsal joints, and the foot gradually drifts into severe valgus deformity. X-rays show osteoporosis and, later, erosion of the tarsal and ankle joints. Soft-tissue swelling may be marked.

Treatment

In the stage of synovitis, splintage is helpful (to allow inflammation to subside and to prevent deformity) while waiting for systemic treatment to control the disease. Initially, tendon sheaths and joints may be injected with triamcinolone, but this should not be repeated more than two or three times. A lightweight below-knee calliper with an inside supporting strap restores stability and may be worn almost indefinitely.

If the synovitis does not subside, operative synovectomy may help. Although tendon replacement is technically feasible, progressive joint erosion will ultimately counteract any improvement this might achieve. In the very late stage, arthrodesis of the ankle and tarsal joints can still restore modest function and abolish pain.

THE FOREFOOT

Pain and swelling of the metatarsophalangeal joints are among the earliest features of rheumatoid arthritis. Shoes feel uncomfortable and the patient walks less and less. Tenderness is at first localized to the metatarsophalangeal joints; later the entire forefoot is painful on pressing or squeezing. With increasing weakness of the intrinsic muscles and joint destruction, characteristic deformities appear: a flattened anterior arch, hallux valgus, claw-toes and prominence of the metatarsal heads in the sole.

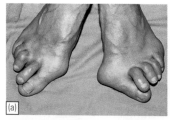

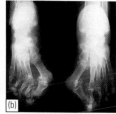

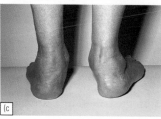

21.13 Rheumatoid arthritis (a,b) Forefoot deformities are similar to those in non-rheumatoid feet but more severe. They are due to a combination of joint erosion and tendon attrition. (c) Swelling and deformity of the hindfoot are due to a combination of arthritis and tenosynovitis. In this case, both the ankle and the subtalar joints were affected.

Subcutaneous nodules are common and may ulcerate. Dorsal corns and plantar callosities also may break down and become infected. In the worst cases the toes are dislocated, inflamed, ulcerated and useless. *X-rays* show osteoporosis and periarticular erosion at the metatarsophalangeal joints.

Treatment

During the stage of synovitis, corticosteroid injections and attention to footwear may relieve symptoms; operative synovectomy is occasionally needed. Once deformity is advanced, treatment is that of the claw-toe deformities and hallux valgus. Shoes can be made to accommodate the toes in greater comfort. If this does not help, the most effective treatment is an excision arthroplasty of the metatarsophalangeal joints in order to relieve pressure in the sole and to correct the toe deformities. For the hallux, metatarsophalangeal fusion is sometimes preferred.

OSTEOARTHRITIS

Osteoarthritis of the ankle is almost always secondary to some underlying disorder: a malunited fracture, recurrent instability, osteochondritis

dissecans of the talus, avascular necrosis of the talus or repeated bleeding with haemophilia.

Symptoms are often quite tolerable, because extremes of range are not required with normal use.

Treatment, in the first instance, is conservative: anti-inflammatory drugs and, sometimes, splintage or simply wearing a strong boot. If operation is required, an arthrodesis is usually the best option. Joint replacement is sometimes used for patients with low functional demands.

GOUT

Swelling, redness, heat and exquisite tenderness of the metatarsophalangeal joint of the big toe ('podagra') is the epitome of gout (see also Chapter 4). The ankle joint, or one of the lesser toes, may be similarly affected – especially following a minor injury. The condition may closely resemble septic arthritis, but the systemic features of infection are absent. The serum uric acid level may be raised.

Treatment with anti-inflammatory drugs will abort the acute attack of gout; until the pain subsides, the foot should be rested and protected from injury.

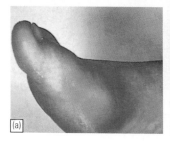

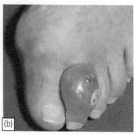

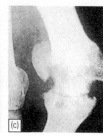

21.14 Gout (a) The classic picture – acute inflammation of the big toe metatarsophalangeal joint. (b) Tophaceous gout of the second toe. (c) X-ray of the first metatarsophalangeal joint; the large excavations are occupied by crystalline tophi.

DISORDERS OF THE TENDO ACHILLIS

PERITENDINITIS

Athletes, joggers and hikers often develop pain and swelling around the tendo Achillis. This is due to local irritation of the paratenon.

Treatment is conservative: rest, ultrasound and a heel raise usually bring relief. For intractable cases, an operation to excise inflamed and degenerate tissue may be successful.

RUPTURE

Rupture probably occurs only if the tendon is degenerate; consequently, most patients are aged over 40 years. While pushing off (running or jumping), the calf muscle contracts, but the contraction is resisted by body weight and the tendon ruptures. The patient feels as if he or she has been struck just above the heel, and is unable to tiptoe. Soon after the tear occurs, a gap can be seen and felt 5 cm above the insertion of the tendon. Plantarflexion of the foot is weak and is not accompanied by tautening of the tendon. Where doubt exists, Simmonds' test is helpful: with the patient prone, the calf is squeezed; if the tendon is intact, the foot is seen to plantarflex; if the tendon is ruptured, the foot remains still.

Treatment

If the patient is seen early, the ends of the tendon may approximate when the foot is passively plantarflexed. If so, plaster is applied with the foot in equinus and is worn for 8 weeks. A shoe with a raised heel is worn for a further 6 weeks. The 're-rupture rate' is about 10 per cent.

Operative repair is probably more reliable, but immobilization in equinus for 8 weeks and a heel raise for a further 6 weeks are still needed. A more sophisticated alternative is a lockable brace which permits early ankle movement yet blocks tension on the newly repaired tendon.

THE DIABETIC FOOT

Foot disorders are common in patients with diabetes and result from:

- *peripheral vascular disease* causing claudication, trophic changes, ulceration and gangrene;
- *neuropathy* with sensory and/or motor impairment leading to trophic changes, ulceration, loss of joint position sense and predisposition to progressive joint destruction (neuropathic joint disease);
- *osteoporosis* and the risk of fracture;
- *infection* following minor trauma or ulceration.

Treatment

Management is a multidisciplinary exercise, involving physician, surgeon, chiropodist and orthotist, all working under the umbrella of a diabetic clinic. The principles of treatment are:

- proper control of the diabetes;
- constant and careful attention to the skin and toenails to prevent infection;
- attention to footwear and pressure-relieving orthoses;
- splintage for unstable joints;
- early attention to signs of gangrene: dry gangrene of the toe can be left to demarcate before amputation; wet gangrene and infection may call for immediate amputation;
- appropriate care of osteoporotic fractures: these should be immobilized only until pain subsides; movement is important.

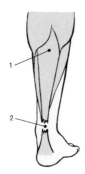
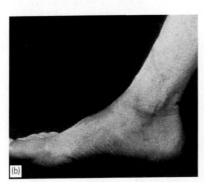
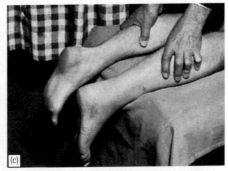

21.15 Rupture of tendo Achillis (a) The soleus may tear at its musculotendinous junction (1), but the tendo Achillis itself ruptures about 5 cm above its insertion (2). (b) There is a visible and palpable depression at the site of rupture just above the heel. (c) Simmonds' test: both calves are being squeezed but only the left foot plantarflexes – the right tendon is ruptured.

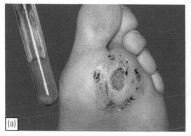
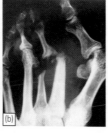
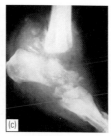

21.16 The diabetic foot (a) Ulceration in a patient with poorly controlled diabetes. (b) Severe toe deformities in a patient with diabetic neuropathy. (c) Neuropathic joint disease is one of the major risks, especially in patients with poorly controlled diabetes. The mid-tarsal joints are the most commonly affected and there is usually a provocative incident, such as a fracture around the ankle or heel. Joint destruction is progressive and severe.

PAINFUL ANKLE

Except after trauma or in rheumatoid arthritis, persistent pain around the ankle usually originates in one of the periarticular structures or the talus rather than the joint itself. Conditions to be looked for are chronic ligamentous instability, tenosynovitis of the tibialis posterior or peroneal tendons, rupture of the tibialis posterior tendon, osteochondritis dissecans of the dome of the talus or avascular necrosis of the talus.

Tenosynovitis

Tenderness and swelling are localized to the affected tendon, and pain is aggravated by active movement – inversion or eversion against resistance. Local injection of corticosteroid usually helps.

Rupture of tibialis posterior tendon

Pain starts quite suddenly and sometimes the patient gives a history of having felt the tendon snap. The heel is in valgus during weight-bearing; the area around the medial malleolus is tender, and active inversion of the ankle is both painful and weak. In physically active patients, operative repair or tendon transfer using the tendon of flexor digitorum longus is worthwhile. For poorly mobile patients, or indeed anyone who is prepared to put up with the inconvenience of an orthosis, splintage may be adequate.

Osteochondritis dissecans of the talus

Unexplained pain and slight limitation of movement in the ankle of a young person may be due to a small osteochondral fracture of the dome of the talus. Tangential x-rays will usually show the tiny fragment. MRI is also helpful and the lesion may be visualized directly by arthroscopy. If the articular surface is intact, it is sufficient to simply restrict activities. If the fragment has separated, it may have to be removed.

Avascular necrosis of the talus

The talus is one of the preferred sites of 'idiopathic' necrosis. The causes are the same as for necrosis at other more common sites, such as the femoral head (see Chapter 5). If pain is marked, arthrodesis of the ankle may be needed.

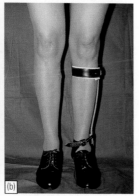

21.17 Rupture of tibialis posterior tendon This patient with rheumatoid arthritis suddenly developed a painful valgus foot on the left. The deformity was well controlled by a light-weight orthosis, and operative repair was unnecessary.

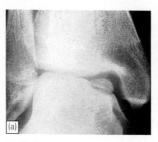
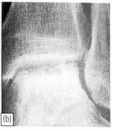

21.18 Osteochondritis dissecans (a) Osteochondritis dissecans at the common site, the anteromedial part of the articular surface of the talus. (b) More extensive lesions can lead to secondary osteoarthritis of the ankle.

THE PAINFUL FOOT

Pain may be felt predominantly in the heel, the midfoot or the forefoot. Common causes are: (1) mechanical pressure (which is more likely if the foot is deformed); (2) joint inflammation or stiffness; (3) a localized bone lesion; (4) peripheral ischaemia; or (5) muscular strain – usually secondary to some other abnormality.

PAINFUL HEEL

Traction 'apophysitis'

This condition usually occurs in young boys. It is not a 'disease', but a mild traction injury. Pain and tenderness are localized to the tendo Achillis insertion. The x-ray may show increased density or irregularity of the apophysis, but often the painless heel looks similar. The heel of the shoe should be raised a little and strenuous activities restricted for a few weeks.

Calcaneal bursitis

Older girls and young women often complain of painful bumps on the backs of their heels. The posterolateral portion of the calcaneum is prominent and shoe friction causes a bursitis. Treatment should be conservative – attention to

21.19 Painful heel (a) Sever's disease – the apophysis is dense and fragmented. (b) Bilateral 'heel bumps'. (c) The usual site of tenderness in plantar fasciitis. (d) X-ray in patients with plantar fasciitis often shows what looks like a spur on the undersurface of the calcaneum. In reality this is a two-dimensional view of a small ridge corresponding to the attachment of the plantar fascia. It is doubtful whether the 'spur' is responsible for the pain and local tenderness.

footwear (open-back shoes are best) and padding of the heel. If symptoms warrant it, removal of the calcaneal prominence may help.

Plantar fasciitis

Pain under the ball of the heel, or slightly forwards of this, is a fairly common complaint in people (mainly men) aged 30–60 years. It is worse on weight-bearing and there is marked tenderness along the distal edge of the heel contact area; a lateral x-ray often shows a bone 'spur' extending distally from this site but it is questionable whether this is the cause of the pain.

The condition is sometimes associated with inflammatory disorders such as gout, ankylosing spondylitis and Reiter's disease. Treatment is conservative: anti-inflammatory drugs or local injection of corticosteroids, and a pad under the heel to off-load the painful area.

Bone lesions

Calcaneal lesions such as infection, tumours and Paget's disease can give rise to unremitting pain in the heel. The diagnosis is usually obvious on x-ray examination.

PAIN OVER THE MIDFOOT

In children, pain in the midtarsal region may be due to osteochondritis of the navicular (Köhler's disease). X-ray shows a flattened navicular, with markedly increased density. Usually no treatment is needed as the condition resolves spontaneously.

In adults, a ridge of bone sometimes develops on the adjacent dorsal surfaces of the medial cuneiform and the first metatarsal (the 'overbone'). The tender bump is irritated by shoe pressure. If shoe adjustment fails to provide relief, the lump may be bevelled off.

PAIN IN THE FOREFOOT (METATARSALGIA)

Any foot abnormality which results in faulty weight distribution may cause nagging pain in the forefoot. It is therefore a common complaint in patients with hallux valgus, claw-toes, pes cavus or flat-foot. However, three specific disorders require special mention.

Freiberg's disease

This is a crushing type of osteochondritis of the second metatarsal head (rarely the third). It usually affects young adults, mostly women. A bony lump (the enlarged head) is palpable and tender and movement of the metatarsophalangeal

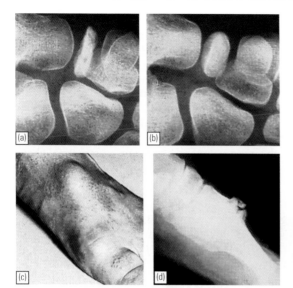

21.20 Pain over the midfoot (a) Köhler's disease compared with (b) the normal foot. (c,d) The bump on the dorsum of the foot due to osteoarthritis of the first cuneiform-metatarsal joint.

joint is painful. X-rays show the head to be wide and flat.

If footwear modifications (moulded insoles) do not relieve symptoms, operative synovectomy, debridement and trimming of the metatarsal head should be considered. Pain relief is usually good and the range of dorsiflexion is improved.

Stress fracture

Stress fractures of the second and third metatarsal bones are seen in young adults after unaccustomed

activity. The affected metatarsal shaft feels thick and tender. The x-ray appearance is at first normal, but later shows fusiform callus around a fine transverse fracture. Rest is all that is needed.

Similar fractures sometimes occur in elderly, osteoporotic patients who (for one reason or another) change their pattern of walking and weight-bearing.

Morton's metatarsalgia

The patient, usually a woman of around 50 years, complains of pain in the forefoot radiating to the toes. Tenderness is localized to one of the intermetatarsal spaces – usually the third – and pressure just proximal to the interdigital web may elicit both the pain and a tingling sensation distally. Squeezing the metatarsal heads together may produce a painful click (Mulder's click).

This is essentially an entrapment or compression syndrome affecting one of the digital nerves, but secondary thickening of the nerve creates the impression of a 'neuroma'. If symptoms do not respond to the use of protective padding and wearing wider shoes, nerve compression can often be released by dividing the tight transverse intermetatarsal ligament. Intractable cases may need excision of the 'neuroma'.

> ⚠ **Sudden forefoot pain: x-ray for metatarsal stress fracture – and x-ray again 2 weeks later when signs are more obvious.**

TOENAIL DISORDERS

The toenail of the hallux may be ingrown, overgrown or undergrown.

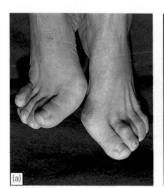
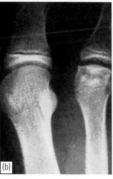
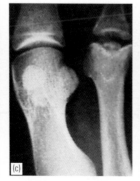
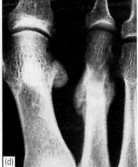

21.21 Pain in the forefoot (a) Long-standing deformities such as dropped anterior arches, hallux valgus, hammer-toe, curly toes and overlapping toes (all of which are present in this patient) can cause metatarsalgia. Localized pain and tenderness suggest a more specific cause. (b,c) Stages in the development of Freiberg's disease. (d) Periosteal new-bone formation along the shaft of the second metatarsal, the classic sign of a stress fracture.

Ingrown toenail

The nail burrows into the nail groove; this ulcerates and its wall grows over the nail, so the term 'embedded toenail' would be better. The patient is taught to cut the nail square, to insert pledgets of wool into the nail groove and always to keep the feet clean and dry. If these measures fail, the portion of germinal matrix which is responsible for the 'ingrow' should be ablated, either by operative excision or by chemical ablation with phenol. Rarely is it necessary to remove the entire nail or completely ablate the nail bed.

Overgrown toenail (onychogryposis)

Sometimes the nail, for no apparent reason, becomes unusually hard, thick and curved. A chiropodist can make the patient comfortable, but occasionally nails need complete excision.

Subungual bone growth

In this condition the nail is gradually lifted from its bed by an 'exostosis' growing on the dorsum of the terminal phalanx. X-ray examination shows the bony protuberance. The 'exostosis' should be removed.

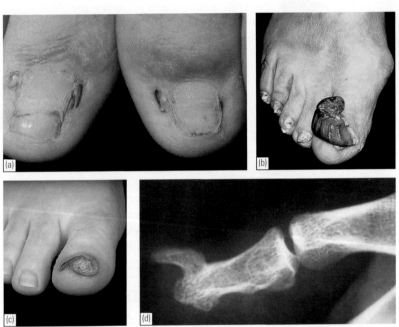

21.22 Toenail disorders
(a) Ingrown toenails.
(b) Overgrown toenail (onychogryposis). (c,d) Exostosis from the distal phalanx, pushing the toenail up.

3 Fractures and Joint Injuries

CHAPTER 22

MANAGEMENT OF MAJOR INJURIES

Trauma is the main cause of death in people under 40. Limb injuries are the commonest, head and visceral injuries are the most lethal; this simple observation determines the priorities in management.

Trauma mortality has a trimodal distribution. (1) Most deaths occur during the first hour after injury, before the patient reaches hospital. (2) A second peak in the death rate occurs between 1 and 4 hours after injury, when patients die mainly because of blood loss; this is the 'golden hour', during which death can and should be prevented by competent treatment. (3) A third peak occurs several weeks later when patients die of late complications and multiple organ failure. The management of severe injuries proceeds in well-defined stages:

1. Emergency treatment immediately after the accident.
2. Resuscitation and evaluation in the hospital accident department.
3. Early treatment of visceral injuries and cardiorespiratory complications.
4. Treatment of musculoskeletal injuries.
5. Long-term rehabilitation.

MANAGEMENT AT THE SCENE OF THE ACCIDENT

The first duty of a doctor arriving at the scene of a major accident is to introduce calm and order into the prevailing chaos. Actions should be swift yet unhurried, cautious yet purposeful. Messages are

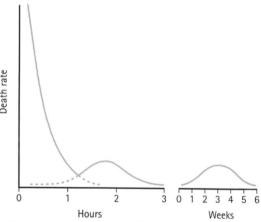

22.1 Death following trauma The trimodal pattern of mortality following severe trauma.

sent to the emergency services, and the nearest accident centre is alerted. Management of the injured follows a disciplined sequence:

■ protect the cervical spine
■ free the airway
■ ensure ventilation
■ arrest haemorrhage
■ put up a drip
■ control pain
■ splint fractures
■ transport to hospital.

The patient's head and neck should be freed by removing the surrounding debris. The neck must be held immobile, with gentle traction. A collar (makeshift if necessary) should be applied as soon as possible.

The upper airway is checked. If the patient is unconscious, the jaw should be pulled forward, *but do not extend the neck.* A finger in the mouth ensures that there is no mechanical obstruction.

If there is still difficulty with breathing, look for a chest wound. Administer oxygen if available.

External bleeding must be stanched by direct pressure.

If facilities are available, intravenous fluids may be given for shock. Intravenous morphine is useful, but should not be administered to patients with abdominal or head injuries.

Injured limbs should be splinted as well as possible, using whatever is available.

The patient is then carefully lifted by at least two and preferably three people so that he or she can be transported with minimal physical manipulation.

MANAGEMENT IN HOSPITAL

Having survived the accident, the patient now faces the second 'mortality peak' – the risk of dying from either hypoxia or hypovolaemic shock. This is the *golden hour* during which effective resuscitation can save life. Assessment and treatment are undertaken in four co-ordinated stages:

1. a rapid primary survey with simultaneous resuscitation,
2. a detailed secondary survey,
3. continual re-evaluation,
4. definitive care.

PRIMARY SURVEY

The patient is stripped and examined rapidly from head to toe. If there are injuries around the head and face, damage to the cervical spine should be assumed and care should be taken *not to flex or extend the neck* until a cervical spine injury has been definitely excluded. The neck must either be supported manually in the neutral position or immobilized by sandbags on either side and a tape across the forehead. Life-threatening conditions should be treated as they are identified. Remember the ABC of primary evaluation and treatment: **A**irway – **B**reathing – **C**irculation. It is also important to record the level of consciousness.

Airway

The priority is to ensure a clear airway. Check for any obstruction due to a decreased level of consciousness, facial trauma, neck trauma or inhalation of vomit or teeth. The sound of an obstructed airway – stridor – is unmistakable. A gloved finger is effective for removing vomitus or foreign matter from the mouth. Suction is used if it is available; a short oropharyngeal airway is a further help.

If there is still no free airway, an orotracheal tube can be inserted, but only if the necessary expertise, drugs and equipment are immediately available.

If all these attempts fail, a high flow of oxygen can be provided via a needle passed through the cricothyroid membrane, with 1 second of insufflation and 3 seconds' deflation. This buys time for some 30 minutes until the carbon dioxide levels begin to rise. A more definitive procedure (e.g. cricothyrotomy) can then be performed.

The airway must be checked frequently throughout the resuscitation phase; one that appears initially to be safe may not remain so.

Breathing

If, despite a clear airway, ventilation is inadequate, the chest should be carefully examined for atelectasis, pneumothorax or a flail segment. *Tension pneumothorax* is a life-threatening complication and should be treated by immediate decompression (see page 260). *Sucking chest wounds* must be closed and a *flail chest* may require endotracheal intubation and positive-pressure ventilation.

It is essential to give all severely injured patients supplemental oxygen and to take a blood sample for measurement of the arterial oxygen tension ($P\text{O}_2$) and carbon dioxide tension ($P\text{CO}_2$).

Circulation

Any major external haemorrhage is controlled by direct pressure. The patient is assessed for signs of shock, and blood specimens are taken for full blood count, estimation of electrolytes and cross-matching (see page 262).

Level of consciousness

The level of consciousness is assessed on the Glasgow Coma Scale (see page 261). All findings are carefully recorded and kept available for comparison with later assessment.

RESUSCITATION

Further examination of the patient should not interfere with resuscitation. Specific problems, such as ineffectual ventilation and shock, are dealt with immediately (see pages 262–264). Fractures

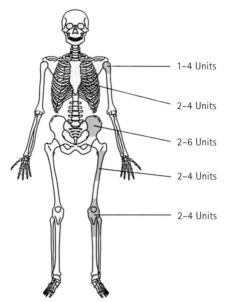

1–4 Units

2–4 Units

2–6 Units

2–4 Units

2–4 Units

22.2 Severe injuries – blood loss Range of blood loss in closed fractures. The patient loses more blood than you think!

must be splinted until the patient is fit for definitive treatment. Pain is controlled by the judicious use of analgesics.

SECONDARY SURVEY

Once the patient has been resuscitated, a head-to-toe survey is carried out. The back can be examined by gently 'log-rolling' the patient onto his or her side.

X-rays of the chest, spine and pelvis are obtained, as well as any other investigations which might be helpful.

RE-EVALUATION

The vital signs should be checked repeatedly to assess the response to treatment. The patient should not leave the emergency department until his or her condition is stable, unless it is to be taken directly to the operating theatre for the control of haemorrhage or some other surgical emergency.

REGIONAL INJURIES

At any stage of the primary or secondary evaluation it may become obvious that the patient has sustained a specific injury which requires immediate treatment. The most important are

chest injuries, abdominal injuries, pelvic injuries and head injuries.

CHEST INJURIES

Chest injuries may damage the rib cage or its contents. Remember that small wounds may hide serious complications.

Clinical assessment

The patient may have chest pain or show obvious signs of respiratory distress. The skin is inspected for bruising (a seat-belt injury) and for open wounds (especially 'sucking' wounds, which communicate with the pleural cavity). The trachea is palpated to see if it is deviated and the chest is examined for signs of pulmonary collapse and mediastinal shift.

X-rays

X-ray examination may reveal a pleural effusion, pneumothorax or lung collapse; widening of the mediastinum suggests a ruptured aortic arch. Search also for fractures of the ribs, sternum or thoracic vertebrae

Management

General approach

Minor chest injuries are common and many require little more than treatment for pain. However, one should always be alert to the danger of complications, which may appear only after several days. For *severe chest injuries,* three measures are essential: (1) blood replacement (but not with crystalloid fluids, which aggravate pulmonary congestion); (2) the administration of oxygen; and (3) adequate analgesics (but not respiratory depressants). Patients should be carefully monitored for signs of acute respiratory distress syndrome (ARDS) (see page 263).

Uncomplicated rib fractures

These usually need no treatment other than analgesics. The patient with multiple fractures and extensive bruising should, however, be kept under observation in hospital until complications have been positively excluded. If pain is marked, infiltration with local anaesthetic may be needed to facilitate breathing and prevent atelectasis and lung infection.

Simple closed pneumothorax

An air leak into the pleural cavity can usually be seen on an x-ray taken with the patient upright. Small collections require no treatment apart from breathing exercises. A large pneumothorax may need drainage (see below).

Tension pneumothorax

This occurs when a pleural tear acts like a valve, allowing air into the pleural cavity during inspiration but preventing it from escaping during expiration. The patient is distressed; chest movements are diminished, the mediastinum is shifted to the unaffected side and breath sounds are absent on the affected side. *This is a lethal emergency: there may be only minutes in which to act before the patient dies.* A large-bore needle should be inserted into the pleural cavity through the second intercostal space in the mid-clavicular line anteriorly. Once the emergency is over, this is replaced by a thoracostomy tube which is inserted through the fourth intercostal space in the mid-axillary line and connected to an underwater seal; this is retained until the lung re-expands.

Surgical emphysema

Air may appear under the skin, extending over the chest wall and into the neck. This happens when a lung perforation (or rupture) communicates with the subcutaneous tissues. If there is a tension pneumothorax, it should be decompressed.

Haemothorax

Bleeding from a torn lung or blood vessel can be diagnosed by withdrawing blood through a needle. The blood is drained by an intercostal catheter through a low intercostal space. Breathing exercises are encouraged.

Stove-in chest

Multiple rib fractures are often associated with underlying lung damage. Sometimes an entire section of the chest wall is isolated as a flail segment, which is sucked inwards during inspiration and blown outwards during expiration. This so-called *paradoxical respiration* is useless for ventilating the lung and it may lead to respiratory failure (particularly if the lung is also damaged).

A stove-in chest with only moderate respiratory difficulty can be treated by strapping a large pack over the mobile segment and administering oxygen. More severe cases require endotracheal intubation and positive-pressure ventilation; a chest drain connected to an underwater seal may be needed if there is lung damage. Positive-pressure ventilation is maintained (if necessary by changing to a tracheostomy until the chest wall is stable).

ABDOMINAL INJURIES

A blow to the abdomen may rupture viscera or blood vessels. A ruptured spleen or liver may be deceptively 'silent', but it should be suspected if there are signs of continuing blood loss; this is a particular problem in unconscious patients. An ultrasound scan may be helpful and abdominal paracentesis may show blood in the peritoneal cavity.

Stab wounds can be missed unless the abdomen is carefully examined. The size of the wound is no guide to the amount of damage: a sharpened bicycle spoke can perforate bowel, spleen, diaphragm and heart in a single blow.

If a serious injury is suspected, laparotomy is essential. A ruptured spleen can sometimes be salvaged but usually has to be removed. Bleeding from a ruptured liver is difficult to control, but an attempt should be made to suture or ligate injured vessels; if this fails, haemorrhage may be controlled by packing. A ruptured bowel can usually be repaired.

PELVIC INJURIES

Fractures of the pelvis are often associated with serious visceral injury and blood loss. This subject is dealt with in Chapter 30.

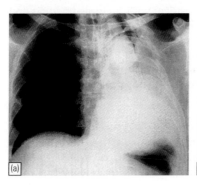

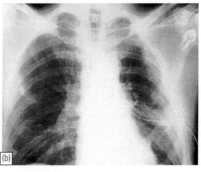

22.3 Tension pneumothorax
(a) This patient with rib fractures became distressed. The x-ray shows 'black-out' of the right side of the chest with the mediastinal contents shifted to the left. (b) The situation after intercostal drainage.

HEAD INJURIES

Most head injuries result from a blow that causes either direct damage or intracerebral movement due to rapid acceleration or deceleration. Damage may consist of: (1) minor contusion causing transient loss of consciousness or amnesia; (2) severe contusion or laceration, due either to direct injury or to shearing forces; (3) localized intracranial bleeding; (4) fractures of the skull; (5) diffuse oedema and a rise in intracranial pressure.

Secondary brain injury also arises from hypoxia (obstructed airway, inadequate ventilation or poor circulation), which may be the last straw for injured brain cells.

Clinical assessment

The history may give important clues to the type and severity of the injury. Did the patient lose consciousness? If so, for how long? Was there a period of amnesia? Did the patient take drugs or alcohol? Is there a previous history of fits or neurological disorder? What other injuries are present? No matter how appalling the head injury may appear, freeing the airway, protecting the cervical spine, ensuring full ventilation and arresting haemorrhage always take precedence.

There may be obvious swelling and/or bruising of the face. The scalp should be examined for cuts or localized swelling (haematoma); open wounds should be gently explored with a gloved finger to exclude underlying fractures. The nose and ears are examined for blood or cerebrospinal fluid leakage; other signs of basal fracture are sub-conjunctival haemorrhage without a posterior margin, localized periorbital haematomas ('racoon eyes') and retromastoid bruising (Battle's sign).

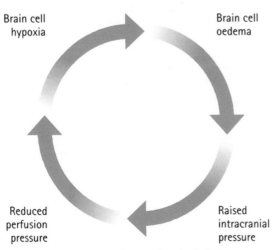

Brain cell hypoxia

Brain cell oedema

Reduced perfusion pressure

Raised intracranial pressure

22.4 The vicious circle of secondary brain injury

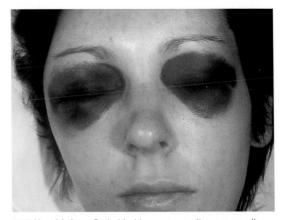

22.5 Head injury Periorbital haematomas ('racoon eyes') should suggest the presence of a basal skull fracture.

The pupils are examined for asymmetrical dilatation and the light reflex is tested on each side. With increased intracranial pressure and tentorial herniation, compression of the third nerve results in dilatation of the pupil and a failure to react to light.

Imaging

X-ray of the skull is mandatory and *CT* is needed for those with persistent subnormal consciousness, depressed skull fractures, penetrating injuries or focal neurological signs. Throughout the examination, great care must be exercised not to flex or extend the neck unless an associated cervical spine injury has been excluded.

The level of consciousness

The level of consciousness should be assessed according to the Glasgow Coma Scale. This is based on descending levels of eye opening and verbal and motor responses (Table 22.1). The maximum score, representing normality, is 15; a score of 8 or less implies severe head injury; absence of eye opening, speech and response to commands is indicative of coma.

Repeated examination will show whether the patient's condition is improving or not. A deterioration of 2 points is highly significant and is an indication for CT.

Management

Most head injuries are fairly trivial and require no more than careful examination and reassurance. The indications for admission to hospital for observation and reassessment are any of the

Table 22.1 Glasgow Coma Scale

	Score
Eye opening	
Spontaneous	4
On command	3
On pain	2
Nil	1
Best motor response	
Obeys	6
Localizes pain	5
Normal flexor	4
Abnormal flexor	3
Extensor	2
Nil	1
Verbal response	
Orientated	5
Confused	4
Words	3
Sounds	2
Nil	1

following: (1) a diminished level of consciousness; (2) a history of transient loss of consciousness or amnesia; (3) a skull fracture; and (4) abnormal neurological signs.

In patients who appear to be comatose, drowsy, restless or merely confused, it may be difficult to distinguish the effects of a head injury from those of hypoglycaemia, alcohol or drugs. All such patients, as well as those whose cerebral dysfunction may be due to shock or hypoxia, should be graded on the Glasgow Coma Scale and kept under observation until the diagnosis is clear. If there is any chance that the patient has suffered an intracranial bleed, a CT scan is urgent.

Concussion

Following a blow, there is a transient loss of consciousness, often associated with amnesia. However brief the period of unconsciousness, the skull should be x-rayed. If the patient was unconscious for only a few minutes and is now fully conscious, and a skull fracture has been excluded, he or she can be allowed to go home in the care of a responsible adult who will be at hand for the next 48 hours. If this cannot be arranged, the patient should be admitted for observation.

Those with either a skull fracture or an impaired level of consciousness will also need a CT scan.

Scalp wounds

Scalp wounds (after thorough cleansing) can be sutured, provided there is no underlying depressed fracture.

Fractures

A linear fracture may be quite harmless, but a CT should be obtained to exclude intracranial damage or haematoma. If there is a cerebrospinal fluid leak (otorrhoea or rhinorrhoea), the patient is given prophylactic benzyl penicillin. A depressed fracture requires exploration, elevation and clearance of damaged tissue.

Extradural haematoma

The classic scenario is of a patient who has a head injury but seems to be perfectly well, is allowed to go home and then rapidly becomes unconscious. There may be a minor fracture which causes bleeding and cerebral compression. Look for a fixed dilated pupil on the affected side. CT shows an extradural haematoma and a shift of the brain (Fig. 22.6). This requires urgent treatment: burr holes and evacuation of the haematoma; if necessary, the middle meningeal artery is ligated.

Severe brain contusion

Patients with severe head injuries (a Glasgow Coma Scale score of 8 or less) should be kept under continuous observation until they recover spontaneously, or develop signs calling for operative treatment, or ultimately show the features of 'brain death'. They are best managed by endotracheal intubation and artificial ventilation. The main indication for craniotomy is the development of an intracranial haematoma.

GENERAL COMPLICATIONS OF TRAUMA

SHOCK

Shock is a generalized state of reduced tissue perfusion; if allowed to persist, it will result in irreversible damage to the life-supporting organs. It may be caused by direct injury to the heart, massive cardiac infarction or acute pulmonary embolism *(cardiogenic shock),* or by sudden loss of venous tone due to spinal cord injury *(neurogenic shock).* Usually, however, it is the result of haemorrhage and reduction of blood volume *(hypovolaemic shock),* the effects of which may be

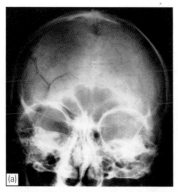 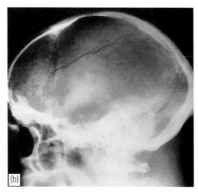 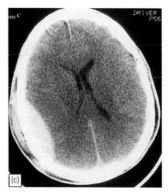

22.6 Head injuries – imaging (a,b) X-rays showing a fracture of the parietal bone. (c) The CT scan shows an extradural haematoma with distortion of the lateral ventricle on that side.

compounded by low haemoglobin, inadequate ventilation and infection. Various compensatory mechanisms come into play, but if blood loss is too great, they will fail: cardiac output falls, the blood pressure drops and decreased tissue perfusion leads to hypoxia, acidosis and progressive cell damage. The greater the degree of hypovolaemia, and the longer it is allowed to persist, the greater the risk of organ failure.

Clinical features and diagnosis

The patient becomes apathetic and thirsty, breathing is shallow and rapid, the lips and skin are pale and the extremities feel cold and clammy. As compensation fails, the pulse becomes rapid and feeble, the blood pressure drops and the patient may become confused. Eventually renal function is impaired and urinary output falls. If it is difficult to measure the blood pressure reliably and repeatedly, continuous intra-arterial pressure monitoring should be instituted. While the diagnosis and monitoring of post-traumatic hypovolaemic shock are usually straightforward, the picture is sometimes complicated by signs of right ventricular failure, requiring more specialized investigations and monitoring systems.

Treatment

The treatment of hypovolaemic shock is urgent: the essentials are to oxygenate the patient, arrest bleeding and replace lost blood. Pneumatic antishock garments (military antishock trousers, or 'MAST' suits) are sometimes used; they work by compressing the capillary bed and increasing vascular resistance. If there are fractures, early reduction and splintage help to reduce the effects of shock.

The essential feature of treatment, however, is the early restoration of blood volume. A practical routine is to start with the rapid infusion of 2 L of crystalloid solution such as Ringer's lactate; the patient's response is checked by measuring the heart rate, blood pressure and central venous pressure, and, later on, urinary output and acid–base balance. If improvement is not sustained and other causes of cardiac embarrassment have been excluded, concealed haemorrhage into the chest or abdomen is probable and should be sought by investigations such as ultrasonography, CT and abdominal paracentesis.

If the patient does not respond quickly to intravenous crystalloids, blood transfusion will be necessary. In an emergency, group O Rh-negative blood may be used until cross-matched blood is available.

It is important not only to give blood but also to give *enough* blood. Even with closed injuries, there is far more bleeding into tissues than is commonly appreciated: two or three units may be lost with a single major limb fracture (see Fig. 22.2).

ADULT RESPIRATORY DISTRESS SYNDROME

During the later stages of shock and septicaemia, endothelial cell damage and increased small-vessel permeability lead to the extravasation of haemorrhagic, protein-rich fluid into the pulmonary interstitial tissue and alveoli. Over a period of a few days the picture may change from pulmonary congestion to diffuse alveolar destruction. The early changes are reversible, but once diffuse alveolar damage occurs, there is usually an inexorable progression to severe hypoxaemia, multiple organ failure and death.

Clinical features

About 36 hours after injury and hypovolaemic shock, the patient develops mild dyspnoea. Even before this, if blood gases are measured, they may show a diminished PO_2. These changes are common after long-bone fractures, and fat embolism is often suspected. By the second or third day, the clinical features are more obvious: the patient is restless, mildly cyanosed and shows signs of respiratory distress. X-rays may now show diffuse pulmonary infiltrates. Special lung function tests are required to show the full extent of the condition. In the most severe cases, pulmonary deterioration is inexorable and the outcome is fatal.

Treatment

The most important aspect of management is the early and effective treatment of shock. There is also evidence that, in patients with multiple injuries, the incidence of pulmonary dysfunction is reduced by early stabilization of fractures.

The treatment of established ARDS is supportive and aims to minimize further lung damage until recovery occurs, whilst optimizing oxygen delivery to the tissues. This requires highly specialized methods of artificial ventilation and continuous cardiopulmonary assessment.

FAT EMBOLISM

Circulating fat globules occur in most young adults after closed fractures of long bones; fortunately, only a few develop the fat embolism syndrome, which is now thought to be part of the wider spectrum of acute post-traumatic respiratory distress.

The source of the fat emboli is probably the bone marrow, and the condition is more common in patients with multiple closed fractures; however, fat embolism has been reported in a variety of disorders other than skeletal trauma (e.g. burns, renal infarction and cardiopulmonary operations); the pathogenesis is still a matter of controversy.

Clinical features

The patient is usually a young adult with a closed long-bone fracture. Clinical features appear within 72 hours of injury; they include shortness of breath, restlessness and mild confusion, with a rise in temperature and pulse rate. In the worst cases the patient develops marked respiratory distress, followed by restlessness, coma and death. Clinical signs are few, but a careful search may reveal petechiae on the chest, in the axillae and in the conjunctival folds.

There is no infallible test for fat embolism, but a fairly constant finding is hypoxaemia; the blood PO_2 should always be monitored during the first 72 hours of any major injury, and values below 8 kPa (60 mmHg) must be regarded with grave suspicion.

Treatment

There is no specific treatment for fat embolism; the most important measure is to counteract the hypoxaemia by giving oxygen, in mild cases by nasal catheter or oxygen mask and in severe cases by tracheal intubation and assisted ventilation; the blood PO_2 is carefully monitored and it should be maintained above 9.3 kPa (70 mmHg).

Supportive therapy includes blood and fluid replacement, with intravenous corticosteroids and heparin, which are thought to reduce pulmonary oedema and intravascular clotting.

DISSEMINATED INTRAVASCULAR COAGULATION

An insidious complication of severe injury and blood loss is a widespread disorder of coagulation and haemostasis. (The same condition sometimes occurs in severe septicaemia.) This is due, at least in part, to the release of tissue thromboplastins into the circulation, endothelial damage and platelet activation. The result is a complex mixture of intravascular coagulation, depletion of clotting factors, fibrinolysis and thrombocytopenia. Microvascular occlusion causes haemorrhagic infarctions and tissue necrosis, while deficient haemostasis leads to abnormal bleeding.

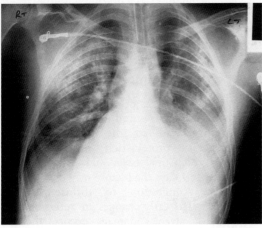

22.7 Adult respiratory distress syndrome (ARDS) X-ray showing diffuse pulmonary infiltrates in both lungs.

Clinical features

The patient, usually after a period of severe blood loss and transfusion, becomes confused and restless; other features of microvascular thrombosis are neurological dysfunction, skin infarcts, oliguria and incipient renal failure. Abnormal haemostasis causes excessive bleeding at operation, oozing drip sites and wounds, spontaneous bruising, gastrointestinal bleeding and haematuria. The diagnosis is confirmed by finding a low haemoglobin concentration, prolonged pro-thrombin and thrombin times, thrombocytopenia, hypofibrinogenaemia and raised levels of fibrinogen degradation products.

Treatment

The best 'treatment' is the prevention or early correction of hypovolaemic shock. If the bleeding is marked, it may help to replace clotting factors and platelets. However, this is a complex problem and it is wise to seek the advice of a haematologist.

CRUSH SYNDROME

The crush syndrome may occur if a large bulk of muscle is crushed, as by fallen masonry, or if a tourniquet has been left on too long. When compression is released, acid myohaematin (cytochrome c) is carried to the kidney and blocks the tubules. An alternative explanation is that renal artery spasm leads to tubular necrosis.

Shock is profound. The released limb is pulseless and later becomes red, swollen and blistered; sensation and muscle power may be lost. Renal secretion diminishes and a low-output uraemia with acidosis develops. If renal secretion returns within a week, the patient survives; most patients become increasingly drowsy and die within 14 days. Renal dialysis may be life saving.

Treatment

To avert disaster, a limb crushed severely and for several hours should be amputated. Likewise, if a tourniquet has been left on for more than 6 hours, the limb must be sacrificed. Amputation is carried out above the site of compression and before compression is released.

If compression has already been released, the limb must be cooled and the patient treated for shock and renal failure.

TETANUS

The tetanus organism flourishes only in dead tissue. It produces an exotoxin which passes to the central nervous system via the blood and the perineural lymphatics from the infected region. The toxin is fixed in the anterior horn cells and thereafter cannot be neutralized by antitoxin.

Established tetanus is characterized by tonic, and later clonic, contractions, especially of the muscles of the jaw and face (trismus, risus sardonicus), those near the wound itself, and later of the neck and trunk. Ultimately, the diaphragm and intercostal muscles may be fixed in spasm and the patient dies of asphyxia.

Prophylaxis

Active immunization of the whole population by tetanus toxoid is an attainable ideal. Patients seen more than 10 years after such immunization will need booster doses of toxoid after all but trivial skin wounding. In non-immunized patients, prompt and thorough wound toilet together with antibiotics may be adequate, but if the wound is contaminated, and particularly with delay before operation, antitoxin is advisable. Horse serum carries a considerable risk of anaphylaxis, and human antitetanus globulin should be used. The opportunity is taken to initiate active immunization with toxoid at the same time.

Treatment

With established tetanus, intravenous antitoxin (again, human for choice) is advisable. Heavy sedation and muscle relaxant drugs may help; tracheal intubation and controlled respiration are employed for the patient with respiratory and swallowing embarrassment.

CHAPTER 23

FRACTURES AND JOINT INJURIES

A fracture is a break in the structural continuity of bone. It may be no more than a crack, a crumpling or a splintering of the cortex; more often the break is complete and the bone fragments are displaced. If the overlying skin remains intact, it is a *closed* (or *simple*) *fracture;* if the skin or one of the body cavities is breached, it is an *open* (or *compound*) *fracture,* liable to contamination and infection.

Inevitably the surrounding soft tissues are involved as well. Changes range from local oedema and inflammatory reactions to severe soft-tissue damage and vascular impairment. Some of the most troublesome complications of fractures arise in joints which themselves appeared not to have been injured at the time.

When the joint itself is injured, this may take the form of *strained ligaments, subluxation* of the joint, *dislocation* or a combination of bone and joint injury – *fracture–dislocation* – with or without *articular cartilage damage.*

PATHOLOGY OF FRACTURES

Bone is relatively brittle, yet it has sufficient strength and resilience to withstand the normal stresses of everyday activities. Fractures result from: (1) a single highly stressful, traumatic incident; (2) repetitive stress of normal degree persisting to the point of mechanical fatigue; or (3) normal stress acting on abnormally weakened bone (a so-called 'pathological' fracture).

CAUSES OF FRACTURES

Fractures due to sudden trauma

Most fractures are caused by sudden and excessive force, which may be direct or indirect. *With direct force* the bone breaks at the point of impact, e.g. fracture of the ulna caused by a blow on the arm. *With indirect force* the bone breaks at a distance from where the force is applied; common examples are spiral fractures of the tibia and fibula due to torsion of the leg, vertebral compression fractures due to sudden, severe spinal flexion, and avulsion fractures due to violent traction by a muscle, tendon or ligament.

Stress or fatigue fractures

Cracks can occur in bone, as in metal and other materials, because of repetitive stress. This is most often seen in the tibia or fibula or metatarsals, especially in athletes, dancers and army recruits who go on long route marches.

Pathological fractures

Common examples of fractures in mechanically abnormal bone are seen in osteoporosis (skeletal insufficiency), Paget's disease (brittle bone) and bone tumours (osteolytic lesions).

TYPES OF FRACTURE

Fractures vary greatly in appearance, but for

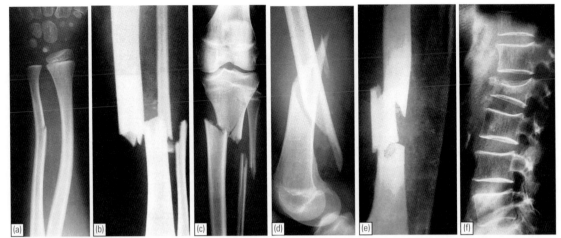

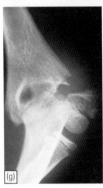

23.1 Common types of fracture (a) Incomplete 'greenstick' fracture of the ulna; (b) displaced transverse fracture; (c) oblique fracture; (d) spiral fracture, due to a twisting force – a typical low-energy fracture; (e) segmental fracture – a typical high-energy injury; (f) compression fracture, typically of an osteoporotic lumbar vertebra; and (g) avulsion fracture – in this case of the lateral humeral condyle, due to severe strain on the lateral ligaments of the elbow.

practical purposes they can be divided into a few well-defined groups.

Complete fractures

The bone is completely broken into two or more fragments. If the fracture is *transverse,* the fragments usually remain in place after reduction; if it is *oblique* or *spiral,* they tend to slip and re-displace even if the bone is splinted. In an *impacted fracture* the fragments are jammed tightly together and the fracture line is indistinct. A *comminuted fracture* is one in which there are more than two fragments; because there is poor interlocking of the fragments, these fractures are often unstable.

Incomplete fractures

Here the bone is incompletely divided and the periosteum remains in continuity. In a *greenstick fracture* the bone is buckled or bent (like snapping a green twig); this is seen in children, whose bones are more springy than those of adults. Reduction is usually easy and healing is quick. *Stress fractures* also may be incomplete, with the break initially appearing in only one part of the cortex; nevertheless, they take just as long to heal as

complete fractures. *Compression fractures* occur when cancellous bone is crumpled. This happens in adults, especially in the vertebral bodies.

Physeal fractures

Fractures through the growing physis are a special case. Damage to the cartilaginous growth plate may give rise to progressive deformity out of all proportion to the apparent severity of the injury.

FRACTURE DISPLACEMENT

After a complete fracture the fragments usually become displaced, partly by the force of the injury, partly by gravity and partly by the pull of muscles attached to them. Displacement is usually described in terms of translation, alignment, rotation and altered length.

Translation (shift)

The fragments may be shifted sideways, backwards or forwards in relation to each other, such that the fracture surfaces lose contact. The fracture will usually unite even if apposition is imperfect, and

267

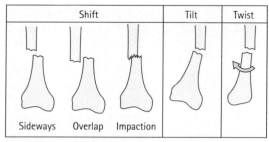

Shift			Tilt	Twist

Sideways   Overlap   Impaction

23.2 Fracture displacements The different types of fracture displacement.

sometimes even if the bone ends lie side by side with the fracture surfaces making no contact at all.

Alignment (angulation)

The fragments may be tilted or angulated in relation to each other. If malalignment is marked, the bend in the limb may be obvious; small degrees of malalignment are detected only by x-ray.

Rotation (twist)

Long-bone fragments may be rotated in relation to each other; the bone looks straight but the limb ends up with a torsional deformity.

Length

The fragments may be distracted and separated, or they may overlap, due to muscle spasm, causing shortening of the bone.

SOFT-TISSUE DAMAGE

Low-energy (low-velocity) fractures cause only moderate soft-tissue damage; the classic example is

a closed spiral fracture. *High-energy (high-velocity) fractures* cause severe damage; examples are segmental and comminuted fractures, no matter whether open or closed. The state of the enveloping soft tissues has a significant effect on fracture healing. A full description of the fracture should therefore include comment on the soft tissues.

FRACTURE HEALING

Fractures heal by two different methods: with callus or without.

Healing by callus

The process of fracture repair varies according to the type of bone involved and the amount of movement at the fracture site. In a tubular bone, and in the absence of rigid fixation, healing proceeds in five stages:

1. *Tissue destruction and haematoma formation.* Vessels are torn and a haematoma forms around and within the fracture. Bone at the fracture surfaces, deprived of a blood supply, dies back for a millimetre or two.
2. *Inflammation and cellular proliferation.* Within 8 hours of the fracture there is an acute inflammatory reaction with proliferation of cells under the periosteum and within the breached medullary canal. The fragment ends are surrounded by cellular tissue, which bridges the fracture site. The clotted haematoma is slowly absorbed and fine new capillaries grow into the area.
3. *Callus formation.* The proliferating cells are potentially chondrogenic and osteogenic; given the right conditions, they will start forming

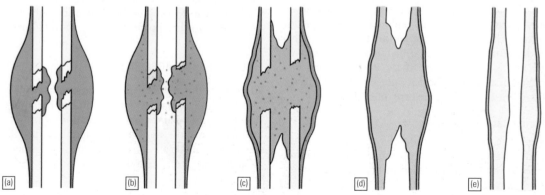

23.3 Fracture healing Five stages of healing. (a) *Haematoma*: tissue damage and bleeding at the fracture site; the bone ends die back for a few millimetres. (b) *Inflammatory reaction*: inflammatory cells appear in the haematoma. (c) *Callus*: the cell population changes to osteoblasts and osteoclasts; dead bone is mopped up and woven bone appears in the fracture callus. (d) *Consolidation*: woven bone is replaced by lamellar bone; the fracture has united. (e) *Remodelling*: the newly formed bone is remodelled to resemble the normal structure.

bone and, in some cases, also cartilage. The cell population now also includes osteoclasts (probably derived from the new blood vessels) which begin to mop up dead bone. The thick cellular mass, with its islands of immature bone and cartilage, forms the callus or splint on the periosteal and endosteal surfaces. As the immature bone (or 'woven' bone) becomes more densely mineralized, movement at the fracture site progressively decreases and the fracture 'unites'. The entire process is driven by inductive proteins, which include fibroblast growth factors, transforming growth factors and bone morphogenic protein.

4. *Consolidation.* With continuing osteoclastic and osteoblastic activity, the woven bone is transformed into lamellar bone. The system is now rigid enough to allow osteoclasts to burrow through the debris at the fracture line, and close behind them osteoblasts fill in the remaining gaps between the fragments with new bone. This is a slow process and it may be several months before the bone is strong enough to carry normal loads.

5. *Remodelling.* The fracture has been bridged by a cuff of solid bone. Over a period of months, or even years, this crude 'weld' is reshaped by a continuous process of alternating bone resorption and formation. Thicker lamellae are laid down where the stresses are high; unwanted buttresses are carved away; the medullary cavity is reformed. Eventually, and especially in children, the bone re-assumes something like its normal shape.

Healing without callus

Callus is the response to movement at the fracture site. It serves to stabilize the fragments as rapidly as possible – a necessary precondition for bridging by

bone. If the fracture site is absolutely immobile – for example an impacted fracture in cancellous bone, or a fracture rigidly immobilized by internal fixation – there is no need for callus. Instead, new-bone formation occurs directly between the fragments. Gaps between the fracture surfaces are invaded by new capillaries and bone-forming cells growing in from the edges. Where the crevices are very narrow (less than 200 μm), osteogenesis produces lamellar bone; wider gaps are filled first by woven bone, which is then remodelled to lamellar bone (gap healing).

Healing by callus, though less direct, ensures mechanical strength while the bone ends heal. With rigid metal fixation, on the other hand, the absence of callus means that there is a long period during which the bone depends entirely upon the metal implant for its integrity. Moreover, the implant diverts stress away from the bone, which may become osteoporotic and not recover fully until the metal is removed.

The time factor

Repair of a fracture is a continuous process and there are no specific events signifying a moment of 'union' or 'consolidation'. The ultimate test is the bone's ability to withstand the stresses placed upon it: fracture 'union' is incomplete repair and it is not safe to subject the unprotected bone to stress; 'consolidation' is also less than complete repair, but it allows unprotected function; only after remodelling and the restoration of normal bone density is the process of repair complete.

The rate of repair depends upon the *type of bone* involved (cancellous bone heals faster than cortical bone), the *type of fracture* (a transverse fracture takes longer than a spiral fracture), the state of the *blood supply* (poor circulation means slow healing), the patient's *general constitution* (healthy bone

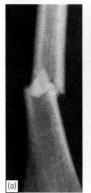 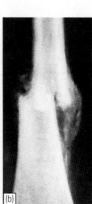 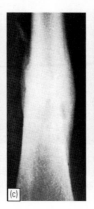 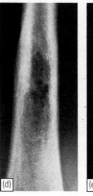 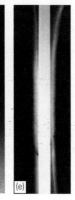

23.4 Fracture repair
(a) Fracture. (b) Union with callus. (c) Consolidation. (d) After bone remodelling. The fracture must be protected until consolidated. (e) Healing with rigid internal fixation (intramedullary nail fitted snugly). Note that no callus is visible on x-ray.

heals faster) and, most of all, the patient's *age* (healing is almost twice as fast in children as in adults). A rough guide for fractures of tubular bones in healthy adults is shown in the box below.

Average times for fracture healing		
	Upper limb	*Lower limb*
Callus visible	2–3 weeks	2–3 weeks
Union	4–6 weeks	8–12 weeks
Consolidation	6–8 weeks	12–16 weeks

FRACTURES THAT FAIL TO UNITE (NON-UNION)

Sometimes the normal process of fracture repair is thwarted and the bone fails to unite. Causes of delayed union and non-union are:

- distraction and separation of the fragments,
- interposition of soft tissues between the fragments,
- excessive movement at the fracture site,
- poor local blood supply,
- severe damage to soft tissues which makes them non-viable (or nearly so),
- infection,
- abnormal bone.

In such cases, cell proliferation is predominantly fibroblastic; the fracture gap is filled by fibrous tissue and the bone fragments remain mobile, creating a false joint or pseudarthrosis. In some cases callus formation starts off quite well: the fragment ends become thickened and even splayed, suggesting that periosteal new-bone formation is florid, but bridging of the fracture gap is prevented *(hypertrophic non-union)*. Union is still possible provided the bone fragments are apposed and held immobile. In other cases, bone formation peters out altogether and what one sees on x-ray are the tapered ends of the fracture fragments with no sign of attempted bridging *(atrophic non-union)*; the fragments will never unite unless they are immobilized and helped along with bone-grafts.

Delayed union and non-union are discussed in more detail in Chapter 25.

CLINICAL FEATURES

History

There is usually a history of *injury*, followed by *inability to use the injured limb*. But beware! The fracture is not always at the site of the injury: a blow to the knee can obviously fracture the patella or the femoral condyles, but it may also fracture the shaft of the femur or even the acetabulum. The patient's age and the mechanism of injury are important. If a

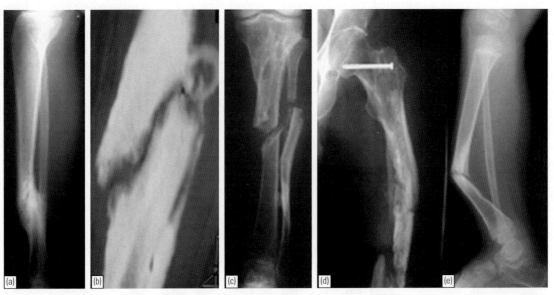

23.5 Fractures that fail to unite Some causes of non-union. (a,b) Excessive movement at the fracture site. Callus forms but the fracture gap cannot be bridged; this is shown more clearly in (b) the CT scan (hypertrophic non-union). (c) Too large a gap between the fracture ends with no attempt at healing (atrophic non-union). (d) Infection. (e) Abnormal bone, as in this case of congenital pseudarthrosis of the tibia.

fracture occurs with trivial trauma, suspect a pathological lesion. *Pain, bruising* and *swelling* are common symptoms, but they do not distinguish a fracture from a soft-tissue injury. *Deformity* is much more suggestive. Remember also that some children with greenstick fractures and elderly people with impacted fractures of the femoral neck may experience little or no pain or loss of function.

Always enquire about symptoms of *associated injuries:* numbness or loss of movement, skin pallor or cyanosis, blood in the urine, abdominal pain, difficulty with breathing or transient loss of consciousness.

Once the acute emergency has been dealt with, ask about *previous injuries, or any other musculoskeletal abnormality* that might cause confusion when the x-ray is seen. Finally, a *general medical history* is important, in preparation for anaesthesia or operation.

Examination

Unless it is obvious from the history that the patient has sustained a purely local injury, *priority must be given to dealing with the general effects of trauma* (see Chapter 20).

Injured tissues must be handled gently. To try to elicit crepitus or abnormal movement is unnecessarily painful; in any case, x-ray diagnosis is more reliable. In other respects, a systematic approach is essential, or damage to arteries, nerves, ligaments and viscera may be overlooked.

1. Examine the most obviously injured part.
2. Check for arterial damage.
3. Test for nerve injury.
4. Look for injuries of local soft tissues and viscera.
5. Look for injuries in distant parts.

Look

Swelling, bruising and deformity may be obvious, but the important point is whether the skin is intact; even the smallest wound which communicates with the fracture makes it an 'open' injury and therefore vulnerable to infection. Check also whether the skin is stretched over a projecting fragment of bone; this needs special protection to prevent a closed fracture from turning into an open one.

Note also the posture of the distal extremity and the colour of the skin (for tell-tale signs of nerve or vessel damage).

Feel

The injured part is gently palpated for localized tenderness. Some fractures would be missed if not specifically looked for, e.g. the classic sign of a fractured scaphoid is tenderness in the anatomical snuff-box. The common and characteristic associated injuries also should be felt for even if the patient does not complain of them, e.g. an isolated fracture of the ulna may be associated with a dislocated head of radius. In high-energy injuries, always examine the spine and pelvis. Vascular and peripheral nerve abnormalities should be tested for both before and after treatment.

Move

Crepitus and abnormal movement should be tested for only in unconscious patients. Usually it is more important to ask if the patient can move the joints distal to the injury.

Imaging

X-ray examination is mandatory. Remember the rule of twos:

- *Two views.* A fracture or a dislocation may not be seen on a single x-ray film; at least two views (anteroposterior and lateral) must be obtained.
- *Two joints.* The joint above and the joint below the fracture must be included on the x-ray films; they may be dislocated or fractured.
- *Two limbs.* In children, the appearance of immature epiphyses may confuse the diagnosis of a fracture; x-rays of the uninjured limb are needed for comparison.
- *Two injuries.* Severe force often causes injuries at more than one level. Thus, with fractures of the calcaneum or femur, it is important also to x-ray the pelvis and spine.
- *Two occasions.* Some fractures are notoriously difficult to detect soon after injury, but another x-ray examination a week or two later may show the lesion. Common examples are undisplaced fractures of the distal end of the clavicle, the scaphoid, the femoral neck and the lateral malleolus, and also stress fractures and physeal injuries wherever they occur.

CT and *MRI* are useful for displaying fracture patterns in 'difficult' sites such as the vertebral column, the acetabulum and the calcaneum. Three-dimensional reconstructed images are even better. *Radioisotope scanning* is helpful in diagnosing a suspected stress fracture or other 'occult' fractures.

Secondary injuries

Certain fractures are apt to cause secondary injuries and *these should always be assumed to have occurred until proved otherwise.*

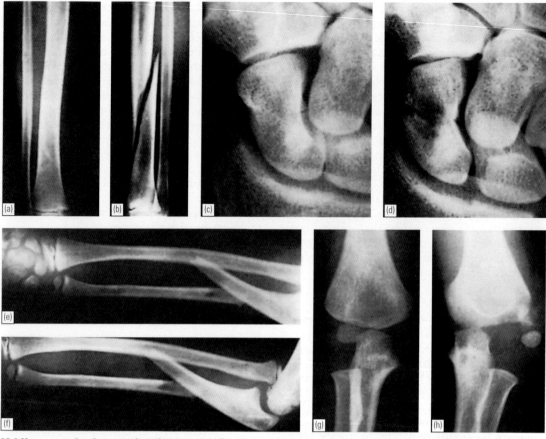

23.6 X-ray examination must be adequate (a,b) Two films of the same tibia; the anteroposterior view fails to show the fracture, which is obvious in the oblique view. (c) A fractured scaphoid is often not visible on the day of injury, but clearly seen (d) 2 weeks later. (e,f) Monteggia fracture–dislocation: failure to include both joints in forearm fractures (e) may result in a radiohumeral dislocation (f) being missed. (g,h) Fractured lateral condyle of the humerus (h); in a child, comparison with the uninjured side (g) is useful.

Thoracic injuries

Fractured ribs or sternum may be associated with injury to the lungs or heart. It is essential to check cardiorespiratory function.

Spinal cord injury

With any fracture of the spine, neurological examination is essential (a) to establish whether the spinal cord or nerve roots have been damaged and (b) to obtain a baseline for later comparison if neurological signs should change.

Pelvic and abdominal injuries

Fractures of the pelvis may be associated with visceral injury. Enquire about urinary function and look for blood at the urethral meatus. Diagnostic urethrograms or cystograms may be necessary.

Pectoral girdle injuries

Fractures and dislocations around the pectoral girdle may damage the brachial plexus or the large vessels at the base of the neck. Neurological and vascular examinations are essential.

Testing for fracture union

Fracture union is a gradual process and it is impossible to tell from clinical and x-ray features precisely when the bone fragments have joined. What is more important – and what the patient wants to know – is (a) whether the fracture shows signs of healing and (b) when the bone is strong enough to withstand normal loading in that area. Encouraging signs of healing are:

■   absence of pain during daily activities,

- absence of tenderness at the fracture site,
- absence of pain on stressing the fracture (a gentle bending movement),
- absence of mobility at the fracture site,
- x-ray signs of callus formation, then bone bridging across the fracture, and finally trabeculation across the old fracture site.

Of course, if the fracture has been internally fixed, all but the last of these criteria may be satisfied and the fracture still not united. Callus formation is usually sparse with internal fixation and one may have to wait for definite x-ray signs of trabecular continuity before declaring the fracture united. Even then, it is wise to wait for several more months before removing the fixation implants.

FRACTURES IN CHILDREN

Fractures in growing bones are subject to influences which do not apply to adult bones.

1. In very young children, the bone ends are largely cartilaginous and therefore do not show up in x-ray images. Fractures at these sites are difficult to diagnose; it helps to x-ray both limbs and compare the appearances on the two sides.
2. Children's bones are less brittle, and more liable to plastic deformation, than those of adults. Hence the frequency of incomplete fractures – torus fractures (buckling of the cortex) and greenstick fractures, injuries which are very rare in adults.

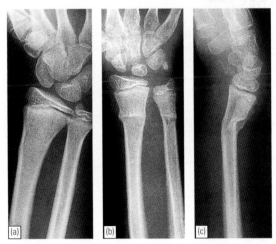

23.7 Fractures in children Childhood fractures are often incomplete: (a) *buckle* or *torus* fracture of the distal third of the radius; (b,c) *greenstick* fractures of the distal ends of the radius and ulna.

3. The periosteum is thicker than in adult bones; this may explain why fracture displacement is more controlled. Cellular activity is also more marked, which is why children's fractures heal so much more rapidly than those of adults. The younger the child, the quicker is the rate of union. Femoral shaft fractures in infants will heal within 3 weeks, and in young children in 4–6 weeks, compared to 14 weeks or longer in adults.
4. Non-union is very unusual.
5. Bone growth involves modelling and remodelling, processes which determine the structure and overall form of the bone. This makes for a considerable capacity to reshape fracture deformities (other than rotational deformities) over time.
6. Injuries of the physis have no equivalent in adults. Damage to the growth plate can have serious consequences however rapidly and securely the fracture might heal.

INJURIES OF THE PHYSIS

More than 10 per cent of childhood fractures involve injury to the physis (or growth plate). Because this is a relatively weak part of the bone, injuries that cause ligament strains in adults are liable to disrupt the physis in children. The fracture usually runs transversely through the hypertrophic (calcified) layer of the growth plate, often veering off towards the shaft to include a triangular piece of the metaphysis. This has little effect on longitudinal growth, which takes place in the germinal and proliferating layers of the physis. However, if the fracture traverses the cellular 'reproductive' layers of the plate, it may result in premature ossification of the injured part and cessation of growth or deformity of the bone end.

Classification

The most widely used classification of physeal injuries is that of Salter and Harris, which distinguishes five basic types of injury.

Type 1

A transverse fracture through the hypertrophic or calcified zone of the plate. Even if the fracture is quite alarmingly displaced, the growing zone of the physis is usually not injured and growth disturbance is uncommon.

Type 2

This is similar to type 1, but towards the edge the fracture deviates away from the physis and splits off a triangular piece of metaphyseal bone. Growth is usually not affected.

Type 3

A fracture running partly along the physis and then veering off through the epiphysis into the joint. Inevitably it damages the reproductive zone of the physis and may result in growth disturbance.

Type 4

As with type 3, the fracture splits the epiphysis, but it continues through the physis into the metaphysis. These fractures are particularly liable to displacement and a consequent misfit between the separated parts of the physis, resulting in asymmetrical growth.

Type 5

A longitudinal compression injury of the physis. There is no visible fracture, but the growth plate is crushed and this may result in growth arrest.

Clinical features

Physeal fractures usually result from falls or traction injuries; they occur mostly in road accidents and during sport or playground activities and are more common in boys than in girls. Deformity is usually minimal, but any injury in a child followed by pain and tenderness near the joint should arouse suspicion, and x-ray examination is essential.

X-rays

The physis itself is radiolucent and the epiphysis may be incompletely ossified; this makes it hard to tell whether the bone end is damaged or deformed. The younger the child, the smaller the 'visible' part of the epiphysis and thus the more difficult it is to make the diagnosis; comparison with the normal side is a great help. Tell-tale features are widening of the physeal 'gap', incongruity of the joint or tilting of the epiphyseal axis. If there is marked displacement, the diagnosis is obvious, but even type 4 fractures may at first be so little displaced that they are hard to see; if there is the faintest suspicion of a physeal fracture, a second x-ray examination after 4 or 5 days is essential. Type 5 injuries are usually diagnosed only in retrospect.

Treatment

Undisplaced fractures

These may be treated by splinting the part in a cast or a close-fitting plaster slab for 2–4 weeks (depending on the site of injury and the age of the child). However, *with type 3 and 4 fractures, a check x-ray after 4 days and again at about 10 days is mandatory in order not to miss late displacement.*

Displaced fractures

Displaced fractures must be reduced as soon as possible. With types 1 and 2, this can usually be done closed; the part is then splinted securely for 3–6 weeks. Type 3 and 4 fractures demand perfect anatomical reduction. An attempt can be made to achieve this by gentle manipulation under general anaesthesia; if this is successful, the limb is held in a cast for 4–8 weeks (the longer periods for type 4 injuries). Here again, check x-rays at about 4 and 10 days are essential to ensure that the position has been retained. If a type 3 or 4 fracture cannot be reduced accurately by closed manipulation, immediate open reduction and internal fixation is called for. The limb is then splinted for 4–6 weeks, but it takes that long again before the child is ready to resume unrestricted activities.

Complications

Premature fusion

Type 1 and 2 injuries, if properly reduced, usually have an excellent prognosis and bone growth is not adversely affected. Exceptions to this rule are injuries involving the distal femoral and proximal tibial physes; both are undulating in shape, so a

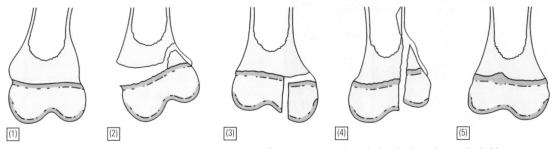

23.8 Physeal injuries *Type 1* – separation of the epiphysis. *Type 2* – fracture through the physis and metaphysis (the commonest type). *Type 3* – here the fracture runs along the physis and then veers off into the joint, splitting the epiphysis. *Type 4* – vertical fracture through the epiphysis and the adjacent metaphysis. *Type 5* – crushing of the physis without visible fracture.

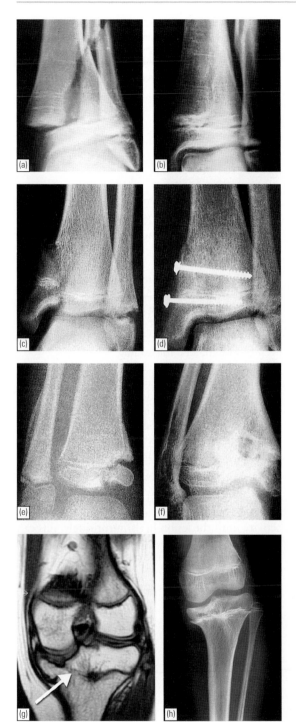

transverse fracture may pass through several zones in the physis and result in a focal point of fusion.

Type 3, 4 and 5 injuries are more likely to cause *premature fusion* of part of the growth plate, resulting in *cessation of growth* or *asymmetrical growth and deformity* of the bone end. The size and position of the bony bridge across the physis can be assessed by CT or MRI (Fig. 23.9g). If it is relatively small (less than half the width of the physis), it can be excised and replaced by a fat-graft, with some prospect of preventing or diminishing the growth disturbance. However, if the bone bridge is more extensive, the operation is contraindicated as it can end up doing more harm than good.

Deformity

Established deformity, whether from asymmetrical growth or from malunion of a displaced fracture (e.g. a valgus elbow due to proximal displacement or non-union of a lateral humeral condylar fracture), should be treated by corrective osteotomy. If further growth is abnormal, the osteotomy may have to be repeated.

'SPONTANEOUS' FRACTURES IN CHILDREN

Fractures following minimal trauma may be due to unusual genetic disorders (e.g. osteogenesis imperfecta, which is described in Chapter 8). It is obvious, however, that infants cannot say what happened to them and one should keep in mind the possibility that they may be victims of deliberate injury (the 'battered baby' syndrome). Suspicious features are an unconvincing history, multiple fractures in different stages of healing and bruises elsewhere on the body. X-rays may show florid callus formation, mimicking the appearances of osteomyelitis or scurvy (Fig. 23.10).

STRESS FRACTURES AND INSUFFICIENCY FRACTURES

A *stress* or *fatigue fracture* is one occurring in the normal bone of a healthy patient. It is caused not by a specific traumatic incident but by unaccustomed, repetitive loading of the bone. This is most likely to occur in new army recruits, athletes in training and

23.9 Physeal injuries – x-ray (a) Typical Type 2 injury; after reduction (b), bone growth is normal. (c,d) This Type 4 fracture of the tibial physis was treated immediately by open reduction and internal fixation, giving an excellent result. (e,f) By contrast, in this case accurate reduction was not achieved and the physeal fragment remained displaced; the end result was partial fusion of the physis and severe deformity of the ankle. (g) MRI showing a localized bony bar across the medial part of the proximal tibial physis. (h) In the plain x-ray one can see the deformity caused by lagging growth in the medial part of the proximal tibia.

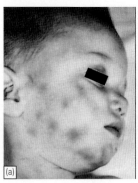
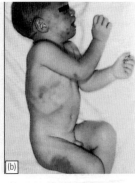
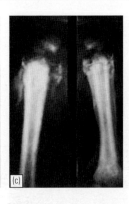

23.10 The 'battered baby' syndrome Note the multiple bruises and bilateral metaphyseal fractures with marked callus formation.

ballet dancers. *Insufficiency fractures* are those that occur following minimal trauma to bones that are significantly weaker than normal, typically osteoporotic and osteomalacic bones.

Sites affected

Sites usually affected are the metatarsal bones *(march fracture),* the distal shaft of fibula *(runner's fracture),* the proximal half of the tibia, the femoral neck, the pubic rami, the pars interarticularis of the fifth lumbar vertebra and the ala of the sacrum.

Clinical features

There may be a history of unaccustomed and repeated activity. A common sequence of events is pain after exercise → pain during exercise → pain without exercise. Occasionally the patient presents only after the fracture has healed, leaving a tender lump on the bone.

X-ray

At first the fracture is difficult to detect, but a bone scan will show increased activity at the painful spot. A few weeks later one may see a small transverse defect in the cortex and, later still, localized periosteal new-bone formation. These appearances can be mistaken for those of an osteosarcoma, a horrifying trap for the unwary.

Diagnosis

Many disorders, including osteomyelitis, scurvy and the battered baby syndrome, may be confused with stress fractures. The great danger, however, is a mistaken diagnosis of osteosarcoma; scanning shows increased uptake in both conditions and even biopsy may be misleading.

Missed diagnosis is even more common than incorrect diagnosis. When dealing with elderly osteoporotic patients, sudden pain in the back, the sacroiliac region or the hip should alert one to the possibility of an insufficiency fracture; likewise with younger individuals who develop pain in the foot, leg or thigh after stressful activity.

Treatment

Most stress fractures need no treatment other than an elastic bandage and avoidance of the painful activity until the lesion heals; surprisingly, this can take many months, and the enforced inactivity is not easily accepted by the hard-driving sportsman or dancer.

An important exception is a stress or

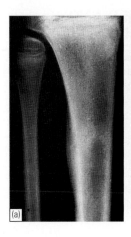
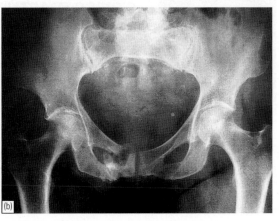

23.11 Stress fractures Stress fractures are often missed or wrongly diagnosed. (a) This tibial fracture was at first thought to be an osteosarcoma; even the biopsy was confusing. (b) Stress fractures and 'insufficiency fractures' in elderly people can be mistaken for metastases (of the pubic rami on the right side in this case).

insufficiency fracture of the femoral neck. If the diagnosis is confirmed by bone scan, CT or MRI, the femoral neck should be pinned as a prophylactic measure.

PATHOLOGICAL FRACTURES

When abnormal bone gives way, this is referred to as a pathological fracture. The causes are numerous and varied (see box). Often the diagnosis is not made until a biopsy is examined.

Causes of pathological fracture
Generalized bone disease
1. Osteogenesis imperfecta
2. Postmenopausal osteoporosis
3. Metabolic bone disease
4. Myelomatosis
5. Polyostotic fibrous dysplasia
6. Paget's disease
Local benign conditions
1. Chronic infection
2. Solitary bone cyst
3. Fibrous cortical defect
4. Chondromyxoid fibroma
5. Aneurysmal bone cyst
6. Chondroma
7. Monostotic fibrous dysplasia
Primary malignant tumours
1. Chondrosarcoma
2. Osteosarcoma
3. Ewing's tumour
Metastatic tumours
Carcinoma from breast, lung, kidney, thyroid and prostate

Clinical features

Bone that fractures spontaneously or after trivial injury must be regarded as abnormal until proved otherwise. Under the age of 20, the common causes are benign bone tumours and cysts. Over the age of 40, the common causes are metabolic bone disease, myelomatosis, secondary carcinoma

and Paget's disease. Ask about previous illnesses or operations: a history of gastrointestinal disease, chronic alcoholism or prolonged corticosteroid therapy should suggest a metabolic bone disorder; a malignant tumour, no matter how long ago it occurred, may be the source of a late metastatic lesion.

Local signs of bone disease should not be missed. *General examination* may show features suggestive of hypercortisonism or Paget's disease, or generalized tissue wasting due to malignant disease.

X-rays

Understandably, the fracture itself attracts most attention. But the surrounding bone must also be examined, and features such as cyst formation, cortical erosion, abnormal trabeculation and periosteal thickening should be sought. The type of fracture, too, is important: vertebral compression fractures may be due to severe osteoporosis or osteomalacia, but they can also be caused by skeletal metastases or myeloma. Radioisotope scans may reveal deposits elsewhere in the skeleton.

Special investigations

Investigations should include a full blood count, ESR and protein electrophoresis. Urinalysis may reveal blood from a tumour, or Bence-Jones protein in myelomatosis.

Biopsy

Some lesions are so typical that a biopsy is unnecessary (solitary cyst, fibrous cortical defect, Paget's disease). Others are more obscure and a biopsy is essential for diagnosis. If open reduction of the fracture is indicated, the biopsy can be done at the same time; otherwise a definitive procedure should be arranged.

Treatment (see also Chapter 9)

The principles are the same as for other fractures, though the choice of method will be influenced by the condition of the bone. The underlying pathological disorder may also need treatment in its own right.

Generalized bone disease

In most of these conditions (including Paget's disease) the bones fracture more easily, but they heal quite well provided the fracture is properly immobilized. Internal fixation is therefore advisable (and for Paget's disease almost essential). Patients with osteomalacia, hyperparathyroidism,

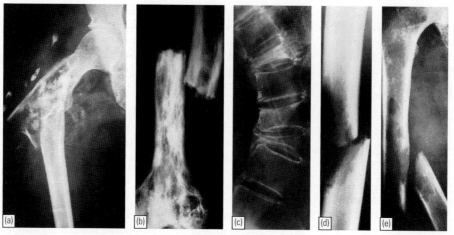

23.12 Pathological fractures Fractures due to (a) primary chondrosarcoma; (b) Paget's disease; (c) vertebral metastases; (d) metastasis in the midshaft of the femur; and (e) myelomatosis.

renal osteodystrophy and Paget's disease may need systemic treatment as well.

Local benign conditions

Fractures through benign cyst-like lesions usually heal quite well and they should be allowed to do so before tackling the underlying lesion. Treatment is therefore the same as for simple fractures in the same area, although in some cases it will be necessary to take a biopsy before immobilizing the fracture. When the bone has healed, the tumour can be dealt with by curettage or local excision.

Primary malignant tumour

The fracture may need splinting, but this is merely a prelude to definitive treatment of the tumour, which by now will have spread to the surrounding soft tissues. The prognosis depends on the type of tumour. Even osteosarcomas are amenable to resection and prosthetic replacement, with long-term survival being reported in more than 60 per cent of patients.

Metastatic tumours

Metastasis is a frequent cause of pathological fracture in older people. Breast cancer is the commonest source and the femur the commonest site. Nowadays cancer patients (even those with metastases) often live for several years, and effective treatment of the fracture will vastly improve their quality of life. Preoperatively, imaging studies should be performed to detect other bone lesions; these may be amenable to 'prophylactic' fixation.

Fracture of a long-bone shaft should be treated by internal fixation; intramedullary nails are more

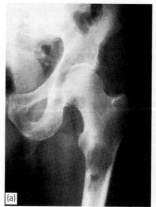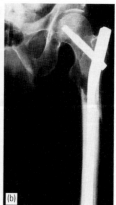

23.13 Pathological fractures – treatment (a) This patient with a secondary deposit below the lesser trochanter was advised to have prophylactic nailing. In the event, the bone actually fractured during the operation (b).

suitable than plates and screws and, if necessary, the site is also packed with acrylic cement. This may be followed by local irradiation.

Fracture near a bone end can often be treated by excision and prosthetic replacement.

Pathological compression fractures of the spine cause severe pain. This is due largely to spinal instability, and treatment should include operative stabilization. If there are clinical or imaging features of actual or threatened spinal cord or cauda equina compression, the affected segment should be decompressed; postoperative irradiation may also be needed.

Pre-emptive surgery

Prophylactic fixation of a localized deposit may forestall the difficulties of dealing with a pathological fracture. Once the wound has healed, local irradiation should be applied to reduce the risk of progressive osteolysis.

JOINT INJURIES

Joints are usually injured by twisting or tilting forces that stretch the ligaments and capsule. If the force is great enough, the ligament will tear, or the bone to which it is attached may be pulled apart. The articular cartilage, too, may be damaged if the joint surfaces are compressed or if there is a fracture into the joint.

As a general principle, forceful angulation will tear the ligaments rather than crush the bone, but in older people with porotic bone the ligaments may hold and the bone on the opposite side of the joint is crushed instead, while in children there may be a fracture–separation of the physis.

SPRAINS AND STRAINS

There is much confusion about the use of the terms 'sprain', 'strain' and 'rupture'. In clinical parlance, a *sprain* is any painful wrenching (twisting or pulling) of a joint, short of actual tearing of the ligaments or capsule. *Strain* is more specific: it implies stretching or microscopic tearing of some fibres in the ligament. If the force is great enough, the ligament may be strained to the point of complete *rupture*.

Sprained joint

A twisted joint is painful but there is little or no swelling and no sign of bruising. In superficial joints, tenderness can sometimes be localized to a particular ligament. In deep joints, and in the neck and back, it is usually impossible to tell whether it is the ligaments or the muscles that have been injured.

Treatment consists of reassurance and, most importantly, encouragement of movement and exercise from the outset.

Strained ligament

The joint is momentarily twisted or bent into an abnormal position. Some of the fibres in the ligament are torn (perhaps only microscopically) but the joint remains stable. The patient presents with pain, swelling and bruising around one or other aspect of the joint. Tenderness is localized to the injured ligament, and stretching the tissues on that side causes a sharp increase in pain.

Treatment

The joint should be firmly strapped and rested until the acute pain subsides. Ice packs and non-steroidal anti-inflammatory medication are helpful if swelling is marked. As soon as pain permits, active movements and muscle strengthening exercises are encouraged.

Following strains around the knee and ankle, there is often a tendency for the joint to give way repeatedly due to unexpected pain rather than true instability. The patient should be warned about this and shown how to protect the ligament during weight-bearing.

RUPTURED LIGAMENT

The ligament is completely torn and the joint is unstable. Hinge joints (the knee, ankle, fingers and thumb) are more vulnerable than others.

As with a strain, the joint is suddenly forced into an abnormal position; sometimes the patient

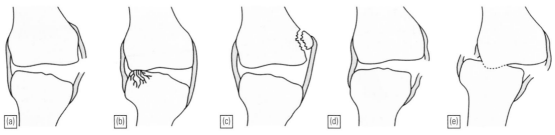

23.14 Joint injuries Severe stress and strain may cause various types of injury. (a) A ligament may rupture, leaving the bone intact. If the soft tissues hold, the bone on the opposite side may be crushed (b), or a fragment of bone may be pulled off by the taut ligament (c). (d) Subluxation. (e) Dislocation.

actually hears a snap. Pain is severe and there may be considerable bleeding under the skin; if the joint is swollen, this is probably due to a haemarthrosis. The patient is unlikely to permit a searching examination, but under general anaesthesia instability can be demonstrated by stressing the joint; it is this that distinguishes the lesion from a strain. If the ligament is avulsed rather than torn, x-ray may show a detached flake of bone.

Treatment

A torn ligament will heal spontaneously by fibrosis if it is held without tension for 4–6 weeks. However, scarring is diminished and strength improved by early movement. Treatment aims to encourage these natural processes.

Non-operative treatment

Most ligament ruptures can be treated non-operatively. Initially, measures will be needed to control pain and swelling: these are splintage of the joint, ice packs and non-steroidal anti-inflammatory medication. A tense haemarthrosis should be aspirated. After a few days the splint can usually be exchanged for a functional brace that allows joint movement but at the same time prevents repeated injury to the ligament. Physiotherapy is applied to maintain muscle strength and later on proprioceptive exercises are added. If residual instability causes a problem, reconstructive surgery can be undertaken at a later stage.

Operative treatment

There are some exceptions to the above routine.

1. If the ligament is avulsed with an attached fragment of bone, the fragment should be re-attached if it is large enough.
2. Complex tears and fracture–dislocations may need early operative treatment to restore joint stability.
3. Joints which rely entirely on ligaments for their anatomical position and stability (e.g. the metacarpophalangeal joint of the thumb) are best treated by early operative repair of the ruptured ligament.

DISLOCATION AND SUBLUXATION

Dislocation means that the joint surfaces are completely displaced and are no longer in contact; *subluxation* implies a lesser degree of displacement, such that the articular surfaces are still partly apposed.

Clinical features

Following an injury, the joint is painful and the patient tries at all costs to avoid moving it. The shape of the joint is abnormal and the bony landmarks may be displaced. The limb is often held in a characteristic position; movement is painful and restricted. X-rays will usually clinch the diagnosis; they will also show whether there is an associated bony injury affecting joint stability – i.e. a fracture–dislocation.

If the dislocation is reduced by the time the patient is seen, the diagnosis may be in doubt. This is where the *apprehension test* is useful. The joint is stressed as if almost to reproduce the suspected dislocation: the patient develops a sense of impending disaster and violently resists further manipulation.

Recurrent dislocation

If the ligaments and joint margins are damaged, repeated dislocation may occur. This is seen especially in the shoulder and the patellofemoral joint.

Habitual (voluntary) dislocation

Some patients acquire the knack of dislocating (or subluxating) the joint by voluntary muscle contraction. Ligamentous laxity may make this easier, but the habit often betrays a manipulative and neurotic personality. It is important to recognize this because such patients are seldom helped by operation.

Treatment

The dislocation must be reduced as soon as possible; usually a general anaesthetic is required, and sometimes a muscle relaxant as well. The joint is rested or immobilized until soft-tissue healing occurs – usually after 3–4 weeks – and this is followed by a course of physiotherapy. If ligaments have been torn, they may have to be repaired.

Complications

Complications such as vascular injury, nerve injury, avascular necrosis of bone, heterotopic ossification, joint stiffness and secondary osteoarthritis are the same as those following fractures and are dealt with in Chapter 25.

CHAPTER 24

FRACTURES – PRINCIPLES OF TREATMENT

General resuscitation is the first consideration: *treat the patient, not only the fracture*. The principles are discussed in Chapter 22.

Treatment of the fracture consists of *manipulation* to improve the position of the fragments, followed by *splintage* to hold them together until they unite; meanwhile, joint *movement* and *function* must be preserved. Fracture healing is promoted by muscle activity and bone loading, so *exercise* and early *weight-bearing* are encouraged. These objectives are covered by three simple injunctions: REDUCE! HOLD! EXERCISE!

The problem is how to hold a fracture adequately and yet use the limb sufficiently. This is a conflict *(Hold v. Move)* which the surgeon seeks to resolve as rapidly as possible (e.g. by internal fixation), but without incurring unnecessary risks. So here is a second conflict *(Speed v. Safety)*. This dual conflict encapsulates four important factors that influence the modern approach to fracture management. (The term 'fracture quartet' was coined by Alan Apley in earlier editions of this book; it is no coincidence that, as an accomplished pianist, he himself was a member of an amateur quartet!)

CLOSED FRACTURES

REDUCE

Although general treatment and resuscitation must always take precedence, there should be no undue delay in attending to the fracture: swelling of the soft parts during the first 12 hours makes reduction increasingly difficult. However, there are some situations in which reduction is unnecessary: (1) when there is little or no displacement; (2) when displacement does not matter (e.g. in some fractures of the clavicle); and (3) when reduction is unlikely to succeed (e.g. with compression fractures of the vertebrae).

Reduction should aim for *adequate apposition* and *normal alignment* of the bone fragments. The greater the contact surface area between fragments, the more likely is healing to occur; a gap between the fragments is a common cause of delayed union or non-union. However, as long as the fragments are in contact and properly aligned, some overlap at the fracture surfaces is permissible; the exception is a fracture involving an articular surface, which should be reduced as near to perfection as possible because any irregularity will predispose to degenerative arthritis.

There are three methods of reduction: manipulation, mechanical traction and open operation.

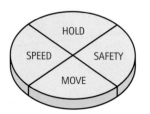

24.1 The fracture quartet

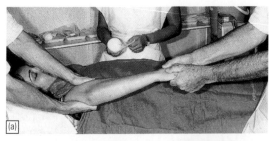

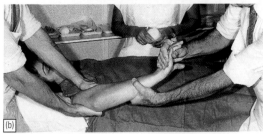

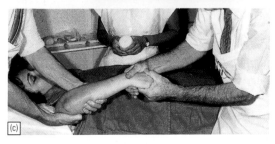

24.2 Closed reduction (a) Traction and counter-traction in the line of the bone. (b) Manipulation to disimpact the fragments. (c) Continued manipulation to press the distal fragment into the reduced position.

Manipulation

Closed manipulation is suitable for all minimally displaced fractures, for most fractures in children and for fractures that are likely to be stable after reduction. Unstable fractures are sometimes reduced 'closed' prior to mechanical fixation.

Under anaesthesia and muscle relaxation, the fracture is reduced by a threefold manoeuvre: (1) the distal part of the limb is pulled in the line of the bone; (2) as the fragments disengage, they are repositioned (by reversing the original direction of force if this can be deduced); and (3) alignment is adjusted in each plane. This is most effective when the periosteum and muscles on one side of the fracture remain intact; the soft-tissue strap prevents over-reduction and stabilizes the fracture after it has been reduced.

Mechanical traction

Some fractures (e.g. of the femoral shaft) are difficult to reduce by manipulation because of powerful muscle pull. Often, however, they can be reduced by sustained mechanical traction, which then serves also to hold the fracture until it starts to unite (see below). In some cases, rapid mechanical traction is applied, under anaesthesia and assisted by image intensification, prior to internal fixation.

Open operation

Operative reduction under direct vision is indicated: (1) when closed reduction fails, either because of difficulty in controlling the fragments or because soft tissues are interposed between them; (2) when there is a large articular fragment that needs accurate positioning; (3) for avulsion fractures in which the fragments are held apart by muscle pull; (4) when an operation is needed for associated injuries (e.g. arterial damage); and (5) when a fracture will anyhow need internal fixation to hold it.

HOLD

The word 'immobilization' is avoided because the objective is seldom complete immobility: usually it

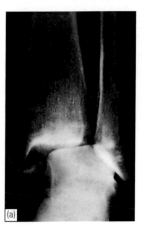

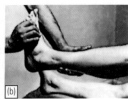

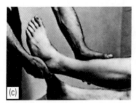

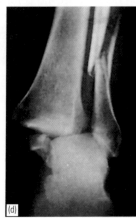

24.3 Countering the mechanism of injury These two ankle fractures look similar but are caused by different forces, which must be reversed to achieve reduction: (a) is an external rotation injury and is reduced by internal rotation (b); (c) rotation plus adduction is needed for (d).

is the prevention of displacement. Some restriction of movement is also needed to alleviate pain, to promote soft-tissue healing and to allow free movement of the unaffected parts. *The aim is to splint the fracture, not the entire limb.*

The available methods of holding reduction are: (1) sustained traction, (2) cast splintage, (3) functional bracing, (4) internal fixation, and (5) external fixation. Closed methods are most suitable for fractures with intact soft tissues (which provide a form of splintage), and are liable to fail if they are used for fractures with severe soft-tissue damage. Other contraindications to non-operative methods are inherently unstable fractures, multiple fractures and fractures in confused or uncooperative patients.

Sustained traction

Traction is applied to the limb distal to the fracture, so as to exert a continuous pull in the long axis of the bone. In most cases a counterforce will be needed to prevent the patient simply being dragged along the bed. The method is particularly useful for spiral fractures of long-bone shafts, which are easily displaced by muscle contraction. The *hold* is obviously not perfect, but traction is *safe* (provided it is not excessive); the bone is gradually pulled out to length and meanwhile the patient can *move* the joints and exercise the muscles. The problem is *speed* (or rather lack of it): not because the fracture unites slowly (it does not), but because sustained lower limb traction keeps the patient in bed for a long time, thus increasing the likelihood of complications such as thromboembolism, respiratory problems and general weakness. For this reason, sustained traction is best avoided in elderly patients, and even in younger patients traction should be replaced by cast splintage or functional bracing as soon as the fracture becomes 'sticky'.

Traction by gravity

Fractures of the humerus are often treated by simply allowing the weight of the arm to supply the traction. The forearm is supported in a wrist sling and movement at the fracture site is reduced by applying a 'sleeve' cast or brace to the upper part of the arm.

Balanced traction

Traction is applied to the limb, either by way of adhesive strapping which is kept in place by bandages *(skin traction)* or via a stiff wire or pin inserted through the bone distal to the fracture *(skeletal traction)*. Skin traction will sustain a pull of no more than 4 or 5 kg. Skeletal traction can be used to apply several times as much force, which is needed to hold lower limb fractures; the transfixing pin passes through the proximal tibia for traction on hip, thigh and knee injuries and through the distal tibia or calcaneum for tibial fractures. Cords are attached and run over pulleys at the end of the bed to hold the weights that supply the traction force. Counter-traction is usually supplied by raising the foot of the bed and relying on the opposing weight of the patient's body. The limb is usually supported, both for comfort and to prevent sagging at the fracture site, in a type of cradle – Thomas's splint for the femur or Braun's frame for the tibia.

Fixed traction

The principle is the same as for balanced traction, except that in this case the limb is held in a Thomas's splint and the traction tapes are tied to the distal end of the splint while the proximal padded ring of the splint abuts firmly against the pelvis. This method is particularly useful when the patient has to be transported.

Note. Sustained traction is sometimes used to treat femoral shaft fractures in very young children. Skin traction is applied and the child's legs are suspended from an overhead beam, the weight of the body supplying the traction force ('gallows traction'). There is risk that the traction tapes and circular bandages may constrict the circulation; for this reason, *gallows traction should never be used for children over 12 kg in weight.*

Cast splintage

Plaster of Paris (or one of the newer lightweight substitutes) is still widely used as a splint, especially for distal limb fractures and for most children's fractures. It is *safe* enough, provided it is not applied too tightly or unevenly. The *speed* of union is neither greater nor less than with traction, but the patient can go home sooner. *Holding* reduction is usually no problem, and patients with tibial fractures can bear weight on the cast. The big

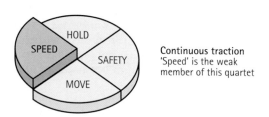

24.4 Continuous traction 'Speed' is the weak member of this quartet.

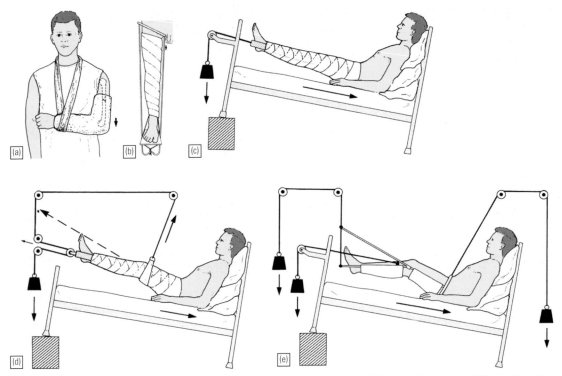

24.5 Methods of traction (a) Traction by gravity. (b–d) Skin traction, which may be (b) fixed, (c) balanced or (d) Russell traction. (e) Skeletal traction with a splint and a knee flexion piece.

drawback is that joints encased in plaster cannot *move* and are liable to stiffen; as the swelling and haematoma resolve, adhesions form which bind muscle fibres to each other and to the bone. This complication can be minimized by: (a) delayed splintage – that is, by using traction until movement has been regained, and only then applying plaster; or (b) starting with a conventional cast but, after a few weeks, when the limb can be handled without too much discomfort, replacing the cast by a functional brace which permits joint movement.

The technique of applying a plaster cast is shown in Figure 24.7. Check x-rays are essential and the

HOLD

SPEED   SAFETY

MOVE

Casts
'Move' is the weakest member of the quartet

24.6 Cast splintage 'Move' is the weakest member of the quartet.

fracture position can be adjusted to some extent by cutting and wedging the cast.

Complications

Complications are liable to appear once the patient has left hospital and is no longer under daily supervision. This carries the added risk of delay before the problem is attended to.

Tight cast   The cast may be put on too tightly, or it may become tight if the limb swells. The patient complains of diffuse pain; only later – sometimes much later – do the signs of vascular compression appear. *The limb should be elevated, but if the pain does not subside during the next hour, the only safe course is to split the cast, ease it open throughout its length and cut through all the padding down to skin.* Whenever swelling is anticipated, the cast should be applied over thick padding and then split before it sets, so as to provide a firm but not absolutely rigid splint.

Pressure sores   Even a well-fitting cast may press upon the skin over a bony prominence (the patella, the heel, the elbow or the head of the ulna). The

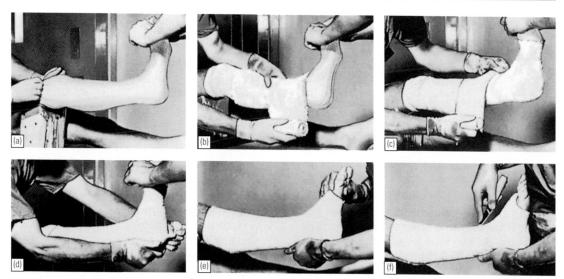

24.7 Plaster technique (a) Stockinette is fitted smoothly on to the limb. (b) For a padded plaster, wool-bandage is rolled on and it must be even. (c) Plaster is next applied smoothly, taking a tuck with each turn, and (d) smoothing each layer firmly on to the one beneath. (e) While still wet, the cast is moulded away from the bony points. (f) With a recent injury, the plaster should then be split to avoid compression by swelling.

patient complains of localized pain precisely over the pressure spot. Such localized pain demands immediate inspection through a window in the cast. But pressure should have been prevented by padding all prominent bony points before applying the cast.

Skin abrasion or laceration This is really a complication of removing plasters, especially if an electric saw is used. Complaints of nipping or pinching during plaster removal should never be ignored; a ripped forearm is a good reason for litigation.

Loose cast Once the swelling has subsided, the cast may no longer hold the fracture securely. If it is loose, the cast should be replaced.

Functional bracing

Functional bracing, using either plaster of Paris or one of the lighter materials, is one way of preventing joint stiffness while still permitting fracture splintage and loading. Segments of a cast are applied only over the shafts of the bones, leaving the joints free; cast segments above and below a joint can be connected by metal or plastic hinges which allow movements in one plane. The splints are 'functional' in that joint movements are less restricted than with conventional casts.

Functional bracing is used most widely for fractures of the femur or tibia, but, since the brace is not very rigid, it is usually applied only when the fracture is beginning to unite, i.e. after 3–6 weeks of traction or restrictive splintage. Used in this way, it comes out well on all four of the basic requirements: the fracture can be *held* reasonably well; the joints can be *moved;* the fracture joins at normal *speed* without keeping the patient in hospital; and the method is *safe.*

Internal fixation

Bone fragments may be fixed with screws, transfixing pins or nails, a metal plate held by screws, a long intramedullary nail (with or without locking screws), circumferential bands, or a combination of these methods.

Properly applied, internal fixation *holds* a fracture securely so that *movements* can begin at once and, with early movement, the 'fracture disease' (stiffness and oedema) is abolished. *Speed* is not an issue; the patient can leave hospital as soon as the wound is healed but must remember that, even though the bone moves in one piece, the fracture is not united – it is merely held by a metal bridge; full weight-bearing is, for some time, unsafe. The greatest *danger*, however, is sepsis; if infection supervenes, all the manifest advantages of internal fixation (precise reduction, immediate

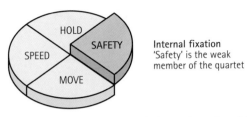

24.8 Internal fixation 'Safety' is the weak member of the quartet.

stability and early movement) may be lost. The risk of infection depends upon: (1) the patient – devitalized tissues, a dirty wound and an unfit patient are all dangerous; (2) the surgeon – thorough training, a high degree of surgical dexterity and adequate assistance are all essential; and (3) the facilities – a guaranteed aseptic routine,

a full range of implants and staff familiar with their use are all indispensable.

Indications for internal fixation

1. Fractures that cannot be reduced except by operation.
2. Fractures that are inherently unstable and prone to re-displacement after reduction.
3. Fractures that unite poorly and slowly, principally fractures of the femoral neck.
4. Pathological fractures, in which bone disease may prevent healing.
5. Multiple fractures, where early fixation reduces the risk of general complications.
6. Fractures in patients who present severe nursing difficulties.

More controversial is the use of internal fixation as a preferred, rather than a necessary, form of treatment. The introduction of reliable image-guided techniques for 'closed' reduction and

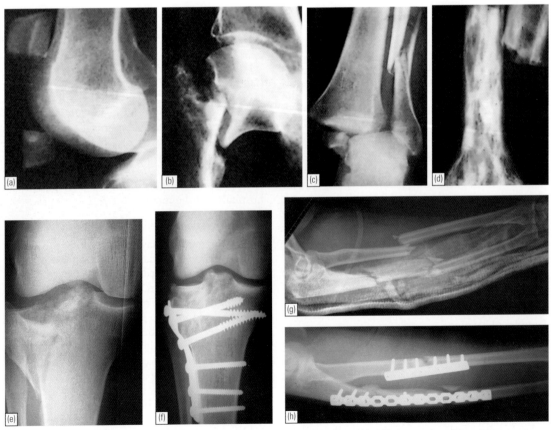

24.9 Indications for open reduction and internal fixation (a) Traction lesions with wide separation of fragments.
(b) Fractures that unite poorly, e.g. of the femoral neck. (c) Fractures that are inherently unstable and prone to re-displacement.
(d) Pathological fractures. (e,f) Large fragments involving a joint surface. (g,h) Fractures that are very difficult to reduce and likely to re-displace after reduction.

nailing of long-bone fractures has gained wide acceptance as an alternative to more difficult and cumbersome non-operative methods.

Types of internal fixation

A variety of materials and methods are available for fixing fractures, and a sound knowledge of the mechanical properties and applications of the different mechanisms is essential. The reader is referred to *AO Principles of Fracture Management* by T.P. Ruedi and W.M. Murphy (Thieme Publishing Group 2000).

Screws   Interfragmentary screws (lag screws) are useful for fixing small fragments onto the main bone.

Wires   Kirschner   wires   (often   inserted percutaneously without exposing the fracture) can hold fracture fragments together. They are used in situations where fracture healing is predictably quick; some form of external splintage (usually a cast) is applied as supplementary support.

Plates and screws   This form of fixation is useful for treating metaphyseal fractures of long bones and diaphyseal fractures of the radius and ulna. When used on tubular bones, firm coaptation of the fragments is achieved by compression devices before tightening the screws.

Intramedullary nails   These are suitable for long bones. A nail (or long rod) is inserted into the medullary canal to splint the fracture; rotational forces are resisted by introducing *locking screws* which transfix the bone cortices and the nail proximal and distal to the fracture. Nails are used with or without prior reaming of the medullary canal; reaming achieves an interference fit in addition to the added stability from interlocking screws, but at the expense of some damage to the intramedullary blood supply.

> Internal fixation: practise before attempting it; plan before operating; check the equipment; check final position before closing the wound.

Complications of internal fixation

Most of the complications of internal fixation are due to poor technique, poor equipment or poor operating conditions.

Infection   Iatrogenic infection is now the most common cause of chronic osteomyelitis; the metal does not predispose to infection, but the quality of the patient's tissues and the open operation do. If the infection is not rapidly controlled by intravenous antibiotic treatment, the implants should be replaced with some form of external fixation.

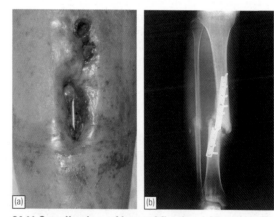

24.11 Complications of internal fixation (a) Postoperative wound infection, which may result in exposure of the metal plate. (b) Implant breakage resulting in non-union.

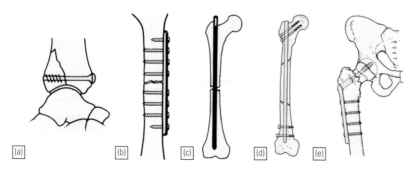

24.10 Types of internal fixation (a) A single interfragmentary screw. (b) Plate and screws. (c) Intramedullary nail. (d) Locked intramedullary nail. (e) Dynamic hip screw.

Non-union Causes of non-union are excessive stripping of the soft tissues, unnecessary damage to the blood supply in the course of operative fixation and rigid fixation with a gap between the fragments.

Implant failure Metal is subject to fatigue, and undue stresses should therefore be avoided until the fracture has united. Pain at the fracture site is a danger signal!

Refracture It is important not to remove metal implants too soon, or the bone may re-fracture; a year is the minimum and 18 or 24 months safer. For several weeks after implant removal the bone is weak, so full weight-bearing should be avoided.

External fixation

The principle of external fixation is simple: the bone is transfixed above and below the fracture with screws or pins or tensioned wires and these are then clamped to a frame, or connected to each other by rigid bars. There are numerous variations in fixation devices and techniques of applying them, providing different degrees of rigidity and stability. All of them permit adjustment of length and angulation, and some allow reduction of the fracture in all three planes. This is especially applicable to the long bones and the pelvis, but the method can be used for fractures of almost any part of the skeleton.

Indications

1. Fractures associated with severe soft-tissue damage where the wound can be left open for inspection, dressing or definitive coverage.
2. Severely comminuted and unstable fractures, which can be held out to length until healing commences.
3. Fractures of the pelvis, which often cannot be controlled quickly by any other method.
4. Fractures associated with nerve or vessel damage.
5. Infected fractures, for which internal fixation might not be suitable.
6. Ununited fractures, where dead or sclerotic fragments can be excised and the remaining ends brought together in the external fixator; sometimes this is combined with elongation in the normal part the shaft.

Complications of external fixation

Modern techniques of external fixation demand a high degree of training and skill. The fact that this method is often used for the most difficult fractures increases the likelihood of complications.

Damage to soft-tissue structures Transfixing pins or wires may injure nerves or vessels, or may tether ligaments and inhibit joint movement. The surgeon must be thoroughly familiar with the

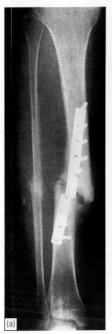
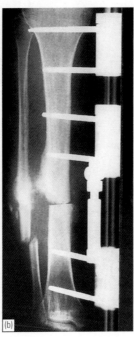
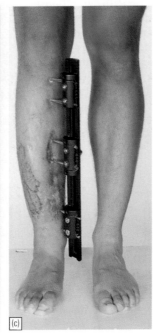

24.12 External fixation (a) The fracture shown here was fixed with a plate and screws but did not unite; (b) this is one of the indications for external fixation and bone transport. (c) The patient was able to walk about while the fracture healed.

local anatomy and the 'safe corridors' for inserting pins.

Over-distraction If there is no contact between the fragments, union may be delayed or prevented.

Pin-track infection This is one of the most troublesome complications of external fixation. Meticulous pin-site care is essential, and antibiotics should be administered immediately if infection occurs.

EXERCISE

More correctly, 'restore function' – not only to the injured parts but also to the patient as a whole. The objectives are to reduce oedema, preserve joint movement, restore muscle power and guide the patient back to normal activity.

Prevention of oedema

Swelling is almost inevitable after a fracture and may cause tissue tension and blistering. It is also an important cause of joint stiffness, especially in the hand, and should be prevented or treated energetically by a combination of elevation and active exercises. If the injury is not severe enough to warrant admission to hospital, the patient should be encouraged to use the limb (within reason) and to keep moving the joints that are free. The essence of soft-tissue care may be summed up thus: *elevate and exercise; never dangle, never force.*

Active exercise

Active movement, in addition to reducing oedema, stimulates the circulation, prevents soft-tissue adhesion and promotes fracture healing. Even a limb encased in plaster is capable of muscle contraction, and the patient should be taught how to do this. When splintage is removed, joint movement is increased and muscle-building exercises encouraged. The unaffected joints also need exercising; it is all too easy to neglect a stiffening shoulder while caring for an injured hand.

Assisted movement

It has long been taught that passive movement can be deleterious, especially with injuries around the elbow where there is a high risk of developing myositis ossificans. Certainly forced movements should never be permitted, but gentle assistance during active exercises helps to retain function or regain movement after fractures involving the articular surfaces. Nowadays this is done with machines that can be set to provide a specified range and rate of movement *(continuous passive motion).*

Functional activity

As the patient's mobility improves, an increasing amount of directed activity is introduced. He or she may need to be taught again how to perform everyday tasks such as walking, getting in and out of bed, bathing, dressing or handling eating utensils. Experience is the best teacher and the patient is encouraged to use the injured limb as much as possible. Those with very severe or extensive injuries may benefit from spending time in a special rehabilitation unit, but the best incentive to full recovery is the promise of re-entry into family life, recreational pursuits and meaningful work.

OPEN FRACTURES

INITIAL MANAGEMENT

Many patients with open fractures have multiple injuries and severe shock; for them, appropriate treatment at the scene of the accident is essential. After splinting the limb, the wound should be covered with a sterile dressing or clean material and left undisturbed until the patient reaches the accident department. This will reduce the risk of further contamination and wound desiccation.

In hospital, a rapid general assessment is the first step, and any life-threatening conditions are addressed (see Chapter 22). Tetanus prophylaxis is administered: toxoid for those previously immunized, human antiserum if not.

The wound is carefully inspected; ideally it should be photographed with a Polaroid or digital camera, so that it can again be kept until the patient is in the operating theatre. Important features to be noted are the site and size of the wound, whether it is tidy or ragged, clean or dirty, and whether it communicates with the fracture. Other important factors are the condition of the soft tissues and the state of the circulation and nerve supply.

CLASSIFYING THE INJURY

Gustilo's classification of open fractures is widely used.

- *Type 1* is a low-energy fracture with a small, clean wound and little soft-tissue damage.
- *Type II* is a moderate-energy fracture with a clean wound more than 1 cm long, but not much soft-tissue damage and no more than moderate comminution of the fracture.

■ *Type III* is a high-energy fracture with extensive damage to skin, soft tissue and neurovascular structures, and contamination of the wound. In *type IIIA* the fractured bone can be adequately covered by soft tissue; in *type IIIB* it cannot and there is also periosteal stripping, as well as severe comminution of the fracture; and the fracture is classified as *type IIIC* if there is an arterial injury which needs to be repaired, regardless of the amount of other soft-tissue damage.

The incidence of wound infection correlates directly with the extent of soft-tissue damage, rising from less than 2 per cent in type I to more than 10 per cent in type III fractures. The risk of infection also rises with increasing delay in obtaining soft-tissue coverage of the fracture.

PRINCIPLES OF TREATMENT

All open fractures, no matter how trivial they may seem, must be assumed to be contaminated; it is important to try to prevent them from becoming infected. The four essentials are:

■ prompt wound debridement,
■ antibiotic prophylaxis,
■ stabilization of the fracture,
■ early definitive wound cover.

Repeated examination of the limb is important: remember that open fractures also can be associated with a compartment syndrome.

Sterility and antibiotic cover

The wound must be kept covered until the patient reaches the operating theatre. Antibiotics are given as soon as possible, no matter how small the laceration, and are continued until the danger of infection has passed. In most cases a combination of benzylpenicillin and flucloxacillin, or better still a second-generation cephalosporin, given 6-hourly for 48 hours will suffice. If the wound is heavily contaminated, it is prudent to cover also for Gram-negative organisms and anaerobes by adding gentamicin or metronidazole and to continue treatment for 4 or 5 days.

Debridement and wound excision

Under general anaesthesia, the patient's clothing is removed while an assistant maintains traction on the injured limb and holds it still. Any dressing is replaced by a sterile pad and the surrounding skin is cleaned and shaved. The pad is then taken off and the wound is irrigated thoroughly with copious amounts of warm normal saline. A tourniquet is not used because it may endanger the circulation still further and make it difficult to recognize which structures are devitalized.

The wound is extended and ragged margins excised to leave healthy skin edges. All foreign material and tissue debris must be carefully removed. The wound is then washed out again with large quantities of warm normal saline: 6–12 L may be needed to irrigate and clean an open fracture of a long bone. Devitalized tissue provides a nutrient medium for bacteria and should be excised. Dead muscle can be recognized by its purplish colour, its failure to contract when stimulated and its failure to bleed when cut; a mushy consistency is a late feature. As a general rule, it is best to leave cut nerves and tendons alone, though if the wound is absolutely clean and no dissection is required – and provided the necessary expertise is available – they can be sutured.

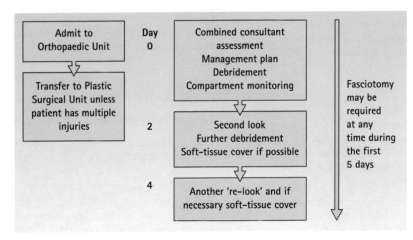

24.13 Management of open fractures Flow chart showing the management of open fractures of the tibia.

> ⚠ A puncture wound is just as liable as a laceration to contamination and infection. If there is any possibility of it communicating with the fracture, it should be extended and debrided in the usual way.

Wound closure

To close or not to close the skin – this can be a difficult decision. Uncontaminated types I and II wounds operated on within a few hours of injury may, after debridement and wound excision, be sutured – *provided this can be done without tension.* All other wounds must be left open, lightly packed with moist, sterile gauze (e.g. soaked in a dilute solution of Betadine) and inspected again after 24–48 hours: if the wound is clean and tidy, it can then be sutured or skin-grafted (provided there is a suitable soft-tissue bed) – this is called delayed primary closure. Type III wounds may occasionally have to be debrided more than once and skin closure may call for plastic surgery.

Skin-grafting is most appropriate if the wound cannot be closed without tension and the recipient bed is clear, free of obvious infection and well vascularized; it is not necessary to wait until the bed is covered with granulation tissue. Partial-thickness grafts can, if necessary, be laid on periosteum or paratenon, but they should not be applied directly over bare bone or tendons or metal implants.

Extensive skin loss over a fracture, or in an open area where the blood supply is suspect, is better dealt with by transposing a *loco-regional fasciocutaneous* or *musculocutaneous flap,* if this can be fashioned without risk to its blood supply. Occasionally the only option is to transfer a *free flap,* with its blood vessels, using microsurgical techniques. Where blood vessels are preserved, they should be sutured outside the zone of injury.

Stabilization of the fracture

It is now recognized that stability of the fracture is important in reducing the likelihood of infection and assisting in recovery of the soft tissues. The method of fixation depends on the degree of contamination, the length of time from injury to operation and the amount of soft-tissue damage. If there is no obvious contamination and the time lapse is less than 8 hours, open fractures of all grades up to IIIA (Gustilo classification) can be treated as for closed injuries: cast splintage, intramedullary nailing, plating or external fixation may be appropriate, depending on the individual characteristics of the fracture and wound. More severe injuries will almost certainly require a combined approach by experienced plastic and orthopaedic surgeons; the precise method of stabilization depends to a large extent on the type of soft-tissue cover that will be employed, although external fixation using a circular frame can accommodate to most problems. (Always consult with the plastic surgeon to avoid placing pins through areas intended for loco-regional flaps.) Plates and screws should be reserved for metaphyseal or articular fractures and for fractures of the smaller tubular bones.

Aftercare

Postoperatively the limb is elevated and the circulation carefully monitored. Antibiotic cover is continued; swab samples will dictate whether a different antibiotic is needed.

If the wound has been left open, it is inspected at 2–3 days. Delayed primary suture is then often safe or, if there has been much skin loss, plastic surgery may be needed.

Teamwork

For optimal results, open fractures with skin and soft-tissue damage are best managed by a partnership of orthopaedic and plastic surgeons, ideally from the outset rather than by later referral. If there is no plastic surgeon on site, it may still be possible to communicate effectively by using a digital camera for image transmission by internet.

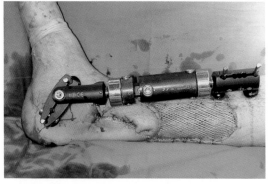

24.14 Combined treatment of open fractures Co-operation between orthopaedic surgeon and plastic surgeon is the ideal. Here, an open tibial fracture has been immobilized in an external fixator, leaving the open wound to be covered by a local flap and skin grafting.

CHAPTER 25

COMPLICATIONS OF FRACTURES

General complications of trauma are dealt with in Chapter 22. *Local complications* can be divided into *early* (those that arise during the first few weeks following injury) and *late*.

EARLY COMPLICATIONS

Early complications may present as part of the primary injury or may appear only after a few days or weeks.

VISCERAL INJURY

Fractures around the trunk are often complicated by injuries to underlying viscera, the most important being penetration of the lung with life-threatening pneumothorax following rib fractures, and rupture of the bladder or urethra in pelvic fractures. These injuries require emergency treatment, before the fracture is dealt with.

NERVE INJURY (See also chapter 11)

Nerve injury is particularly common with fractures of the humerus or injuries around the elbow or knee. The tell-tale signs should be looked for *(and documented!)* during the initial examination and again after reduction of the fracture.

In closed injuries the nerve is seldom severed, and spontaneous recovery should be awaited – it occurs in 90 per cent of cases within 4 months. If recovery has not occurred by the expected time, and if nerve conduction studies fail to show evidence of recovery, the nerve should be explored.

Local complications of fractures		
Urgent	**Less urgent**	**Late**
Local visceral injury	Fracture blisters	Delayed union
Vascular injury	Plaster sores	Malunion
Nerve injury	Pressure sores	Non-union
Compartment syndrome	Nerve entrapment	Avascular necrosis
Haemarthrosis	Myositis ossificans	Muscle contracture
Infection	Ligament injury	Joint instability
Gas gangrene	Tendon lesions	Osteoarthritis
	Joint stiffness	
	Algodystrophy	

Common nerve injuries	
Injury	**Nerve**
Shoulder dislocation	Axillary
Humeral shaft fracture	Radial
Humeral supracondylar fracture	Radial or median (anterior interosseous)
Elbow medial condyle	Ulnar
Elbow dislocation	Ulnar
Monteggia fracture–dislocation	Posterior interosseous
Hip dislocation	Sciatic
Knee dislocation	Peroneal

Common vascular injuries	
Injury	**Vessel**
First rib fracture	Subclavian
Shoulder dislocation	Axillary
Humeral supracondylar fracture	Brachial
Elbow dislocation	Brachial
Pelvic fracture	Presacral and internal iliac
Femoral supracondylar fracture	Femoral
Knee dislocation	Popliteal
Proximal tibial fracture	Popliteal or its branches

In open fractures any nerve lesion is more likely to be complete; the nerve should be explored during wound debridement and repaired, either then or as a 'secondary' procedure.

Early exploration should also be considered if signs of a nerve injury appear *after manipulation of the fracture.*

VASCULAR INJURY

Fractures most often associated with damage to a major artery are those around the knee and elbow and those of the humeral and femoral shafts. The artery may be cut, torn, compressed or contused, either by the initial injury or subsequently by jagged bone fragments. Even if its outward appearance is normal, the intima may be detached and the vessel blocked by thrombus, or a segment of artery may be in spasm. The effects vary from transient diminution of blood flow to profound ischaemia, tissue death and peripheral gangrene.

Clinical features

The patient may complain of paraesthesia or numbness in the toes or the fingers. The injured limb is cold and pale, or slightly cyanosed, and the pulse is weak or absent. X-rays may show one of the 'high-risk' fractures mentioned above. If a vascular injury is suspected, an angiogram should be performed immediately; if it is positive, emergency treatment must be started without further delay.

Treatment

All bandages and splints should be removed. The fracture is re-x-rayed and, if the position of the bones suggests that the artery is being compressed

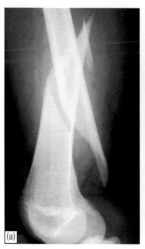
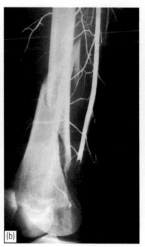
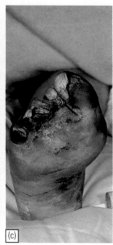

25.1 Vascular injury (a) X-ray of a patient with a fractured femur and early signs of vascular insufficiency. The point of the proximal fragment seems to be dangerously close to the popliteal vessels. Angiography (b) shows that the artery is interrupted at precisely that point. (c) Despite vein-grafting, the patient ended up with peripheral gangrene.

or kinked, prompt reduction is necessary. The circulation is then reassessed repeatedly over the next half hour. If there is no improvement, the vessels must be explored by operation – preferably with the benefit of preoperative or peroperative angiography. A torn vessel can be sutured, or a segment may be replaced by a vein-graft; if it is thrombosed, endarterectomy may restore the blood flow. If vessel repair is undertaken, stable fixation is imperative; where it is practicable, the fracture should be fixed internally.

COMPARTMENT SYNDROME

Fractures of the arm or leg can give rise to severe ischaemia even if there is no damage to a major vessel. Bleeding, oedema or inflammation (infection) may increase the pressure within one of the osteofascial compartments; there is reduced capillary flow which results in muscle ischaemia,

further oedema, still greater pressure and yet more profound ischaemia – a vicious circle that ends, after 12 hours or less, in necrosis of nerve and muscle within the compartment. Nerve is capable of regeneration but muscle, once infarcted, can never recover and is replaced by inelastic fibrous tissue *(Volkmann's ischaemic contracture)*. A similar cascade of events may be caused by swelling of a limb inside a tight plaster cast.

Clinical features

High-risk injuries are fractures of the elbow, the forearm bones and the proximal third of the tibia. Other precipitating factors are operation (usually for internal fixation) or infection.

The classic features of ischaemia are the five Ps: pain, paraesthesia, pallor, paralysis and pulselessness. But it is criminal to wait until they are all present: the diagnosis can be made long before that. The earliest symptoms are pain

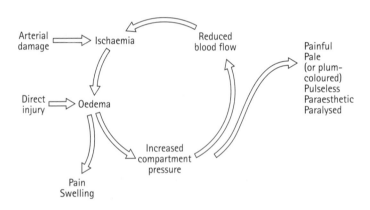

25.2 The vicious circle of Volkmann's ischaemia

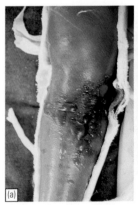
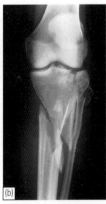
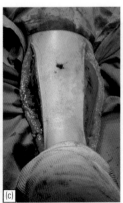
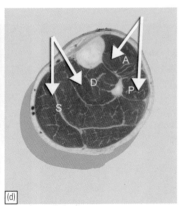

25.3 Compartment syndrome (a,b) A fracture at this level is always dangerous. This man was treated in plaster; pain became intense and when the plaster was split (which should have been done immediately after its application), the leg was swollen and blistered. (c) Tibial compartment decompression is best done through two separate incisions and requires fasciotomies of all compartments (d). A = anterior, P = peroneal, S = superficial posterior, D = deep posterior.

(usually described as a 'bursting' sensation) and altered sensibility. Skin sensation should be carefully and repeatedly checked. Remember that *the presence of a pulse does not exclude the diagnosis.*

Ischaemic muscle is highly sensitive to stretch. When the toes or fingers are passively hyper-extended, there is increased pain in the calf or forearm.

In doubtful cases, the diagnosis can be confirmed by measuring the pressure in the fascial compartment. A catheter is introduced into the compartment and the pressure is measured close to the level of the fracture. A differential pressure (ΔP) – the difference between diastolic pressure and compartment pressure – of less than 30 mmHg (4.00 kPa) is an indication for immediate compartment decompression.

 Don't wait for the obvious signs of ischaemia to appear. If you *suspect* an impending compartment syndrome, start treatment straightaway.

Treatment

The threatened compartment (or compartments) must be promptly decompressed. Casts, bandages and dressings must be completely removed – merely splitting the plaster is utterly useless – and the limb should be nursed flat (elevating the limb causes a further decrease in end-capillary pressure and aggravates the muscle ischaemia). The ΔP should be carefully monitored; if it falls below 30 mmHg, immediate open fasciotomy is performed. *In the case of the leg, 'fasciotomy' means opening all four compartments through medial and lateral incisions.* The wounds should be left open and inspected 2 days later: if there is muscle necrosis, debridement can be done; if the tissues are healthy, the wound can be sutured (without tension), or skin-grafted or simply allowed to heal by secondary intention.

If facilities for measuring compartmental pressures are not available, the decision to operate will have to be made on clinical grounds. The limb should be examined at 15-minute intervals and, if there is no improvement within 2 hours of splitting the dressings, fasciotomy should be performed. Muscle will be dead after 4–6 hours of total ischaemia – there is no time to lose!

HAEMARTHROSIS

Fractures involving a joint may cause acute haemarthrosis. The joint is swollen and tense and the patient resists any attempt at moving it. The blood should be aspirated before dealing with the fracture.

INFECTION

Open fractures may become infected; closed fractures hardly ever do unless they are opened by operation. Post-traumatic wound infection is now the most common cause of chronic osteomyelitis. This does not necessarily prevent the fracture from uniting, but union will be slow and the chance of re-fracturing is increased.

Clinical features

Following an open fracture or operation, the wound becomes inflamed and starts draining sero-purulent fluid. A sample should be submitted immediately for microbiological investigation; while awaiting the result, intravenous antibiotic administration can be started.

Treatment

All open fractures should be regarded as potentially infected and treated by giving prophylactic antibiotics and meticulously excising all devitalized tissue. If there are signs of acute infection and pus formation, the tissues around the fracture should be opened and drained; the choice of antibiotic is dictated by tests for bacterial sensitivity.

If internal fixation has been used, this does not necessarily have to be removed; even worse than an infected fracture is one that is both infected and unstable. However, if the infection does not respond to antibiotic treatment, it may be necessary to remove the implants and replace them with external fixation.

The further treatment of postoperative osteomyelitis is discussed in Chapter 2.

GAS GANGRENE

This terrifying condition is produced by clostridial infection (especially *Clostridium welchii*). These are anaerobic organisms that can survive and multiply only in tissues with low oxygen tension; the prime site for infection, therefore, is a dirty wound with dead muscle that has been closed without adequate debridement. Toxins produced by the organisms destroy the cell wall and rapidly lead to tissue necrosis, thus promoting the spread of the disease.

Clinical features appear within 24 hours of the injury: the patient complains of intense pain and swelling around the wound and a brownish discharge may be seen; gas formation is usually not very marked. There is little or no pyrexia, but the pulse rate is increased and a characteristic smell becomes evident (once experienced, this is never forgotten). Rapidly, the patient becomes toxaemic and may lapse into coma and death.

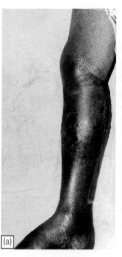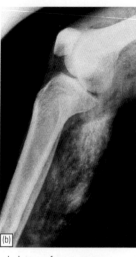

25.4 Gas gangrene (a) Clinical picture of gas gangrene. (b) X-rays show diffuse gas in the muscles of the calf.

PLASTER SORES AND PRESSURE SORES

Plaster sores occur where skin is pressed directly onto bone. They should be prevented by padding the bony points and by moulding the wet plaster so that pressure is distributed to the soft tissues around the bony points. While a plaster sore is developing, the patient feels localized burning pain. A window must immediately be cut in the plaster, or warning pain quickly abates and skin necrosis proceeds unnoticed.

Pressure sores may be produced by splints and other appliances. These should be checked at frequent intervals to ensure that they fit correctly and comfortably.

Bed sores are liable to occur in elderly or paralysed patients. The skin over the sacrum and heels is especially vulnerable. Bed sores can usually be prevented by careful nursing and early activity; once they have developed, treatment is difficult and it may be necessary to excise the necrotic tissue and repair the defect by means of plastic surgery.

It is essential to distinguish gas gangrene, which is characterized by myonecrosis, from anaerobic cellulitis, in which superficial gas formation is abundant but toxaemia usually slight. Failure to recognize the difference may lead to unnecessary amputation for the non-lethal cellulitis.

Prevention

Deep, penetrating wounds in muscular tissue are dangerous; they should be explored, all dead tissue should be completely excised and, if there is the slightest doubt about tissue viability, the wound should be left open. Unfortunately there is no effective antitoxin against *C. welchii*.

Treatment

The key to life-saving treatment is early diagnosis. General measures, such as fluid replacement and intravenous antibiotics, are started immediately. Hyperbaric oxygen has been used as a means of limiting the spread of gangrene. However, the mainstay of treatment is prompt decompression of the wound and removal of all dead tissue. In advanced cases, amputation may be essential.

FRACTURE BLISTERS

These are due to elevation of the superficial layers of skin by oedema, and can sometimes be prevented by firm bandaging. They should be covered with a sterile, dry dressing.

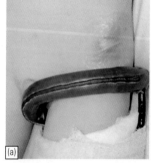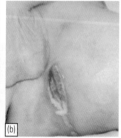

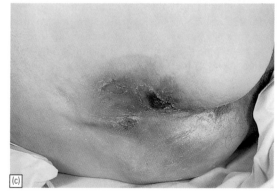

25.5 Pressure sores Pressure sores are a sign of carelessness. (a,b) Sores from poorly supervised treatment in a Thomas' splint. (c) Bed-sores in an elderly patient, which kept her in hospital for months.

LATE COMPLICATIONS

DELAYED UNION

The timetable on page 270 is no more than a rough guide to the period in which a fracture may be expected to unite and consolidate. It must never be relied upon in deciding when treatment can be discontinued. If the time is unduly prolonged, the term 'delayed union' is used.

Causes

Factors causing delayed union are either *biological* or *biomechanical*.

Poor blood supply

A badly displaced fracture will cause tearing of the periosteum and interruption of the intramedullary blood supply. The fracture surface may become necrotic and the normal healing process will take longer than usual.

Severe soft-tissue damage

Severe soft-tissue damage is the most important cause of delayed union and non-union.

Periosteal stripping

Over-enthusiastic stripping of periosteum during internal fixation is an avoidable cause of non-union.

Imperfect splintage

Excessive traction (creating a fracture gap) or excessive movement at the fracture site will delay ossification in the callus. In forearm or leg fractures, an intact fellow bone may actually hold the adjacent fracture fragments apart.

Over-rigid fixation

Contrary to popular belief, rigid fixation delays rather than promotes fracture union. It is only because the fixation device holds the fragments securely that the fracture seems to 'unite'. Union by primary bone healing is slow, but provided stability is maintained throughout, the fracture does eventually unite.

Infection

Tissue healing is severely hampered by bone lysis, necrosis and pus formation. In addition, fixation implants tend to loosen and fracture stability is lost.

Clinical features

Fracture tenderness persists and, if the bone is subjected to stress, pain may be acute.

X-ray

The fracture line remains visible and there is very little callus formation or periosteal reaction. However, the bone ends are not sclerosed or atrophic. The appearances suggest that, although the fracture has not united, it eventually will.

Treatment

Conservative

The two important principles are (1) to eliminate any possible cause of delayed union (see above), and (2) to promote healing by providing the most appropriate biological environment. Immobilization (whether by cast or by internal fixation) should be sufficient to prevent movement at the fracture site; but fracture loading is an important stimulus to union and this can be enhanced by encouraging muscular exercise and weight-bearing in the cast or brace. The watchword is patience; however, there comes a point with every fracture at which the ill-effects of prolonged immobilization outweigh the advantages of non-operative treatment, or at which the risk of implant breakage begins to loom.

Operative

Each case should be treated on its merits; however, if union is delayed for more than 6 months and there is no sign of callus formation, internal fixation and bone-grafting are indicated. The operation should be planned in such a way as to cause the least possible damage to the soft tissues.

NON-UNION

In a minority of cases, delayed union gradually turns into non-union, i.e. it becomes apparent that the fracture will never unite without intervention. Movement can be elicited at the fracture site and pain diminishes; the fracture gap turns into a pseudarthrosis.

On x-ray, the fracture is clearly visible and the bone on either side of it may be either exuberant or rounded off. This contrasting appearance has led to non-unions being divided into hypertrophic and atrophic types. In *hypertrophic non-union* the bone ends are enlarged, suggesting that osteogenesis is still active but not quite capable of bridging the gap. In *atrophic non-union* osteogenesis seems to have ceased; the bone ends are tapered or rounded, with no suggestion of new-bone formation.

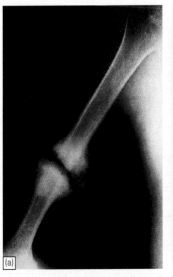
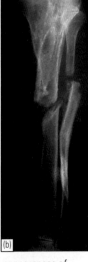

25.6 Non-union X-rays showing typical appearances of (a) hypertrophic non-union and (b) atrophic non-union.

Treatment

Conservative

Non-union is occasionally symptomless, needing no treatment or, at most, a removable splint. Even if symptoms are present, operation is not the only answer; with hypertrophic non-union, functional bracing may be sufficient to induce union, but treatment often needs to be prolonged. Pulsed electromagnetic fields and low-frequency pulsed ultrasound can also be used to stimulate union.

Operative

With hypertrophic non-union and in the absence of deformity, rigid fixation alone (internal or external) may lead to union. With atrophic non-union, fixation alone is not enough. Fibrous tissue in the fracture gap, as well as the hard, sclerotic bone ends, should be excised and bone-grafts packed around the fracture. If there is significant 'die-back', this will require more extensive excision and the gap is then dealt with by interposition graft or bone advancement using the Ilizarov technique (see Chapter 12).

MALUNION

When the fragments join in an unsatisfactory position (unacceptable angulation, rotation or shortening), the fracture is said to be malunited. Causes are failure to reduce a fracture adequately, failure to hold reduction while healing proceeds, or gradual collapse of comminuted or osteoporotic bone.

Clinical features

The deformity is usually obvious, but sometimes the true extent of malunion is apparent only on x-ray. Rotational deformity of the femur, tibia, humerus or forearm may be missed unless the limb is compared with its opposite fellow.

X-rays are essential to check the position of the fracture while it is uniting. This is particularly important during the first 3 weeks, when the situation may change without warning (and when deformity can still be easily corrected). At this stage it is sometimes difficult to decide what constitutes 'malunion'; acceptable norms differ from one site to another, and these are discussed under the individual fractures.

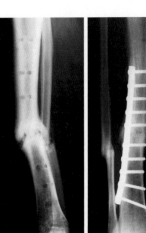
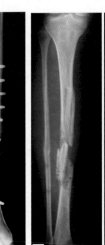
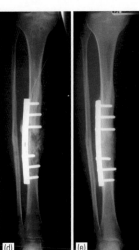

25.7 Non-union – treatment
(a) This patient with fractures of the tibia and fibula was initially treated by internal fixation with a plate and screws. The fracture failed to heal, and developed the typical features of hypertrophic non-union. (b) After a further operation, using more rigid fixation (and no bone-grafts), the fractures healed solidly.
(c,d) This patient with atrophic non-union needed both internal fixation and bone-grafts to stimulate bone formation and union (e).

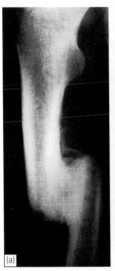

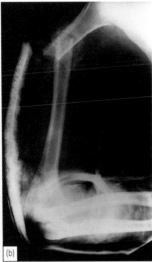

25.8 Malunion (a) Malunion with overlap, but at least the fragments are well aligned. (b) Fractured shaft of humerus treated in a hanging cast, the proximal edge of which lay directly over the fracture site; this acted as a fulcrum over which the fracture could bend. Callus is already visible and the fracture is well on the way to malunion.

Treatment

Incipient malunion may call for treatment even before the fracture has fully united; the decision about the need for re-manipulation or correction may be extremely difficult. A few guidelines are offered.

1. In adults, fractures should be reduced as near to the anatomical position as possible; apposition is important for healing, whereas alignment and rotation are important for function. Angulation of more than 10–15 degrees in a long bone, or a noticeable rotational deformity, may need correction by re-manipulation, or by osteotomy and internal fixation.

2. In young children, angular deformities near the bone ends will often remodel with time; rotational deformities will not.

3. In the lower limb, shortening of more than 2 cm is seldom acceptable to the patient and a shoe raise may be indicated; in cases of severe discrepancy, limb lengthening should be considered.

4. The patient's expectations (often prompted by cosmesis) may be quite different from the surgeon's: they should not be ignored. Early discussion with the patient, and a guided view of the x-rays, will help in deciding on the need for treatment and may prevent later misunderstanding.

5. Little is known of the long-term effects of small angular deformities on joint function. However, it seems likely that malalignment of more than 15 degrees in any plane may cause asymmetrical loading of the joint above or below and the late development of secondary osteoarthritis; this applies particularly to the large weight-bearing joints.

AVASCULAR NECROSIS (See also chapter 6)

Certain regions are notorious for their propensity to develop ischaemia and bone necrosis after injury. They are: (1) the head of the femur (after fracture of the femoral neck or dislocation of the hip); (2) the proximal part of the scaphoid (after fracture through its waist); (3) the lunate (following dislocation); and (4) the body of the talus (after fracture of its neck).

This is really an early complication of bone injury, because ischaemia occurs during the first few hours following fracture or dislocation. However, the clinical and radiological effects are not seen until weeks or even months later.

Clinical features

There are no symptoms associated with avascular necrosis, but if the fracture fails to unite or if the bone collapses, the patient may complain of pain. X-ray shows the characteristic increase in bone density (the consequence of new-bone ingrowth in

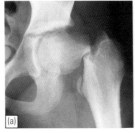

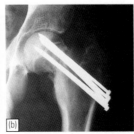

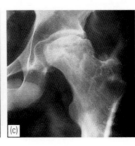

25.9 Avascular necrosis
(a) Displaced fractures of the femoral neck are at considerable risk of developing avascular necrosis. Despite internal fixation within a few hours of the injury (b), the head-fragment developed avascular necrosis. (c) X-ray after removal of the fixation screws.

the necrotic segment and disuse osteoporosis in the surrounding parts).

Treatment

Treatment usually becomes necessary when joint function is threatened. In old people with necrosis of the femoral head, an arthroplasty is the obvious choice; in younger people, realignment osteotomy (or even arthrodesis) may be wiser. Avascular necrosis in the scaphoid or talus may need no more than symptomatic treatment, but arthrodesis of the wrist or ankle is sometimes needed.

GROWTH DISTURBANCE

In children, damage to the physis may lead to abnormal or arrested growth of the bone. This problem is dealt with on page 273.

JOINT INSTABILITY

Bone loss or malunion close to a joint may lead to instability or recurrent dislocation. The commonest sites are the shoulder, the elbow and the patella.

A more subtle form of instability is seen after injuries around the wrist. Patients complaining of persistent discomfort or weakness after wrist injury should be fully investigated for *chronic carpal instability* (see page 164).

OSTEOARTHRITIS

A fracture involving a joint may damage the articular cartilage and give rise to post-traumatic osteoarthritis within a period of months. Even if the cartilage heals, irregularity or incongruity of the joint surfaces may cause localized stress and so predispose to secondary osteoarthritis years later. Little can be done to prevent this once the fracture has united.

LATE SOFT-TISSUE COMPLICATIONS

Joint stiffness

Joint stiffness after a fracture commonly occurs in the knee, the elbow, the shoulder and (worst of all) the small joints of the hand. Sometimes the joint itself has been injured; a haemarthrosis forms and leads to synovial adhesions. More often, the stiffness is due to oedema and fibrosis of the capsule, the ligaments and the muscles around the joint, or adhesions of the soft tissues to each other or to the underlying bone. All these conditions are made worse by prolonged immobilization; moreover, if the joint has been held in a position in which the ligaments are at their shortest, no amount of exercise will afterwards succeed in stretching these tissues and restoring the lost movement completely.

Treatment

The best treatment is prevention: elevation to minimize oedema, functional bracing rather than full-cast immobilization, and exercises that keep the joints mobile from the outset. If a joint has to be splinted, make sure that it is held in the 'position of safe immobilization' (see page 334). Joints that are already stiff take time to mobilize, but prolonged and patient physiotherapy can work wonders. However, surgical release of tight structures is sometimes necessary.

Heterotopic ossification

Heterotopic ossification in the muscles sometimes occurs after an injury, particularly around the elbow. The patient (usually a fit young man) complains of pain and local swelling. X-ray is normal at first but a bone scan may show increased activity. Over the next 2–3 weeks the pain gradually subsides, but joint movement is limited and x-ray may show fluffy calcification in the soft tissues. By 8 weeks, bony mass is easily palpable and is clearly defined in the x-ray.

Heterotopic ossification sometimes occurs spontaneously in unconscious patients.

Treatment

This condition was much more common in bygone years when joints, after plaster immobilization, were treated by vigorous muscle-stretching exercises. Forceful passive movements must be avoided; active movements should be introduced gently and gradually, alternating with rest periods in the position of function. If heterotopic bone has already appeared and is blocking movement, it may be helpful to excise the bony mass. Indomethacin or radiotherapy should be given to help prevent recurrence.

Muscle contracture

Following arterial injury or a compartmental syndrome, the patient may develop ischaemic contractures of the affected muscles (*Volkmann's ischaemic contracture*). Nerves injured by ischaemia sometimes recover, at least partially; thus the patient presents with deformity and stiffness, but numbness is inconstant. The sites most commonly affected are the forearm and hand, the leg and the

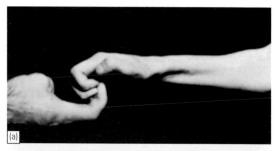

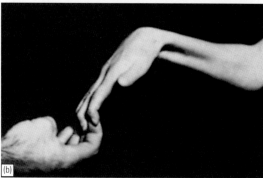

25.10 Muscle contracture (a) Typical claw-finger deformity due to Volkmann's ischaemic contracture of the forearm muscles. With the wrist extended, the fingers are drawn into flexion; (b) when the wrist is allowed to flex, the fingers can be straightened, thus indicating that the deformity is due to muscle shortening.

foot. In a severe case affecting the forearm, there will be muscle wasting and clawing of the fingers.

Treatment

Detachment of the flexor muscles at their origin and along the interosseous membrane in the forearm may improve the deformity, but function

is no better if sensation and active movement are not restored. Nerve-grafts may provide protective sensation in the hand, and tendon transfers (wrist extensors to finger and thumb flexors) will allow active grasp. In less severe cases, median nerve sensibility may be quite good and, with appropriate tendon releases and transfers, the patient regains a considerable degree of function.

Tendon rupture

Rupture of the extensor pollicis longus tendon may occur after a fracture of the lower radius. Direct suture is seldom possible, and the resulting disability is treated by transferring the extensor indicis proprius tendon to the distal stump of the ruptured thumb tendon. Late rupture of the long head of biceps after a fractured neck of humerus usually requires no treatment.

Nerve compression

Nerve compression may damage the lateral popliteal nerve if an elderly or emaciated patient lies with the leg in full external rotation. Radial palsy may follow the faulty use of crutches. Both conditions are due to lack of supervision.

Nerve entrapment

Bone or joint deformity may result in local nerve entrapment with typical features such as numbness or paraesthesia, loss of power and muscle wasting in the distribution of the affected nerve. Common sites are the *ulnar nerve*, due to a post-traumatic valgus deformity of the elbow, and the *median nerve*, following injuries around the wrist. Treatment is by early decompression of the nerve.

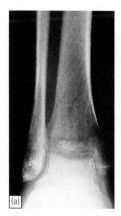
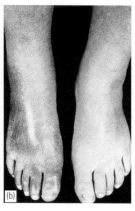
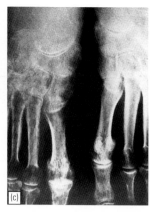

25.11 Complex regional pain syndrome (algodystrophy) Following a fracture of the tibia, this patient developed the typical features of complex regional pain syndrome affecting the right ankle and foot. The skin is atrophic and shiny; the x-ray shows marked regional osteoporosis above and below the ankle.

COMPLEX REGIONAL PAIN SYNDROME

Sudeck, in 1900, described a condition characterized by pain, stiffness and osteoporosis of the hand. The same condition sometimes occurs after fractures of the extremities and for many years it was called *Sudeck's atrophy*. More recently the disorder was held to be due to some type of neurovascular dysfunction and it came to be known variously as *reflex sympathetic dystrophy* or *algodystrophy*. Because of continuing un-certainty about its nature, these names have been replaced by the term *complex regional pain syndrome*.

The patient complains of continuous pain, often described as 'burning' in character. At first there is local swelling, redness and warmth, as well as tenderness and moderate stiffness of the joints near the site of injury. As the weeks go by, the skin becomes pale and atrophic, movements are increasingly restricted and the patient may develop fixed deformities. X-rays characteristically show patchy rarefaction of the bone.

Treatment

The earlier the condition is recognized and treatment begun, the better the prognosis. Elevation and active exercises are important after all injuries, but in this condition they are essential. During the early stage, anti-inflammatory drugs and amitriptyline are helpful. Sympathetic block or sympatholytic drugs have been advocated for this condition. They do sometimes appear to help, but their effect is unpredictable. Prolonged and dedicated physiotherapy will usually be needed.

CHAPTER 26

INJURIES OF THE SHOULDER AND UPPER ARM

The great bugbear of upper limb injuries is stiffness. In elderly patients especially, it is as important to preserve movement as it is to treat the fracture.

FRACTURES OF THE CLAVICLE

A fall on the shoulder or the outstretched hand may fracture the clavicle; the lateral fragment is pulled down by the weight of the arm, while the medial fragment is held up by the sternomastoid muscle.

Special features

The fracture is almost always displaced, producing a lump along the 'collar-bone'. Fractures of the outer third are easily mistaken for acromioclavicular injuries. Vascular and neurological complications are rare.

X-ray

The fracture is usually in the middle third of the bone and the lateral fragment lies below the medial. Outer-third injuries need special views to define any fracture.

Treatment

For the usual middle-third fracture, accurate closed reduction is neither possible nor essential. In most cases all that is needed is to support the arm in a sling until the pain subsides (usually 2–3 weeks). Thereafter, active shoulder exercises should be encouraged; this is particularly important in older patients.

By contrast, outer-third fractures are quite troublesome and may need open reduction and internal fixation.

Complications

Malunion is inevitable; in children the bone is soon remodelled, but in adults the slight deformity has to be accepted.

FRACTURES OF THE SCAPULA

The *body of the scapula* is fractured by a crushing force, which usually also fractures ribs and may dislocate the sternoclavicular joint. The *neck of the scapula* may be fractured by a blow or by a fall on the shoulder.

Special features

Shoulder movements are painful but possible. If breathing also is painful, thoracic injury must be excluded.

X-ray

The films may show a comminuted fracture of the *body* of the scapula, or a fractured *scapular neck*

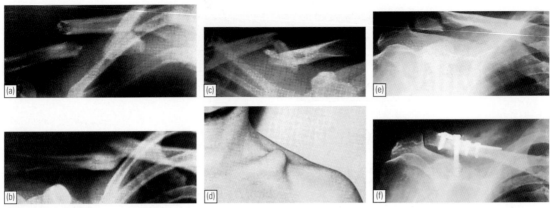

26.1 Fractured clavicle (a) The common site and displacement. (b) Often the fracture unites in a somewhat faulty position. (c) Comminuted fracture which united in this position leaving (d) a large lump. (e) Fracture of the outer (lateral) third with elevation of the shaft of the clavicle due to rupture of the medial part of the coracoclavicular ligament. This was treated by open reduction and internal fixation (f), using a long screw to fix the clavicle to the coracoid process.

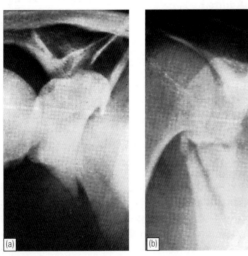

26.2 Scapular fractures (a) Fracture of the neck of the scapula, and (b) of the body of the scapula.

with the outer fragment pulled downwards by the weight of the arm. Occasionally a crack is seen in the *acromion* or the *coracoid process*. CT is useful for demonstrating glenoid fractures.

Treatment

Reduction is usually unnecessary. The patient wears a sling for comfort and from the start practises active exercises of the shoulder, elbow and fingers. Check repeatedly for dislocation of the shoulder; a large glenoid fragment may need to be fixed with a screw.

ACROMIOCLAVICULAR JOINT INJURIES

A fall on the shoulder tears the acromioclavicular ligaments, and upward subluxation of the clavicle may occur; more severe injury also tears the coracoclavicular (conoid and trapezoid) ligaments and results in complete dislocation of the joint.

Special features

The patient can usually point to the site of injury. If there is tenderness but no deformity (or very little deformity), it is probably a strain or a subluxation. With dislocation, the patient is in more pain and a prominent 'step' can be seen and felt.

X-ray

The films show either a subluxation with only slight elevation of the clavicle, or dislocation with considerable separation. A stress view, taken with the patient holding a 5 kg weight in each hand, may reveal the displacement more clearly.

Treatment

Subluxation does not affect function and does not require any special treatment; the arm is rested in a sling until pain subsides (usually no more than a week), and shoulder exercises are then begun.

Dislocation is poorly controlled by padding and strapping. However, surgery is controversial and it is doubtful whether it improves the outcome except in those whose work or hobbies involve using the arm above shoulder height for long periods.

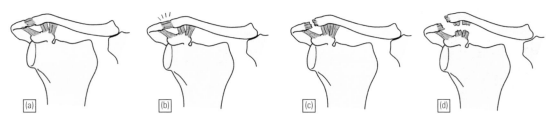

26.3 Acromioclavicular joint injuries (a) Normal joint. (d) Sprained acromioclavicular joint; no displacement. (c) Torn capsule and subluxation but coracoclavicular ligaments intact. (d) Dislocation with torn coracoclavicular ligaments.

One of the more reliable techniques is to reduce the dislocation by open operation, repair the torn ligaments and hold the reduction with a screw inserted downwards from the clavicle into the coracoid process; the screw is removed after 8 weeks.

Complications

Long-standing, unreduced dislocation of the acromioclavicular joint, though still compatible with reasonably good function, may leave the patient with an ill-defined feeling of discomfort and weakness of the shoulder, especially when attempting strenuous overhead activities. If the symptoms warrant active treatment, reconstructive surgery can be advised, but the patient must be warned that improvement cannot be guaranteed. One approach is to excise a small segment of the lateral end of the clavicle and then to tether the 'floating' clavicle by transferring the coraco-acromial ligament to the lateral end of the clavicle; the structure is further stabilized by holding the clavicle down with a screw between the clavicle and the coracoid process.

A very late complication is osteoarthritis of the acromioclavicular joint; this can usually be managed conservatively, but if pain is marked, the outer end of the clavicle can be excised.

STERNOCLAVICULAR DISLOCATION

Anterior dislocation

This uncommon injury is caused by a fall on the shoulder. The inner end of the clavicle springs forward, producing a visible and palpable prominence. The joint can usually be reduced quite easily by direct pressure on the prominent clavicle while the shoulders are relaxed. The problem is keeping it there. Splintage is unsatisfactory and internal fixation carries unnecessary risks (great vessels and pericardium are too close for comfort!). The patient should be persuaded to accept the slight residual deformity and mild discomfort during strenuous activity.

Posterior dislocation

This is very rare, but it can cause compression of the large vessels in the neck and should be reduced as a matter of urgency. Closed reduction can sometimes be achieved by lying the patient supine with a sandbag between the shoulder blades and then pulling on the arm with the shoulder abducted and extended; the joint reduces with a snap. The shoulders are braced backwards with a figure-of-eight bandage, which is kept in place for

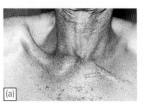

26.4 Acromioclavicular dislocation (a) X-ray showing complete separation of the acromioclavicular joint. (b) The clinical picture is unmistakable: a definite step in the contour at the outer end of the clavicle.

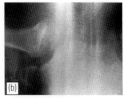

26.5 Sternoclavicular dislocation (a) The bump over the sternoclavicular joint may be obvious, though this is difficult to demonstrate on plain x-ray. (b) Tomography (or, better still, CT) will show the lesion.

3 weeks. If closed reduction fails, operative reduction is called for. The displaced clavicle is pulled forward with a hook.

DISLOCATION OF THE SHOULDER

The glenohumeral joint is very shallow and stability is maintained largely by the glenoid labrum (which slightly deepens the socket) and the surrounding ligaments and muscles. Traumatic dislocation is common; humeral head displacement is usually anterior, less often posterior.

ANTERIOR DISLOCATION

Anterior dislocation is caused either by a fall on the backward-stretching hand or by forced abduction and external rotation of the shoulder. The head of the humerus is driven forward, tearing the capsule or avulsing the glenoid labrum, and usually ends up just below the coracoid process. There may be an associated fracture of the proximal end of the humerus.

Special features

Pain is severe. The patient supports the arm with the opposite hand and is loath to permit any kind of examination. The lateral outline of the shoulder is flattened and a small bulge may be seen and felt just below the clavicle. The arm must always be examined for nerve and vessel injury.

X-ray

This will show the overlapping shadows of the humeral head and glenoid fossa, with the head usually lying below and medial to the socket.

Treatment

Reduction is most easily carried out under general anaesthesia and full relaxation, so as to minimize the risk of further damage. The simplest method is to pull on the arm in slight abduction while the body is stabilized in counter-traction. If anaesthesia is contraindicated, the prone position with the arm hanging may facilitate reduction.

Kocher's method is sometimes used. The elbow is bent to 90 degrees and held close to the body; no traction should be applied. The arm is slowly rotated 75 degrees laterally, then the point of the elbow is lifted forwards and adducted, and finally the arm is rotated medially.

An x-ray is taken to confirm reduction and exclude a fracture. When the patient is fully awake, active abduction is gently tested to exclude an axillary nerve injury.

The arm is rested in a sling for a week or two and active movements are then begun, but combined abduction and lateral rotation must be avoided for at least 3 weeks.

Complications

Rotator cuff tear

The rotator cuff is often torn, particularly in older people. This may later require surgical repair (see page 143).

Nerve injury

The axillary nerve may be injured; the patient is unable to contract the deltoid muscle and there may be a small patch of anaesthesia over the muscle. The lesion is usually a neuropraxia, which recovers spontaneously after a few weeks.

Occasionally the posterior cord of the brachial plexus, the median nerve or the musculocutaneous

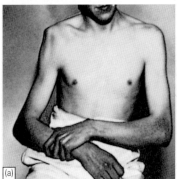
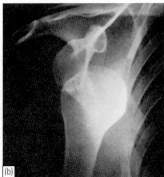
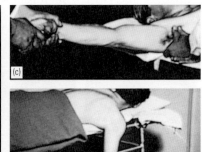

26.6 Anterior dislocation of the shoulder (a) The prominent acromion process and flattening of the contour over the deltoid are typical signs. (b) X-ray confirms the diagnosis of anterior dislocation. (c,d) Two methods of reduction.

nerve may be injured. This is alarming, but these injuries usually recover with time.

Vascular injury

The axillary artery may be damaged. The limb should always be examined for signs of ischaemia. Management is described on page 293.

Fracture–dislocation

If there is an associated fracture of the proximal humerus, open reduction and internal fixation will be necessary.

Recurrent dislocation

If the glenoid labrum has been damaged or detached, recurrent dislocation is likely (see page 149).

POSTERIOR DISLOCATION

This commonly missed injury is not a complete dislocation but a fracture–subluxation. It is usually caused by forced internal rotation of the abducted arm or by a direct blow on the front of the shoulder. It should always be suspected after an epileptic fit or a severe electric shock.

Special features

The diagnosis is frequently missed because, in the anteroposterior x-ray, the humeral head may seem to be in contact with the glenoid. However, clinically the condition is unmistakable because the arm is held in medial rotation and is locked in that position.

X-ray

In the anteroposterior projection, the humeral head, because it is medially rotated, looks somewhat globular. A lateral film is essential; it shows posterior subluxation and, sometimes, indentation of the humeral head.

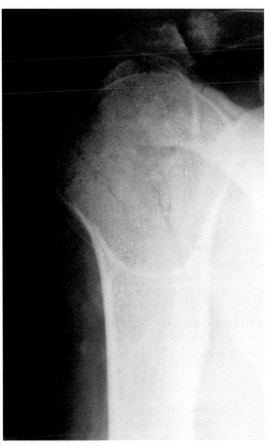

26.8 Posterior dislocation of the shoulder Posterior dislocation produces a characteristic x-ray appearance: because the head of the humerus is internally rotated, the anteroposterior x-ray shows a head-on projection giving the classic 'electric light-bulb' appearance.

Treatment

The arm is pulled and rotated laterally, while the head of the humerus is pushed forwards. After reduction, the management is the same as for anterior dislocation.

RECURRENT DISLOCATION (See also page 149)

Once a shoulder has been dislocated, this may happen repeatedly – and with increasing ease – over the ensuing months or years. In these cases the capsule and labrum may have been stripped from the margin of the glenoid and the humeral head may be indented. In the vast majority of cases, recurrence is anterior, but occasionally it is posterior; the distinction is not as easy as it may seem, because often by the time the patient is examined the head is back in the socket and there is only the history to go by.

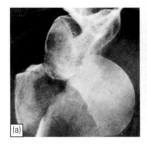 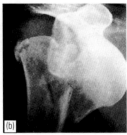

26.7 Fracture–dislocation of the shoulder Two examples of dislocation associated with fracture, (a) of the greater tuberosity, and (b) of the neck of the humerus. This injury may need both reduction and internal fixation of the fracture.

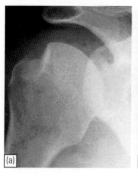
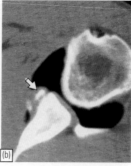
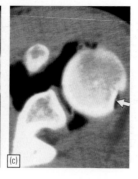

26.9 Recurrent dislocation of the shoulder (a) The classic x-ray sign is a depression in the posterosuperior part of the humeral head (the Hill–Sachs lesion). (b,c) MRI showing both the Hill–Sachs lesion and a Bankart lesion of the glenoid rim (arrows).

With recurrent anterior dislocation, the patient complains that the shoulder 'slips out' when the arm is lifted into abduction and lateral rotation, as in swimming or dressing or reaching backwards and upwards. At first it has to be 'put back' by someone; as time goes by, reduction becomes easier and often patients learn to do it themselves. The *apprehension test* is positive: if the shoulder is passively manipulated into abduction, extension and lateral rotation, the patient tenses up and anxiously resists further movement.

X-ray

An anteroposterior view with the shoulder in internal rotation will often show a posterolateral defect of the humeral head (Hill–Sachs lesion) where the bone has been damaged by the rim of the glenoid fossa. CT may show the damaged glenoid labrum (Bankart lesion).

 Direct blow to the shoulder: x-ray for associated cervical spine injury.

Treatment

If the patient is disabled, an operation will be needed: for anterior dislocation, some form of anterior capsular reconstruction is usually successful; recurrent posterior dislocation is more difficult and may require soft-tissue reconstruction combined with a bone operation to block abnormal movement at the back of the shoulder.

FRACTURES OF THE PROXIMAL HUMERUS

Fractures of the proximal humerus usually occur after middle age and are most common in osteoporotic individuals. The patient falls on the outstretched hand, fracturing the surgical neck; one or both tuberosities may also be fractured.

Special features

Pain may not be very severe because the fracture is often firmly impacted. However, the appearance of a large bruise in the upper arm is very suspicious. The patient should be examined for signs of axillary nerve or brachial plexus injury.

X-ray

In the elderly, a transverse fracture extends across the surgical neck, and often the greater tuberosity also is fractured. The shaft is usually impacted into the head in an abducted position. In younger patients, the proximal end of the humerus may be broken into several pieces. According to *Neer's classification,* a one-part fracture is one in which the fragments are undisplaced or firmly impacted (i.e. the humerus appears to be 'in one piece'); a two-part fracture is one in which the neck fracture is displaced (i.e. there are only two fragments, the humeral head and the rest of the bone); three-part or four-part fractures are those in which, in addition to the neck fracture, one or both of the tuberosities is also fractured. This sounds systematic and straightforward, but it is not easy to distinguish the radiographic outlines of comminuted fractures.

Treatment

Impacted or minimally displaced fractures need no treatment apart from a short period of rest with the arm in a sling. Active movements are begun as soon as practicable, but the sling is retained until the fracture has united (usually after 6 weeks).

Two-part fractures can usually be reduced closed; the arm is then bandaged to the chest for 3 or 4 weeks, after which shoulder exercises are commenced (the elbow and hand are, of course, exercised throughout).

Three-part fractures in young, active individuals usually require open reduction and internal fixation

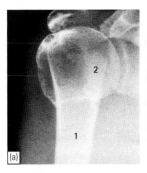
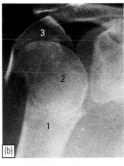
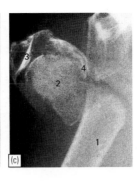

26.10 Fractures of the proximal humerus Neer's classification of proximal humeral fractures. (a) Two-part fracture. (b) Three-part fracture involving the neck and the greater tuberosity. (c) Four-part fracture. 1 = shaft of humerus; 2 = head of humerus; 3 = greater tuberosity; 4 = lesser tuberosity.

with a plate and screws. In elderly patients with osteoporotic bone, the results are less certain and manipulative reduction followed by physiotherapy may be equally satisfactory in the long term.

Four-part fractures, which carry additional risks of incomplete reduction, non-union and avascular necrosis of the humeral head, are best treated by prosthetic replacement, particularly in elderly patients.

Complications

Shoulder dislocation

Combined fracture and dislocation of the shoulder is difficult to manage. The dislocation should be reduced (this may require an operation) and the fracture can then be tackled in the usual way.

Vascular and nerve injuries

These may occur with three-part and four-part fractures and should be sought at the initial examination.

Stiffness

Shoulder stiffness is common. It can be minimized by starting exercises as early as possible.

FRACTURES OF THE SHAFT OF THE HUMERUS

A fall on the hand may twist the humerus, causing a spiral fracture. A fall on the elbow with the arm abducted may hinge the bone, causing an oblique or transverse fracture. A direct blow to the arm causes a fracture which is either transverse or comminuted. A fracture of the shaft in an elderly patient may be through a metastasis.

Special features

The arm is painful, bruised and swollen. Active extension of the wrist and fingers should be tested *before and after treatment* because the radial nerve may be damaged.

X-ray

The fracture is usually obvious, but don't forget to look for features suggesting a pathological lesion (e.g. fracture through a bone cyst or metastasis).

Treatment

Fractures of the humerus require neither perfect reduction nor total immobilization; the weight of the arm with an external cast is usually enough to pull the fragments into alignment. The cast is applied from the shoulder to the wrist with the elbow flexed to 90 degrees; after 2–3 weeks, it may be replaced by a shorter cast (shoulder to elbow) or by a removable brace. Exercises of the shoulder can be started within a week, but abduction is avoided until the fracture has united.

If the fracture is very unstable and difficult to control or if it is a pathological fracture, fixation is preferable. In most cases a plate and screws or a long intramedullary nail with locking screws will suffice. However, high-energy segmental fractures and open fractures are better treated by external fixation.

Complications

Nerve injury

Radial nerve palsy (wrist-drop and paralysis of the metacarpophalangeal extensors) may occur with shaft fractures. In closed injuries the nerve is very seldom divided, so there is no hurry to operate. Passive and active movements of the wrist and hand are encouraged while recovery is awaited.

If there is no sign of recovery by 12 weeks, the nerve should be explored. In complete lesions (neurotmesis), nerve suture is often unsatisfactory, but function can be largely restored by tendon transfers: pronator teres to extensor carpi radialis brevis for wrist extension; flexor carpi radialis or ulnaris to extensor digitorum for metacarpophalangeal extension; and palmaris longus to abductor pollicis longus for thumb abduction.

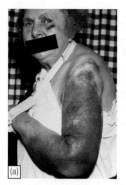
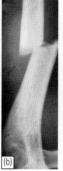
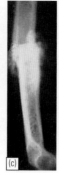
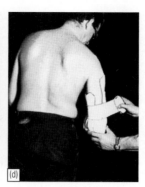
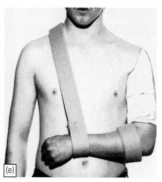

26.11 Fractured shaft of humerus (a) Bruising is always extensive. (b,c) Closed transverse fracture with moderate displacement. (d) Applying a U-slab of plaster (after a few days in a shoulder-to-wrist hanging cast) is usually adequate. (e) Ready-made braces are simpler and more comfortable, though not suitable for all cases. These conservative methods demand careful supervision if excessive angulation and malunion are to be prevented.

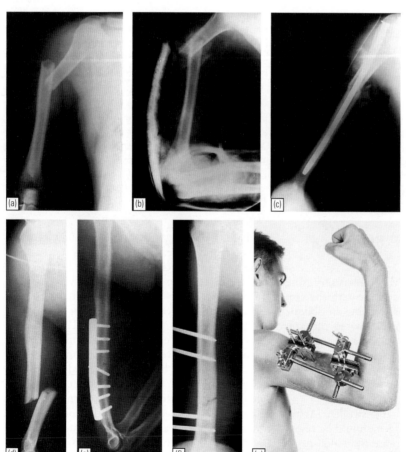

26.12 Fractured shaft of humerus – treatment
(a,b) Most shaft fractures can be treated in a hanging cast or functional brace, but beware the upper-third fracture, which tends to angulate at the proximal border of the cast (b). This particular fracture would have been better managed by (c) intramedullary nailing (and, better still, with a locking nail). Other methods of fixation, especially for (d) lower-third fractures, are (e) compression plating or (f,g) external fixation.

Non-union

Mid-shaft fractures sometimes fail to unite. This is treated by bone-grafting and internal fixation. Care must be taken not to injure the radial nerve.

FRACTURES OF THE DISTAL HUMERUS IN CHILDREN

The elbow is second only to the distal forearm for frequency of fractures in children. Most of these injuries are supracondylar fractures, the remainder being divided between condylar, epicondylar and proximal radial and ulnar fractures. Boys are injured more often than girls and more than half the patients are under 10 years old.

The usual accident is a fall directly on the point of the elbow or onto the outstretched hand with the elbow forced into valgus or varus. Pain and swelling are often marked and examination is difficult. X-ray interpretation also has its problems: the bone ends are largely cartilaginous and therefore radiographically incompletely visualized. *A good knowledge of the normal anatomy is essential if fracture displacements are to be recognized.*

Points of anatomy

The elbow is a complex hinge. Its stability is due largely to the shape and fit of the bones that make up the joint and this is liable to be compromised by any break in the articulating structures. The surrounding soft-tissue structures also are important, especially the capsular and collateral ligaments.

With the elbow extended, the forearm is normally in slight valgus in relation to the upper arm, the average carrying angle in children being about 15 degrees. When the elbow is flexed, the forearm comes to lie directly upon the upper arm. Malunion of a supracondylar fracture will inevitably disturb this relationship.

Since the epiphyses are in some part cartilaginous, only the secondary ossific centres can be seen on x-ray; they should not be mistaken for fracture fragments! The average ages at which they appear are easily remembered by the mnemonic CITE: **C**apitulum – 2 years; **I**nternal (medial) epicondyle – 6 years; **T**rochlea – 8 years; **E**xternal (lateral) epicondyle – 12 years. Epiphyseal displacements will not be detectable on x-ray before these ages, but they are inferred from radiographic indices such as *Baumann's angle* (see Figure 26.14).

SUPRACONDYLAR FRACTURES

These are among the commonest fractures in children. The distal fragment may be displaced and/or tilted either posteriorly or anteriorly, medially or laterally; sometimes it is also rotated.

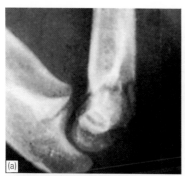
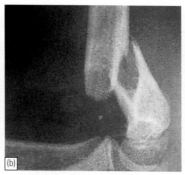
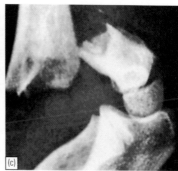
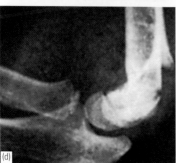

26.13 Supracondylar fractures X-rays showing supracondylar fractures of increasing severity. (a) Undisplaced. (b) Distal fragment posteriorly angulated but in contact. (c) Distal fragment completely separated and displaced posteriorly. (d) A rarer variety with anterior angulation.

Posterior displacement and tilt is the commonest (95 per cent of all cases), suggesting a hyperextension injury, usually due to a fall on the outstretched hand. The jagged end of the proximal fragment pokes into the soft tissues anteriorly, sometimes injuring the brachial artery or median nerve. *Anterior displacement* is rare, but may result from over-reduction of the usual posterior displacements.

Special features

Following a fall, the child is in pain and the elbow is swollen; with a posteriorly displaced fracture, the S-deformity of the elbow is usually obvious. It is essential to feel the pulse and check the capillary return.

X-ray

Undisplaced fractures are easily missed; there may be no more than subtle features of a soft-tissue haematoma. In the common *posteriorly displaced fracture* the distal fragment is tilted backwards and/or shifted backwards. In the rare *anteriorly displaced fracture* the fragment is tilted forwards.

The anteroposterior x-ray is often difficult to interpret because it is taken with the elbow flexed. The degree of sideways tilt (angulation) may therefore not be appreciated. This is where Baumann's angle is most helpful; wherever possible it should be accurately measured and compared with that of the uninjured side (Figure 26.14).

> Beware of leaving residual varus angulation of the distal fragment. Double-check the position and measure Baumann's angle.

Treatment

If there is even a suspicion of a fracture, the elbow is gently splinted in 30 degrees of flexion to prevent movement and possible neurovascular injury during the x-ray examination.

Undisplaced fractures

The elbow is immobilized at 90 degrees and neutral rotation in a light-weight splint or cast and the arm is supported by a sling. *It is essential to obtain an x-ray 5–7 days later to check that there has been no displacement.* The splint is retained for 3 weeks and supervised movement is then allowed.

Posteriorly angulated fracture

Swelling is usually not severe and the risk of vascular injury is low. If the posterior cortices are in continuity, the fracture can be reduced under general anaesthesia by the following step-wise manoeuvre: (1) traction for 2–3 minutes in the length of the arm with counter-traction above the elbow; (2) correction of any sideways tilt or shift and rotation (in comparison with the other arm); (3) gradual flexion of the elbow to 120 degrees, and pronation of the forearm, while maintaining traction and exerting finger pressure behind the distal fragment to correct posterior tilt. *Then feel the pulse and check the capillary return* – if the distal circulation is suspect, immediately relax the amount of elbow flexion until it improves.

X-rays are taken to confirm reduction, checking carefully to see that there is no varus or valgus angulation and no rotational deformity. If the acutely flexed position cannot be maintained without disturbing the circulation, or if the

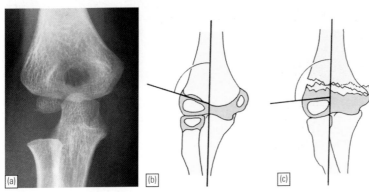

26.14 Baumann's angle Anteroposterior x-rays are sometimes difficult to make out, especially if the elbow is held flexed after reduction of the supracondylar fracture. Measurement of Baumann's angle is helpful. This is the angle subtended by the longitudinal axis of the humeral shaft and a line through the coronal axis of the capitellar physis, as shown in (a) the x-ray of a normal elbow and the accompanying diagram (b). Normally this angle is less than 80 degrees. If the distal fragment is tilted in varus, the increased angle is readily detected (c).

reduction is unstable, the fracture should be fixed with percutaneous crossed Kirschner wires (take care not to skewer the ulnar nerve!).

Following reduction, the arm is held in a collar and cuff; the circulation should be checked repeatedly during the first 24 hours. An x-ray is obtained after 3–5 days to confirm that the fracture has not slipped. If it has, do not delay – a further attempt at reduction is still possible. If reduction is satisfactory, the splint is retained for 3 weeks, after which movements are begun.

Posteriorly displaced fractures

These are usually associated with severe swelling, are difficult to reduce and are often unstable; moreover, there is a considerable risk of neurovascular injury or circulatory compromise due to swelling. The fracture should be reduced under general anaesthesia as soon as possible, by the method described above, and then held with percutaneous crossed Kirschner wires; this obviates the necessity to hold the elbow acutely flexed. Care should be taken not to injure the ulnar and radial nerves. Postoperative management is the same as for simple angulated fractures.

Anteriorly displaced fractures

The fracture is reduced by pulling on the forearm with the elbow semi-flexed, applying thumb pressure over the front of the distal fragment and then extending the elbow fully. A posterior slab is bandaged on and retained for 3 weeks. Thereafter, the child is allowed to regain flexion gradually.

Complications

Vascular injury

The great danger of supracondylar fracture is injury to the brachial artery, which, before the introduction of percutaneous pinning, was reported as occurring in more than 5 per cent of cases. Nowadays the incidence is probably less than 1 per cent. Peripheral ischaemia may be immediate and severe, or the pulse may fail to return after reduction. More commonly, the injury is complicated by forearm oedema and a mounting *compartment syndrome*, which leads to necrosis of the muscle and nerves without causing peripheral gangrene. Undue pain plus one positive sign (pain on passive extension of the fingers, a tense and tender forearm, an absent pulse, blunted sensation or reduced capillary return on pressing the finger pulp) demands urgent action. The flexed elbow must be extended and all dressings removed. If the circulation does not promptly improve, angiography (on the operating table if it saves time) is carried out, the vessel repaired or grafted and a forearm fasciotomy performed. If angiography is not available, or would cause much delay, Doppler imaging should be used. In extreme cases, operative exploration would be justified on clinical criteria alone.

Nerve injury

The median nerve may be injured. Fortunately, loss of function is usually temporary and recovery can be expected in 6–8 weeks.

Malunion

Malunion is common. However, backward or sideways shifts are gradually smoothed out by modelling during growth and they seldom give rise to visible deformity. Forward or backward tilt may limit flexion or extension, but consequent disability is slight.

By contrast, uncorrected sideways tilt (angulation) and rotation may lead to serious deformity of the elbow which will not improve with growth. Cubitus varus is disfiguring and

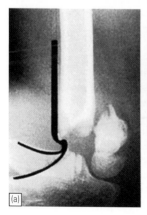 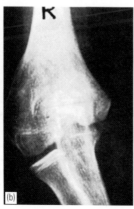 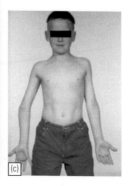

26.15 Supracondylar fractures – complications
The most serious complication is arterial damage (a) leading to Volkmann's ischaemia.
(b,c) Varus deformity of the right elbow following poor reduction.

cubitus valgus may cause late ulnar palsy. If deformity is marked, it will need correction by supracondylar osteotomy.

Elbow stiffness

Full movement may take months to return and must not be hurried. Forced movement will only make matters worse and may contribute to the development of heterotopic ossification (see page 300).

FRACTURE–SEPARATION OF THE LATERAL CONDYLE

The distal humeral epiphysis begins to ossify at the age of about 2 years and fuses with the shaft at about 16; between these ages, the condylar or epicondylar parts of the epiphysis may be sheared off or avulsed by the sudden pull of the forearm muscles during a fall on the hand. Only two of these injuries are at all common: fracture–separation of the entire condyle on the lateral side, and separation of the epicondyle on the medial side.

Special features

If the child falls with the elbow stressed in varus, a large fragment including the lateral condyle can be avulsed by the attached wrist extensors. The fracture line usually runs along the physis to enter the joint through the trochlea or (less often) through the capitulatrochlear groove.

The extent of the injury is often not appreciated because the capitellar epiphysis is largely cartilaginous and only the ossific centre in the fragment is visible on x-ray. If the fracture runs through the trochlea, the elbow joint can dislocate. The fragment may be grossly displaced and capsized.

 The condylar fragment is always larger than the image shown on x-ray.

Treatment

An undisplaced fracture can be treated by splinting the elbow for 2 weeks and then starting exercises. A check x-ray should be obtained after 5 days to make sure that the fracture has not displaced.

A displaced fracture may be reduced by manipulation, but if this fails, operative reduction must be carried out and the fragment fixed in position with a screw or Kirschner wires; the arm is immobilized in a cast. The wires are moved after 3 or 4 weeks and the cast can then be discarded.

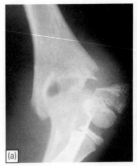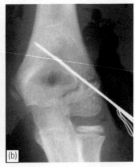

26.16 Fractured lateral condyle (a) A large fragment of bone and cartilage is avulsed; even with reasonable reduction, union is not assured and open reduction with fixation (b) is wise.

Complications

Non-union and malunion

If the condyle is left capsized, *non-union* is inevitable; with growth, the elbow becomes increasingly valgus, and ulnar nerve palsy is then likely to develop. *Malunion,* likewise, can result in cubitus valgus. If deformity is marked, it should be corrected by supracondylar osteotomy.

Recurrent dislocation

Occasionally condylar displacement results in *recurrent posterolateral dislocation* of the elbow. The only effective treatment is reconstruction of the bony and soft tissues on the lateral side.

SEPARATION OF THE MEDIAL EPICONDYLAR APOPHYSIS

If the wrist is forced into extension, the medial epicondylar apophysis is avulsed by the attached wrist flexors; if the elbow opens up on that side, the epicondylar fragment may be pulled into the joint. The inner side of the elbow is swollen and acutely tender. The x-ray has to be studied very carefully to detect the tiny ossific centre which marks the epicondylar fragment.

Treatment

Minor displacement may be disregarded; the elbow is splinted for 2 or 3 weeks to relieve pain, and exercises are then encouraged. However, if the epicondyle is markedly displaced, it should be sutured back in position. If it is trapped in the joint, it must be freed. Manipulation with the elbow in valgus and the wrist hyperextended (to pull on the flexor muscles) may be successful; if this fails, the joint must be opened and the fragment retrieved before being replaced.

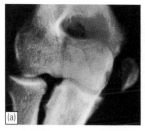
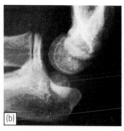

26.17 Fractured medial epicondyle (a) Avulsion of the medial epicondyle following valgus strain. Sometimes the epicondylar fragment is trapped in the joint (b); the serious nature of the injury is liable to be missed unless the surgeon specifically looks for the trapped fragment.

FRACTURE–SEPARATION OF THE ENTIRE DISTAL HUMERAL EPIPHYSIS

Up to the age of 7 years, the distal humeral epiphysis is a solid cartilaginous segment with maturing centres of ossification. With severe injury it may separate *en bloc*. This is likely to occur with fairly severe violence, such as a birth injury or child abuse.

Special features

The child is distressed and the elbow is markedly swollen. The history may be deceptively uninformative.

X-ray

In a very young child, in whom the bony outlines are still unformed, the x-ray may look normal. Medial displacement of either the capitellar ossification centre or the proximal radius and ulna is very suspicious. In older children the deformity is usually obvious.

Treatment

The injury is treated like a supracondylar fracture. If the diagnosis is uncertain, the elbow is merely splinted in flexion for 2 weeks; any resulting deformity (which is rare) can be dealt with at a later age.

FRACTURES OF THE DISTAL HUMERUS IN ADULTS

There are three types of distal humeral fracture: extra-articular supracondylar fracture, intra-articular unicondylar fracture and bicondylar fractures.

SUPRACONDYLAR FRACTURES

Supracondylar fractures are rare in adults. When they do occur, they are usually displaced and unstable or severely comminuted (high-energy injuries).

Treatment

Closed reduction is unlikely to be stable and Kirschner wire fixation is not strong enough to permit early mobilization. Open reduction and internal fixation is therefore the treatment of choice. The distal humerus is approached through a posterior exposure and reflection of the triceps tendon. A transverse or oblique fracture can usually be reduced and fixed with a single contoured plate and screws. Comminuted fractures may require double plates and transfixing screws.

CONDYLAR FRACTURES

Except in osteoporotic individuals, intra-articular condylar fractures should be regarded as high-energy injuries with soft-tissue damage. A severe blow on the point of the elbow drives the olecranon process upwards, splitting the condyles apart. Swelling is considerable and the bony landmarks are difficult to feel. *The patient should be carefully examined for evidence of vascular or nerve injury;* vascular insufficiency must be addressed as a matter of urgency.

X-ray

The fracture extends from the lower humerus into the elbow joint; it may be difficult to tell whether one or both condyles are involved, especially with an undisplaced condylar fracture. Sometimes the fracture extends into the metaphysis as a T-shaped or Y-shaped break, and the bone between the condyles may be comminuted.

Treatment

These are usually severe injuries associated with joint damage; prolonged immobilization will certainly result in a stiff elbow. Early movement is therefore a prime objective.

Undisplaced fractures

These can be treated by applying a posterior slab with the elbow flexed almost 90 degrees; gentle movements are commenced after a week, but only after obtaining another x-ray to exclude late displacement.

Displaced condylar fractures

Open reduction and internal fixation through a posterior approach is the treatment of choice. The best exposure is obtained by performing an intra-articular olecranon osteotomy. The ulnar nerve should be identified and protected throughout. The fragments are reduced and held temporarily with Kirschner wires. A unicondylar fracture without comminution can then be fixed with screws; if the fragment is large, a contoured plate is added to prevent re-displacement. Bicondylar and comminuted fractures will require double plate and screw fixation, and sometimes also bone-grafts in the gaps. Postoperatively, the elbow is held at 90 degrees with the arm supported in a sling. Movement is encouraged but should never be forced.

The fracture heals in about 8 weeks but the elbow often does not regain full movement; in severe injuries, movement may be markedly restricted, however beautiful the postoperative x-ray.

Complications

Vascular injury

Always check the circulation (repeatedly!). Vigilance is required to make the diagnosis and institute treatment as early as possible.

Nerve injury

There may be damage to either the median or the ulnar nerve. It is important to examine the hand and record the findings before treatment is commenced and again after treatment.

Stiffness

Comminuted fractures of the elbow always result in some degree of stiffness. However, the disability may be reduced by encouraging an energetic exercise programme. Late operations to improve elbow movement are difficult but can be rewarding.

Heterotopic ossification

Severe soft-tissue damage may lead to heterotopic ossification. Forced movement should be avoided.

FRACTURED CAPITULUM

This is an articular fracture which occurs only in adults. The patient falls on the hand, usually with the elbow straight. The anterior part of the capitulum is sheared off and displaced.

Fullness in front of the elbow is the most notable feature. The lateral side of the elbow is tender and flexion is grossly restricted.

X-ray

In the lateral view the capitulum (or part of it) is seen in front of the lower humerus, and the radial head is not opposed to it.

Treatment

Undisplaced fractures can be treated by resting the arm in a sling for 4 or 5 days and then starting movement.

Displaced fractures should be treated by operative reduction and fixation with small buried screws. If this proves too difficult, the fragment is best excised. Movements are commenced as soon as discomfort permits.

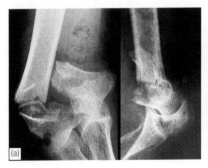
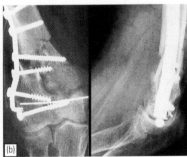

26.18 Bicondylar fractures in adults X-rays taken (a) before and (b) after open reduction and internal fixation. An excellent reduction was obtained in this case; however, often the elbow ends up with marked loss of movement, even though the general anatomy has been restored.

CHAPTER 27

INJURIES OF THE ELBOW AND FOREARM

DISLOCATION OF THE ELBOW

A fall on the outstretched hand may dislocate the elbow. In 90 per cent of cases the forearm bones are pushed backwards and dislocate posteriorly or posterolaterally. Provided there is no associated fracture, reduction will usually be stable and recurrent dislocation unlikely.

Special features

Deformity is usually obvious and the bony landmarks are displaced. In very severe injuries, pain and swelling are so marked that examination of the elbow is impossible; however, the hand should be examined for signs of vascular or nerve damage.

X-ray

X-ray examination is essential (a) to confirm the presence of a dislocation and (b) to identify any associated fractures.

Treatment

Uncomplicated dislocation

The patient should be fully relaxed under anaesthesia. The surgeon pulls on the forearm while the elbow is slightly flexed. With one hand, sideways displacement is corrected, then the elbow is further flexed while the olecranon process is pushed forward. Unless almost full flexion can be obtained, the olecranon is not in the trochlear groove.

After reduction, the elbow should be put through a full range of movement to see whether it is stable. Nerve function and circulation are checked again and the x-ray is repeated to confirm that the joint is reduced and that there are no associated fractures.

The arm is held in a light cast with the elbow flexed to just above 90 degrees and the wrist supported in a collar and cuff. After a week the cast can be removed and gentle exercises begun; at 3 weeks the collar and cuff are discarded. Elbow movements are allowed to return spontaneously and should never be forced.

Fracture–dislocation

Associated fractures of the humeral condyles or epicondyles, or the olecranon process, will need internal fixation. In cases where the elbow remains unstable after the bone and joint anatomy has been restored, a hinged external fixator can be applied in order to maintain mobility while the tissues heal.

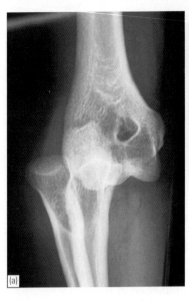

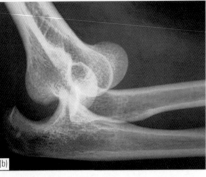

27.1 Dislocation of the elbow X-rays showing (a) lateral and (b) posterior displacement.

Complications

Vascular injury

The brachial artery may be damaged. Absence of the radial pulse is a warning. If there are other signs of ischaemia, this should be treated as an emergency. Splints must be removed and the elbow should be straightened somewhat. If there is no improvement, an arteriogram is performed; the brachial artery may have to be explored.

Nerve injury

The median or ulnar nerve is sometimes injured. Spontaneous recovery usually occurs after 6–8 weeks.

Stiffness

Loss of 20–30 degrees of extension is not uncommon after elbow dislocation. Physiotherapy may help, but forceful manipulation must be avoided.

Heterotopic ossification

Heterotopic bone formation may occur in the damaged soft tissues in front of the joint. In former years 'myositis officans' was a fairly common complication, usually associated with forceful reduction and over-enthusiastic passive movement of the elbow. Nowadays it is rarely seen, but one should be alert for signs such as excessive pain, tenderness, and tardy recovery of active movements. X-rays may show soft-tissue ossification as early as 4–6 weeks after injury. If the condition is suspected, exercises are stopped and the elbow is splinted in comfortable flexion until

pain subsides; gentle active movements and continuous passive motion are then resumed. Anti-inflammatory drugs may help to reduce stiffness; they are also used prophylactically to reduce the risk of heterotopic bone formation.

A bone mass which markedly restricts movement and elbow function should be excised once the bone is 'mature', i.e. has well-defined cortical margins and trabeculae.

Osteoarthritis

Secondary osteoarthritis is a late complication. Symptoms can usually be treated conservatively, but if pain and stiffness are intolerable, total elbow replacement can be considered.

ISOLATED DISLOCATION OF THE RADIAL HEAD

Isolated dislocation of the radial head is very rare; if it is seen, search carefully for an associated fracture of the ulna (the Monteggia injury), which may be difficult to detect in a child because the fracture is often incomplete. Even a minor deformity of the ulna may prevent full reduction of the radial head dislocation.

PULLED ELBOW

In young children the elbow is sometimes injured by a sharp tug on the wrist. The child is in pain; the elbow is held in extension and he or she will not allow it to be moved. There are no x-ray changes. What has happened is that the radius has been pulled distally and the orbicular ligament has slipped up over the head of the radius. A dramatic cure is achieved by forcefully supinating and then flexing the elbow; the ligament slips back with a snap.

FRACTURES OF THE PROXIMAL END OF THE RADIUS

Fractures of the proximal end of the radius are fairly common in young adults and children. A fall on the outstretched hand with the elbow extended and the forearm pronated causes impaction of the radial head against the capitulum. In adults this may fracture the *head of the radius;* in children, it is more likely to fracture the *neck of the radius* (possibly because the head is largely cartilaginous). In addition, the articular cartilage of the capitulum may be bruised or chipped; this cannot be seen on x-ray but is an important complication.

Special features
Following a fall on the oustretched arm, the patient complains of pain and local tenderness posterolaterally over the proximal end of the radius. A further clue is a marked increase in pain on pronation and supination of the forearm.

X-ray
Adults

The typical adult fracture is a vertical split through the radial head; less often there is a marginal fragment, and sometimes the head is crushed or comminuted. Impacted fractures are easily missed unless several views are obtained. The wrist also should be x-rayed to exclude a concomitant injury of the distal radioulnar joint.

Children

In children the fracture is through the neck; the proximal fragment may be tilted forwards and outwards.

Treatment
Adults

Undisplaced fractures of the radial head can be treated by supporting the elbow in a collar and cuff for 3 weeks; active flexion, extension and rotation are encouraged.

Displaced fractures are treated by open reduction and fixation with small screws.

Comminuted fractures have in the past been treated by excising the radial head. However, if there are associated forearm injuries or disruption of the distal radioulnar joint, the risk of proximal migration of the radius is considerable and the patient may develop intractable symptoms of pain and instability in the forearm. In such cases, every effort should be made to reconstruct the radial head or, if it has to be excised, it should be replaced by a silicone or metal prosthesis.

Children

In fractures of the radial neck, up to 30 degrees of radial head tilt and up to 3 mm of transverse displacement are acceptable. The arm is rested in a collar and cuff, and exercises are commenced after a week.

Displacement of more than 30 degrees should be corrected. With the patient's elbow extended, traction and varus force are applied; the surgeon then pushes the displaced radial fragment into position with his or her thumb. If this fails, open reduction is performed; there is no need for

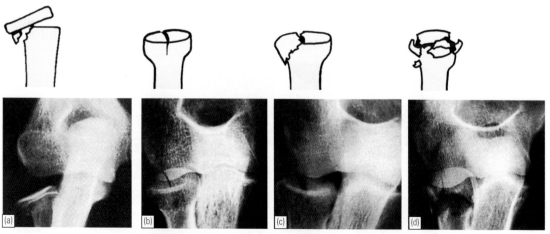

27.2 Fractures of the proximal radius (a) In children, the injury usually causes a fracture of the neck of the radius. (b–d) In adults, the injury is usually a vertical split (b), a marginal fragment (c) or a comminuted fracture of the head of the radius (d).

internal fixation. Following operation, the elbow is splinted in 90 degrees of flexion for a week or two and then movements are encouraged. *The head of the radius must never be excised in children because this will interfere with the synchronous growth of radius and ulna.*

Fractures that are seen a week or longer after injury should be left untreated (except for light splintage).

Complications

Joint stiffness is common and may involve both the elbow and the radioulnar joints.

Recurrent instability of the elbow can occur if the medial collateral ligament was injured and the radial head then excised.

Osteoarthritis of the radiocapitellar joint is a late complication of adult injuries. This may call for excision of the radial head.

FRACTURES OF THE OLECRANON PROCESS

Two types of injury are seen: (1) a *comminuted fracture,* which is due to a direct blow or a fall on the elbow; and (2) a *clean transverse fracture,* due to traction when the patient falls onto the hand while the triceps muscle is contracted.

Special features

A graze or bruise over the elbow suggests a comminuted fracture: the triceps is intact and the elbow can be extended against gravity. With a transverse fracture there may be a palpable gap and the patient is unable to extend the elbow against resistance.

X-ray

A properly orientated lateral view is essential to show details of the fracture, as well as the associated joint damage. The position of the radial head should be checked: it may be dislocated.

Treatment

A comminuted fracture with the triceps intact should be treated conservatively. Many of these patients are old and osteoporotic; internal fixation is impracticable and immobilizing the elbow will lead to stiffness. The arm is rested in a sling until the pain subsides; a further x-ray is obtained to ensure that there is no displacement, and the patient is then encouraged to start active movements.

An undisplaced transverse fracture that does not separate when the elbow is flexed can be treated by immobilizing the elbow in a cast in about 60 degrees of flexion for a week; then exercises are begun.

Displaced transverse fractures can, theoretically, be held by splinting the arm absolutely straight – but stiffness in that position would be disastrous. Operative treatment is therefore preferred. The fracture is reduced under vision and held by one of two methods: (a) fixation with a long cancellous screw inserted from the tip of the olecranon (make sure that the screw does not penetrate the ulnar cortex distally); or (b) tension-band wiring – two stiff wires driven across the fracture, leaving their ends protruding proximally and distally to anchor a tight loop of wire which will pull the fragments together. Early mobilization should be encouraged.

Complications

Stiffness used to be common, but with secure internal fixation and early mobilization the residual loss of movement should be minimal.

Non-union sometimes occurs after inadequate reduction and fixation of a transverse fracture. If elbow function is good, it can be ignored; if not,

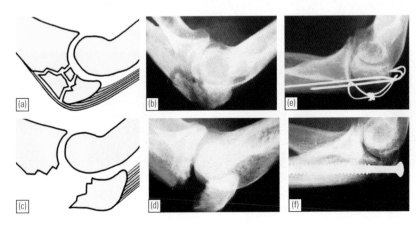

27.3 Fractured olecranon
(a,b) Comminuted fracture – best treated by activity. (c,d) Gap fracture – the extensor mechanism is disrupted and should be reconstituted by reduction and internal fixation using either (e) tension-band wiring or (f) a long screw.

rigid internal fixation and bone-grafting will be needed.

Osteoarthritis is a late complication, especially if the articular surface in the trochlear notch is poorly reduced. This can usually be treated symptomatically.

FRACTURES OF THE RADIUS AND ULNA

A twisting force (usually a fall on the hand) produces spiral fractures with the bones broken at different levels. A direct blow or an angulating force causes transverse fractures of both bones at the same level. The bone fragments are easily displaced by contraction of strong muscles attached to the radius. Bleeding and swelling in the muscle compartments of the forearm may cause circulatory impairment.

Special features

The diagnosis is usually quite obvious, but the wrist and hand must be carefully examined for signs of nerve damage or circulatory impairment.

X-ray

In adults the fractures are easy to see; in children they are often incomplete and the bones may appear bent rather than broken.

Treatment

Children

In children, closed reduction is usually successful and the fragments can be held in a well-moulded, full-length cast extending from the axilla to the metacarpal shafts (to control rotation). The cast is applied with the elbow at 90 degrees. If the radial fracture is proximal to pronator teres, the forearm is supinated; if it is distal to pronator teres, the forearm is held in neutral. The position is checked by x-ray after a week and, if it is satisfactory, splintage is retained until both fractures are united (usually 6–8 weeks). Throughout this period, hand and shoulder exercises are encouraged.

Adults

Unless the fragments are in close apposition, reduction is difficult and re-displacement in the cast almost inevitable. Consequently, most surgeons opt for open reduction and internal fixation from the outset. The fragments are held by plates and screws. The deep fascia is left open to prevent a build-up of pressure in the muscle compartments, and only the skin and subcutaneous tissues are sutured.

After the operation, the arm is kept elevated until the swelling subsides, and during this period active exercises of the hand are encouraged. If the fracture is not comminuted and the patient is reliable, early range-of-movement exercises are commenced, but lifting and sports are avoided. It takes 8–12 weeks for the bones to unite.

Complications

Nerve injury

Nerve injuries are rarely caused by the fracture, but they may be caused by the surgeon! Exposure of the radius in its proximal third risks damage to the posterior interosseous nerve where it is covered by the superficial part of the supinator muscle.

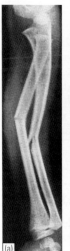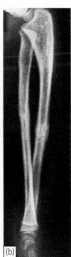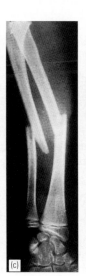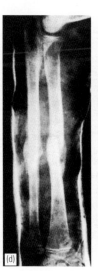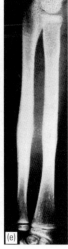

(a) (b) (c) (d) (e)

27.4 Fractured radius and ulna in children Greenstick fractures (a) need only correction of angulation (b) and plaster splintage. Complete fractures (c) are harder to reduce; however, provided alignment is corrected and the arm held in plaster (d), remodelling will restore the anatomy (e).

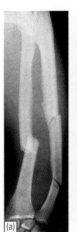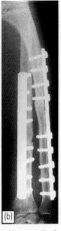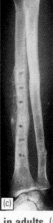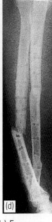

(a) (b) (c) (d)

27.5 Fractured radius and ulna in adults (a,b) Forearm fractures in adults have a strong tendency to re-displace after closed reduction and are therefore usually treated by internal fixation with sturdy plates and screws. Removal of the implants is not without risk. In this case (c,d) the radius fractured through one of the screw holes.

Surgical technique is particularly important here; the anterior Henry approach is safest.

Compartment syndrome

Fractures (and operations) of the forearm bones are always associated with swelling of the soft tissues, with the attendant risk of a compartment syndrome. The threat is even greater, and the diagnosis more difficult, if the forearm is wrapped up in plaster. The byword is 'watchfulness'; if there are any signs of circulatory embarrassment, treatment must be prompt and uncompromising (see page 294).

Delayed union and non-union

Most fractures of the radius and ulna heal within 8–12 weeks. However, one of the bones may take longer than usual, and immobilization may have to be continued beyond the usual time. High-energy and open fractures are at risk of developing non-union, which will require bone-grafting and internal fixation.

Malunion

With closed reduction there is always a risk of malunion, resulting in angulation or rotational deformity of the forearm, cross-union of the fragments, or shortening of one of the bones and disruption of the distal radioulnar joint. If pronation or supination is severely restricted, and there is no cross-union, mobility may be improved by a correctional osteotomy.

Complications of plate removal

Removal of plates and screws is often regarded as a fairly innocuous procedure. Beware! Complications are common, and they include damage to vessels and nerves, infection, and fractures through screw holes.

FRACTURE OF A SINGLE FOREARM BONE

Fracture of either the radius or the ulna alone is uncommon. Its importance lies in the fact that deformity or shortening of one bone (while the partner bone remains intact) usually involves a concomitant disruption of either the proximal or distal radioulnar joint. This associated injury must always be looked for by obtaining a full-length x-ray of the forearm, including the elbow and wrist.

Special features

Ulnar fractures are easily missed – even on x-ray. If there is local tenderness, a further x-ray a week or two later is wise. Always examine the elbow and wrist.

X-ray

The fracture may be anywhere in the radius or ulna. The fracture line is transverse and displacement is slight. In children, the intact bone sometimes bends without actually breaking ('plastic deformation').

Treatment

Isolated fracture of the ulna

The fracture is rarely displaced; a forearm brace leaving the elbow free is usually sufficient. It takes about 8 weeks before full activity can be resumed.

Isolated fracture of the radius

Radial fractures are prone to rotary displacement; to achieve reduction, the forearm needs to be supinated for upper-third fractures, neutral for middle-third fractures and pronated for lower-third fractures. The position is usually difficult to hold; if so, internal fixation with a compression plate and screws is better. With rigid fixation, early movement is encouraged.

MONTEGGIA FRACTURE-DISLOCATION OF THE ULNA

The injury originally described by Monteggia was a fracture of the shaft of the ulna associated with disruption of the proximal radioulnar joint and dislocation of the radiocapitellar joint. Nowadays, the term includes also fractures of the olecranon combined with radial head dislocation.

Special features

Usually the cause is a fall on the hand and forced pronation of the forearm. The radial head usually dislocates forwards and the upper third of the ulna fractures and bows forwards. The forearm deformity is obvious but the radial head dislocation may be missed.

X-ray

Any apparently isolated fracture of the ulna should raise the suspicion of a proximal radial dislocation. A good lateral view of the elbow will confirm the diagnosis: normally the head of the radius points directly to the capitulum; if it is dislocated, it lies in a plane anterior to the capitulum.

Treatment

The secret of successful treatment is to restore the length of the fractured ulna; only then can the dislocated joint be fully reduced and remain stable. In adults, this means an operation. The ulnar fracture must be accurately reduced, with the bone restored to full length, and then fixed with a plate and screws. The radial head usually reduces once the ulna has been fixed. Stability must be tested through a full range of movement. If the radial head does not reduce, or is not stable after reduction, open reduction should be performed.

If the elbow is completely stable, flexion/extension and rotation can be started after 10 days. If there is doubt, the arm should be immobilized in plaster with the elbow flexed for 6 weeks.

Complications

Unreduced dislocation

If the diagnosis has been missed or the dislocation imperfectly reduced, the radial head remains dislocated and limits elbow flexion. In children, no treatment is advised until the end of growth, and then only if function is significantly impaired. In adults, operative reduction or excision of the radial head may be needed.

GALEAZZI FRACTURE–DISLOCATION OF THE RADIUS

The counterpart of the Monteggia injury is a fracture of the distal third of the radius and dislocation or subluxation of the distal radioulnar joint.

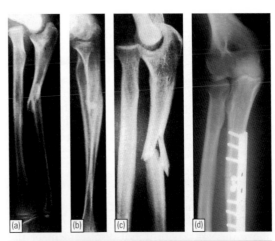

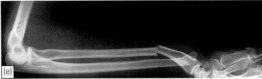

27.6 Monteggia and Galeazzi fracture–dislocations of the radius and ulna (a–d) The Monteggia injury is a fracture of the ulna and dislocation of the proximal end of the radius. X-rays that include the elbow joint will show that the head of the radius no longer points to the capitulum. In a child, closed reduction and plaster (b) is usually satisfactory; in the adult (c), the crucial step is to restore the ulna to its full length by reducing the fracture and holding it with internal fixation (d); in most cases the radial head will then reduce by itself, but if it does not, open reduction is required. (e) By contrast, the Galeazzi injury is a fracture of the radius with dislocation of the distal radioulnar joint. Here, again, the important step is to restore the length of the fractured bone (the radius); in adults this usually means open reduction and internal fixation. (See also Fig. 23.6e,f).

Special features

The Galeazzi fracture is much more common than the Monteggia. Prominence or tenderness over the lower end of the ulna is the striking feature. It is important also to test for an ulnar nerve lesion, which is common.

X-ray

The displaced fracture in the lower third of the radius is obvious; check the inferior radioulnar joint for subluxation or dislocation.

Treatment

As with the Monteggia fracture, the important step is to restore the length of the fractured bone. In children, closed reduction is often successful; in adults, reduction is best achieved by open operation and compression plating of the radius.

An x-ray is taken to ensure that the distal radioulnar joint is reduced and stable. If it is, no further action is needed; the arm is rested for a few days, after which gentle active movements are encouraged. If it is reduced but unstable, the radioulnar joint should be fixed with a Kirschner wire and the forearm splinted in an above-elbow cast for 6 weeks. If there is a large ulnar styloid fragment, it should be reduced and fixed.

COLLES' FRACTURE

The injury which Abraham Colles described in 1814 is a transverse fracture of the radius just above the wrist, with dorsal displacement of the distal fragment. It is the most common of all fractures in older people, the high incidence being related to the onset of postmenopausal osteoporosis. Thus the patient is usually an older woman who gives a history of falling on her outstretched hand.

Special features

With undisplaced fractures, there may be pain and swelling but little or no deformity. Displaced fractures produce a distinctive dorsal tilt just above the wrist – the so-called 'dinner-fork deformity'.

X-ray

The radius is fractured at the corticocancellous junction, about 2 cm from the wrist; often the ulnar styloid is also fractured. Characteristically, the distal fragment is shifted and tilted both dorsally and towards the radial side; in some cases the fracture is impacted, in others it may be severely comminuted.

Treatment

Undisplaced fractures

If the fracture is undisplaced (or only very slightly displaced), a dorsal splint is applied for a day or two until the swelling has resolved, then the cast is completed. The fracture is stable and the cast can usually be removed after 4 weeks to allow mobilization.

Displaced fractures

Displaced fractures must be reduced under anaesthesia (haematoma block, Bier's block or axillary block). The hand is grasped and traction is applied in the length of the bone to disimpact the fragments; the distal fragment is then pushed into place by pressing on the dorsum while manipulating the wrist into moderate flexion,

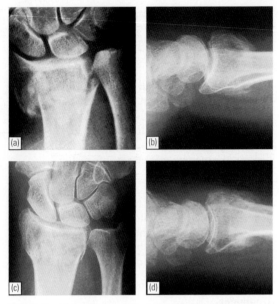

27.7 Colles' fracture (a,b) The typical Colles' fracture is both displaced and angulated towards the dorsum and towards the radial side of the wrist. (c,d) After successful reduction, the radial articular surface faces correctly slightly volarwards.

ulnar deviation and pronation. The position is then checked by x-ray. If it is satisfactory, a dorsal plaster slab is applied, extending from just below the elbow to the metacarpal necks and two-thirds of the way round the circumference of the wrist. It is held in position by a crepe bandage. Extreme positions of flexion and ulnar deviation must be avoided: 20 degrees in each direction is adequate.

The arm is kept elevated for the next day or two; shoulder and finger exercises are started as soon possible. If the fingers become swollen, cyanosed or painful, there should be no hesitation in splitting the bandage.

It is essential to check the position again by x-ray 10 days later. Often the fracture re-displaces in the cast; if re-manipulation is needed, this should be done within the first 2 weeks.

The fracture usually unites in about 5 weeks and, even in the absence of radiological proof of union, the slab may then be discarded and exercises begun.

Comminuted and unstable Colles' fractures

If plaster immobilization alone cannot hold the fracture, this can be supplemented by percutaneous Kirschner wire fixation; the plaster and wires are removed after 5 weeks and exercises begun. For very unstable fractures, external

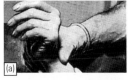
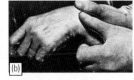
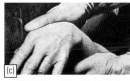
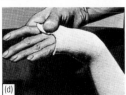
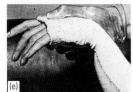
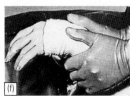
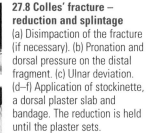

27.8 Colles' fracture – reduction and splintage
(a) Disimpaction of the fracture (if necessary). (b) Pronation and dorsal pressure on the distal fragment. (c) Ulnar deviation. (d–f) Application of stockinette, a dorsal plaster slab and bandage. The reduction is held until the plaster sets.

fixation is the best option. Proximal pins are placed through the radius and distal pins through the shaft of the second metacarpal. Bone-grafts may be added if the radius has markedly collapsed.

Complications

Circulatory impairment

Circulation in the fingers must be checked; the bandage holding the slab may need to be split or loosened.

Nerve injury

The median nerve may be compressed by swelling in the carpal tunnel. If the symptoms are mild, they may resolve with release of the dressings and elevation of the arm. If symptoms are severe or persistent, the transverse carpal ligament should be divided.

Malunion

Malunion is common, either because reduction was not complete or because displacement within the plaster was overlooked. In most cases, treatment is not necessary. However, if disability is marked, the radial deformity can be corrected by osteotomy.

Associated radioulnar and carpal injuries

Ligament strains around the wrist are more common than generally recognized and may be a source of pain and weakness long after the fracture has healed.

Tendon rupture

Rupture of extensor pollicis longus tendon occasionally occurs several weeks after the fracture. The frayed fibres cannot easily be sutured; a tendon transfer, using one of the extensor tendons of the index finger, will restore lost function.

Joint stiffness

Stiffness of the shoulder, elbow and fingers can be avoided by encouraging active movement.

Complex regional pain syndrome

This troublesome condition used to be called Sudeck's atrophy. Early signs are swelling and tenderness of the finger joints – a warning not to neglect the daily exercises. By the time the plaster is removed, the hand is stiff and painful and there are signs of vasomotor instability. X-rays show osteoporosis and there is increased activity on the bone scan. Treatment is discussed on page 301.

SMITH'S FRACTURE

Smith (a Dubliner, like Colles) described a similar fracture about 20 years later. However, in this injury the distal fragment is displaced and tilted anteriorly (which is why it is sometimes called a 'reversed Colles'). It is caused by a fall on the back of the hand.

Treatment

The fracture is reduced by traction and extension of the wrist, and the forearm is immobilized in a cast for 6 weeks.

FRACTURE OF THE RADIAL STYLOID PROCESS

This injury is caused by forced radial deviation of the wrist, usually the result of a fall. The fracture line is transverse, just proximal to the radial styloid process.

Treatment

If the styloid fragment is displaced, it should be reduced and held with screws or Kirschner wires.

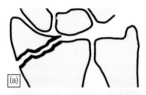

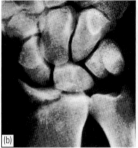

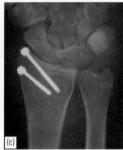

27.9 Fracture of the radial styloid process (a,b) The fracture inevitably involves the wrist joint and it is therefore important to obtain accurate reduction. This can be done by fixation with Kirschner wires or (c) one or two screws.

FRACTURE–SUBLUXATION OF THE WRIST (BARTON'S FRACTURE)

Barton's injury is an oblique fracture which runs from the volar surface of the distal end of the radius into the wrist joints. The fragment is often displaced anteriorly, carrying the carpus with it as a fracture–dislocation. The significance of recognizing this fracture is that it can be expected to be unstable.

Treatment

The fracture may be easily reduced, but it is just as easily re-displaced. Internal fixation, using a small anterior buttress plate, is recommended.

COMMINUTED INTRA-ARTICULAR FRACTURES IN YOUNG ADULTS

In the young adult, a comminuted intra-articular fracture is a high-energy injury. A poor outcome will result unless intra-articular congruity, fracture alignment and length are restored and movements started as soon as possible.

Treatment

The simplest option is a manipulation and cast immobilization. If the anatomy is not restored, an open reduction may be necessary. The medial (ulnar side) complex must be anatomically reconstituted, which may require open reduction

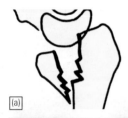

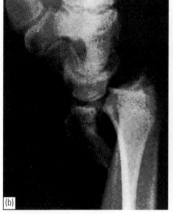

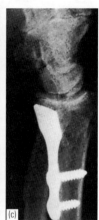

27.10 Barton's fracture (a,b) The true Barton's fracture runs across the volar aspect of the distal radius into the joint. The entire carpus moves volarwards with the small fragment, thus making it a fracture–subluxation of the wrist (c). The fracture has been reduced and held (c) with a small anterior plate.

through dorsal and palmar approaches and a combination of wires, plates, screws, bone-grafts and external fixation.

Complications of radiocarpal fractures

Carpal instability

Any serious injury of the distal radius and ulna, and especially those involving the wrist joint, may be associated with unsuspected injuries of the carpus. These can be excluded only by careful clinical and x-ray examination. If they are overlooked, the patient may return months or years later with symptoms and signs of carpal instability (see page 164).

Secondary osteoarthritis

Injuries around the wrist joint may eventually lead to secondary osteoarthritis. It is difficult to predict when (or even whether) this is likely to occur: symptoms develop slowly and disability is often not severe. If pain and weakness interfere significantly with function, arthrodesis of the wrist may be needed.

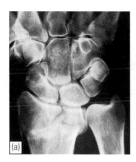
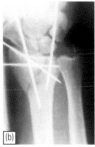
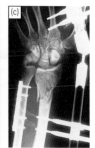

27.11 Comminuted fracture of the distal radius and ulna These fractures are difficult to reduce and even more difficult to hold. In some cases (a,b) this can be achieved with the use of Kirschner wires. (c) High-energy fractures may require more complex surgery, including a combination of internal and external fixation.

DISTAL FOREARM FRACTURES IN CHILDREN

The distal radius and ulna are among the commonest sites of childhood fractures. The break may occur through the distal radial physis or in the metaphysis of one or both bones. Metaphyseal fractures are often incomplete or greenstick.

The usual injury is a fall on the outstretched hand with the wrist in extension; the distal fragment is usually forced posteriorly (this is often called a 'juvenile Colles' fracture'). Lesser force may do no more than buckle the metaphyseal cortex (a type of compression fracture, or torus fracture).

Special features

The wrist is painful, and often quite swollen; sometimes there is an obvious 'dinner-fork deformity'.

X-ray

Physeal fractures are almost invariably Salter–Harris type 1 or 2, with the epiphysis shifted and tilted backwards and radially. Metaphyseal injuries may appear as mere buckling of the cortex, as angulated greenstick fractures, or as complete fractures with displacement and shortening. If only the radius is fractured, the ulna may be bent though not fractured.

Treatment

Physeal fractures are reduced, under anaesthesia, by pressure on the distal fragment. The arm is immobilized in a full-length cast with the wrist slightly flexed and ulnar deviated, and the elbow at 90 degrees. The cast is retained for 4 weeks. These fractures do not interfere with growth. Even if reduction is not absolutely perfect, further growth and modelling will obliterate any deformity within a year or two.

Buckle fractures require no more than 2 weeks in plaster, followed by another 2 weeks of restricted activity.

Greenstick fractures are usually easy to reduce – but apt to re-displace in the cast! Some degree of angulation can be accepted: in children under the age of 10, up to 30 degrees, and in children over 10, up to 15 degrees. If the deformity is greater, the fracture is reduced by thumb pressure and the arm is immobilized in a full-length cast with the wrist and forearm in neutral and the elbow flexed 90 degrees. The cast is changed and the fracture re-x-rayed at 1 week; if it has re-displaced, a further gentle manipulation can be carried out. The cast is finally discarded after 6 weeks.

Complete fractures can be difficult to reduce – especially if the ulna is intact. The fracture is manipulated in much the same way as a Colles' fracture; the reduction is checked by x-ray and a full-length cast is applied with the wrist neutral

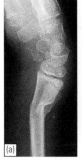
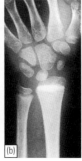
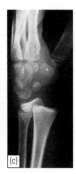
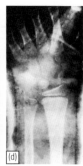
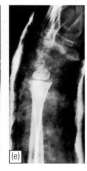

27.12 Distal forearm fractures in children (a) In older children it is usually a greenstick fracture about 2 cm above the wrist. (b,c) Physeal fractures are usually a Salter–Harris type 1 or 2. Here, accurate reduction was achieved (d,e).

and the forearm supinated. After 1 week, a check x-ray is obtained; the cast is kept on for 6 weeks. If the fracture slips, especially if the ulna is intact, it should be stabilized with a percutaneous Kirschner wire.

Complications

Forearm swelling and a threatened compartment syndrome are prevented by avoiding over-forceful or repeated manipulations, splitting the plaster, elevating the arm for the first 24–48 hours and encouraging exercises.

Malunion as a late sequel is uncommon in children under 10 years of age. Deformity of as much as 30 degrees will straighten out with further growth and remodelling over the next 5 years. This should be carefully explained to the worried parents.

CHAPTER 28

INJURIES OF THE WRIST AND HAND

INJURIES OF THE WRIST

Injuries of the wrist comprise soft-tissue strains and fractures or dislocations of individual carpal bones. However, they should never be regarded as isolated injuries: the entire carpus suffers, and sometimes, long after the fracture has healed, the patient still complains of pain and weakness in the wrist.

Clinical assessment

Following a fall, the patient complains of pain in the wrist, perhaps accompanied by swelling. Tenderness can often be localized to a particular spot, providing a clue to the diagnosis. Movements are likely to be restricted and painful.

X-ray

Fractures are often quite obvious, but sometimes multiple views – and examination on multiple occasions – are needed to detect an undisplaced crack.

Study the shape of the carpus and the relationship of the bones to each other. Familiarity with the normal anatomy is essential. Unusual gaps suggest disruption of ligaments; more subtle changes appear in the alignment of the bones. In the lateral x-ray, the axes of the radius, lunate, capitate and third metacarpal are co-linear, and the scaphoid projects at an angle of about 45 degrees to this line. With traumatic instability, the linked carpal segments collapse (like the buckled carriages of a derailed train). Two patterns are recognized: dorsal intercalated segment instability (DISI), in which the lunate is torn from the scaphoid and tilted backwards; and volar intercalated segment instability (VISI), in which the lunate is torn from the triquetral and turns towards the palm. Motion studies may reveal a subluxation.

Principles of management

'Wrist sprain' should not be diagnosed until a more serious injury has been excluded with certainty. Even with apparently trivial injuries, ligaments are sometimes torn and the patient may later develop carpal instability.

If the initial x-rays seem to be normal but the clinical signs suggest a carpal injury, a splint or plaster should be applied and the x-ray examination repeated 2 weeks later; a fracture or dislocation may then be more obvious.

If splintage is needed, the fingers should be left free so that movements are not unnecessarily impeded.

FRACTURE OF THE SCAPHOID

Scaphoid fractures account for almost 75 per cent of all carpal fractures. The usual mechanism is a fall on the hand with wrist extended. The critical movement is probably a combination of dorsiflexion and radial deviation, with the force passing between the two rows of carpal bones; the scaphoid, lying partly in each row, fractures across its waist. There may also be disruption of the scapholunate ligaments. The injury is rare in children and in the elderly.

The blood supply of the scaphoid diminishes proximally. This accounts for the fact that 1 per cent of distal-third fractures, 20 per cent of

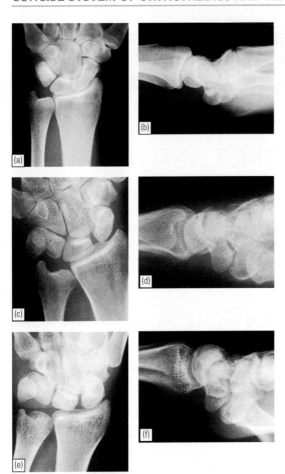

28.1 Carpal injuries (a,b) Normal appearances in anteroposterior and lateral x-rays. (c,d) 'Sprained wrist' followed by pain and weakness. In the anteroposterior view (c) the scaphoid image is foreshortened (compared with the normal) and there is an unusually large gap between the scaphoid and the lunate (scapholunate dissociation). In the lateral view (d) the lunate is seen to be dorsally tilted. This is the typical dorsal intercalated segment instability (DISI) pattern. (e,f) This patient also had a sprained wrist. The anteroposterior x-ray again shows foreshortening of the scaphoid and in the lateral view (f) the lunate is tilted volarwards (volar intercalated segment instability (VISI) pattern).

middle-third fractures and 40 per cent of proximal fractures result in non-union or avascular necrosis of the proximal fragment.

Special features

There may be slight fullness in the anatomical snuffbox; precisely localized tenderness in the same place is an important diagnostic sign.

X-ray

Anteroposterior, lateral and two oblique views are all essential; even then, the fracture may not be seen in the first few days after the injury. Two weeks later, the break will be much clearer; it is usually transverse through the narrowest part of the bone (the waist), but it may be more proximal or more distal. Always look for signs of associated carpal displacement.

Treatment

If the clinical features are suggestive of a fracture but the x-ray looks normal, the patient must be told to return for a second x-ray 2 weeks later. Meanwhile, the wrist is immobilized in a cast extending from the upper forearm to just short of the metacarpophalangeal joints of the fingers, but incorporating the proximal phalanx of the thumb; the wrist is held dorsiflexed and the thumb forwards in the 'glass-holding' position (the so-called scaphoid plaster). *If a fracture is confirmed,* treatment will depend on the type of fracture and the degree of displacement.

Fracture of the scaphoid tubercle needs no splintage and should be treated as a wrist sprain; a crepe bandage is applied and movement is encouraged.

Undisplaced fractures of the waist need no reduction and are treated in plaster; 90 per cent should heal. After 8 weeks, the plaster is removed and the wrist examined clinically and radiologically. If there is no tenderness and the x-ray shows signs of healing, the wrist is left free; however, complete radiographic union may take several months.

If the scaphoid is tender, or the fracture still visible on x-ray, the cast is re-applied and retained for a further 6 weeks. If, at that stage, there are signs of *delayed union* (bone resorption and cavitation around the fracture), healing can be hastened by bone-grafting and internal fixation.

Displaced fractures can be manipulated and treated in plaster, but the outcome is less predictable. It is better to reduce the fracture openly and to fix it with a compression screw.

Complications

Avascular necrosis

X-ray examination at 2–3 months may show increased density of the proximal fragment. This is pathognomonic of avascular necrosis. Although revascularization and union are theoretically possible, they take years and meanwhile the wrist collapses and arthritis develops. Bone-grafting as

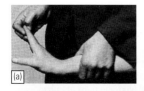
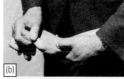
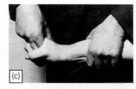

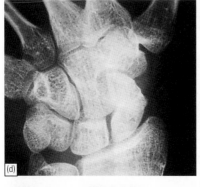
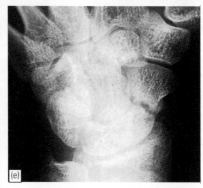

28.2 Scaphoid fractures – diagnosis (a–c) *Clinical signs.* Pain on dorsiflexion of the wrist, tenderness in the anatomical snuffbox, and pain on gripping.

X-ray signs: (d) The anteroposterior view often fails to show the fracture; always ask for an oblique 'scaphoid' view (e). The fracture may be through (f) the proximal pole, (g) the waist, or (h) the scaphoid tubercle. If at first the x-ray shows no fracture (i), repeat the examination at 2 weeks (j); now the fracture is obvious.

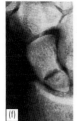
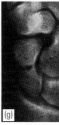
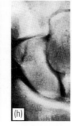
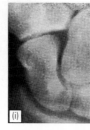
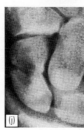

for delayed union may be successful, in which case the bone, though abnormal, is structurally intact. If the wrist becomes painful, the dead fragment can be excised. However, the wrist tends to collapse after this procedure; a better option may be to remove the entire proximal row of carpal bones, or else to remove the scaphoid and fuse the proximal to the distal row.

Non-union

By 3 months it may be obvious that the fracture will not unite. Bone-grafting may still be attempted, because this reduces the chance of secondary osteoarthritis. However, patients who are completely asymptomatic may prefer to accept the situation, at least until osteoarthritis supervenes.

Osteoarthritis

Non-union or avascular necrosis may lead to secondary osteoarthritis of the wrist. If the arthritis is confined to the distal pole, excising the radial styloid may help. As the arthritis progresses, changes appear in the scaphocapitate joint. Salvage procedures include proximal row carpectomy, intercarpal fusion and radiocarpal fusion.

FRACTURES OF OTHER CARPAL BONES

Carpal fractures, other than those of the scaphoid, can be difficult to diagnose on the usual x-ray views. However, the diagnosis, if suspected, can usually be confirmed by special carpal tunnel views, CT or MRI.

Undisplaced fractures are treated by splintage for a week or two. Displaced fractures may need open reduction and internal fixation.

ULNAR-SIDE WRIST INJURIES

The distal radioulnar joint is often injured with fractures of the radius; less often as an isolated event. Injuries comprise tears of the triangular fibrocartilage complex (TFCC), avulsion of the ulnar styloid process and articular fractures of the head of the ulna.

Special features

There is tenderness over the distal radioulnar joint and pain on rotation of the forearm. The distal ulna may be unstable; the *piano-key sign* is elicited by holding the patient's forearm pronated and pushing sharply on the prominent head of the ulna.

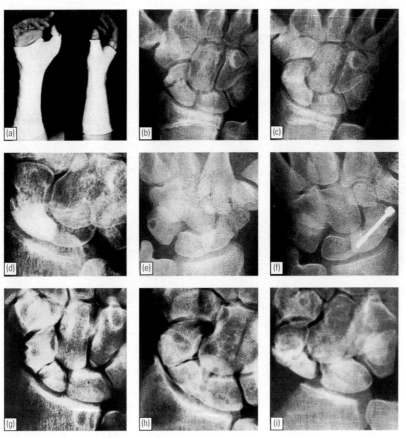

28.3 Scaphoid fractures – treatment and complications
(a) Scaphoid plaster.
(b,c) Fracture going on to union at 10 weeks. (d) Avascular necrosis of the proximal half.
(e) Non-union, treated by
(f) inserting a Herbert screw.
(g) Established non-union.
(h) Non-union with osteoarthritis at the fracture site. (i) Treatment by excising the radial styloid process.

Investigations

X-ray examination may show a fracture or signs of incongruity of the distal radioulnar joint. Arthrography, MRI and arthroscopy help to confirm the diagnosis.

Treatment

Dislocation of the distal radioulnar joint can usually be reduced by closed manipulation; the arm and wrist are then immobilized in an above-elbow cast (to prevent rotation) for 4 weeks. If the joint is still unstable, operative reduction and pinning may be needed.

A TFCC tear should be repaired and the ulnocarpal capsule reefed.

SCAPHOLUNATE DISSOCIATION

What is thought to be a sprain giving rise to persistent tenderness over the dorsum of the wrist may be shown by x-ray to be a much more significant injury: subluxation of the scaphoid and disruption of the ligaments between scaphoid and lunate. The pathognomonic features are foreshortening of the scaphoid and the appearance of a large gap between scaphoid and lunate.

Treatment

If the condition is diagnosed less than 4 weeks after injury, the bones should be repositioned by

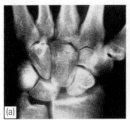
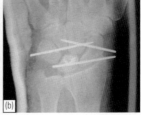

28.4 Scapholunate dissociation (a) After a fall, this patient complained of pain and tenderness in the anatomical snuffbox. X-ray (a) shows that the scaphoid is intact, but the image is markedly foreshortened and there is a wide gap between the scaphoid and the lunate. After open reduction and repair of the dorsal ligaments, the scaphoid was held in position with Kirschner wires (b).

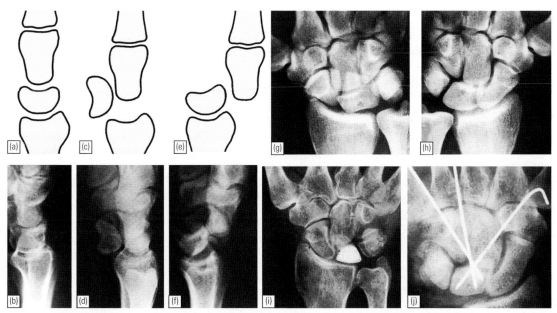

28.5 Lunate and perilunate dislocations (a,b) Lateral view of normal wrist; (c,d) Lunate dislocation; (e,f) Perilunar dislocation. (g,h) Anteroposterior view of both wrists: dislocated lunate on the left side, giving a triangular image instead of the usual cuboidal image seen in the right wrist. (i) Avascular necrosis following reduction of a dislocated lunate. (j) Wire fixation following reduction of lunate dislocation.

open operation and held in place with Kirschner wires; it may be possible at the same time to repair the ligaments with interosseous sutures. The wrist is immobilized in a cast for 8 weeks.

If the diagnosis is missed, the patient may end up with chronic carpal instability (see Chapter 15).

LUNATE AND PERILUNATE DISLOCATIONS

A fall with the hand forced into dorsiflexion may tear the tough ligaments that normally bind the carpal bones. The lunate usually remains attached to the radius, and the rest of the carpus is displaced backwards *(perilunate dislocation)*. Usually the hand immediately snaps forwards again but, as it does so, the lunate may be levered out of position to be displaced anteriorly *(lunate dislocation)*. Sometimes the scaphoid remains attached to the radius and the force of the perilunar dislocation causes it to fracture through the waist *(transscaphoid perilunate dislocation)*.

Special features

The wrist is painful and swollen and is held immobile. If the carpal tunnel is compressed, there may be paraesthesia or blunting of sensation in the territory of the median nerve, and weakness of palmar abduction of the thumb.

X-ray

Most dislocations are *perilunate*. In the anteroposterior view, the carpus is diminished in height and the bone shadows overlap abnormally. One or more of the carpal bones may be fractured (usually the scaphoid). *Lunate* dislocation can be recognized by the abnormal shape of the lunate image – triangular instead of quadrilateral.

In the lateral view, it is easy to distinguish a lunate from a perilunate dislocation. The dislocated lunate is tilted forwards and is displaced in front of the radius, while the capitate and metacarpal bones are in line with the radius. With a perilunate dislocation, the lunate is not displaced forwards.

Treatment

Closed reduction

Pulling on the hand with the wrist in extension and applying thumb pressure to the displaced bones may succeed. A plaster slab is applied, holding the wrist neutral. Percutaneous Kirschner wires may be needed to hold the reduction.

Open reduction

If closed reduction fails, open reduction is imperative. The carpus is exposed by an anterior approach, which has the advantage of decompressing the carpal tunnel. While an assistant pulls on the hand, the lunate is levered into place and kept there by a Kirschner wire which is inserted through the lunate into the capitate. If the scaphoid is fractured, this too can be reduced and fixed with a screw or Kirschner wires. Torn ligaments should be repaired through palmar and dorsal approaches. At the end of the procedure, the wrist is splinted. Fingers, elbow and shoulder are exercised throughout this period. The splint and Kirschner wires are removed at 8 weeks.

Complications

Avascular necrosis of the lunate may follow disruption of its blood supply. The x-ray shows progressive increase in bone density. Treatment is required only if symptoms demand it. If the wrist is stiff and painful, removal of the lunate and partial arthrodesis may be preferable.

HAND INJURIES

Hand injuries are important out of all proportion to their apparent severity, because of the need for perfect function. Local oedema and stiffness of the joints – common accompaniments of all injuries – are more threatening in the hand than anywhere else. Fractures may heal and joints re-stabilize, and yet the patient may still be left with a useless hand because of insufficient attention to splintage, the prevention of swelling, the preservation of movement and rehabilitation.

The patient should be examined in a clean environment with the hand displayed on sterile drapes. The history should include details of the accident, as well as the patient's age, occupation, leisure activities and 'handedness'. Examination should establish (1) the degree of mutilation, (2) the presence of any deformity, (3) the state of the circulation, (4) nerve function and (5) tendon function.

Closed injuries and small wounds can often be treated under regional block anaesthesia. Large wounds and multiple fractures are better dealt with under general anaesthesia.

Definitive treatment is dictated by the nature of the injury, but common to all injuries are three important requirements: safe splintage, the prevention of swelling, and dedicated rehabilitation.

Safe splintage

Splintage must be kept to a minimum. If only one finger is injured, it alone should be splinted – either by strapping it to its neighbour so that both move as one ('buddy-strapping'), or by fashioning a splint that does not impede movement in the uninjured fingers. If the whole hand is splinted or bandaged, this must always be in the *'position of safe immobilization'* – with the knuckle joints flexed at least 70 degrees and the finger joints straight. That way the ligaments are at full stretch, so if they do become adherent it is still possible to regain movement with physiotherapy.

Prevention of swelling

Swelling must be controlled by elevating the hand and by early and repeated active exercises.

Rehabilitation

Long-term physiotherapy and rehabilitation are best carried out in a special hand therapy unit under the supervision of both physiotherapists and occupational therapists.

CARPOMETACARPAL DISLOCATION

Dislocation below the wrist is caused by forceful dorsiflexion of the wrist combined with a longitudinal impact. Thus it is seen typically in boxers and in motorcyclists.

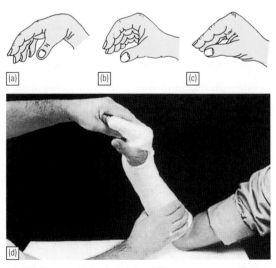

28.6 Splintage of the hand (a–c) Three common positions of the hand: (a) relaxed, (b) ready for action (the position of function) and (c) the position of safe immobilization. (d) *If splintage is needed, this should always be with the hand in the position of safe immobilization.*

The dislocation is reduced by traction, manipulation and thumb pressure. A protective slab is worn for 6 weeks, during which time the fingers are kept moving. If reduction is unstable (usually in the thumb carpometacarpal joint), it may need to be held with a Kirschner wire until the soft tissues heal.

FRACTURED METACARPALS

The metacarpal bones are vulnerable to blows and falls upon the hand, or the force of a boxer's punch. The bones may fracture at their base, in the shaft or through the neck.

In the mid-shaft, angular deformity is usually not marked, and even if it persists it does not interfere much with function. Rotational deformity, however, is serious and may result in malposition of the entire ray when the hand is closed in a fist.

In fractures of the neck – and particularly the neck of the fifth metacarpal – the small distal fragment may be tilted markedly towards the palm.

Special features

If the fragments are displaced, there may be a bump on the back of the hand, or one of the knuckles may be flattened. There is considerable swelling and local tenderness.

X-ray

Fractures of the base of the metacarpal are usually impacted. Fractures of the shaft are either transverse or oblique; there may be shortening or angulation of the fragments. Fractures of the metacarpal neck may result in forward tilting of the distal fragment.

Treatment

Undisplaced fractures

Fractures that are undisplaced (or only slightly displaced) require only a firm crepe bandage (for comfort), which is worn for 2 or 3 weeks. This should not be allowed to interfere with active movements of the fingers, which must be practised assiduously.

Displaced fracture of the shaft

If there is marked displacement or shortening of the bone, open reduction and internal fixation with mini-plates and screws is the best option. Careful attention should be given to correcting rotation, otherwise the finger will go awry during flexion. A useful guide is to remember that in flexion every finger should point towards the scaphoid. After operation, movements are started as soon as possible.

Displaced fracture of the neck

With fractures of the metacarpal neck, angulation of up to 40 degrees in the fourth and fifth metacarpals and 20 degrees in the second and third can be accepted. All other displaced metacarpal fractures should be reduced by traction and pressure. Reduction can be held by a plaster slab extending from the forearm over the fingers (only the damaged ones); the slab is maintained for 3 weeks and the undamaged fingers are exercised. However, because of the risk of stiffness in the splinted finger, fixation with percutaneous wires or a low-profile plate is usually preferred.

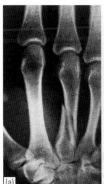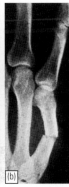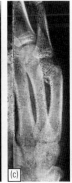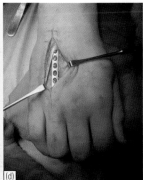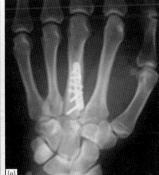

28.7 Metacarpal fractures (a) A spiral fracture of a single metacarpal is usually held adequately by neighbouring bones and muscles. (b) A displaced transverse fracture will often require internal fixation. (c) Angulated fracture of the fifth metacarpal neck: this does not need any particular treatment. (d) Internal fixation of a fractured metacarpal shaft using a low-profile plate and screws. (e) Postoperative x-ray following internal fixation.

Complications

Malunion

Angulation may result in a visible bump or a flattened knuckle, but function is usually good. Rotational deformity is much more serious because the patient cannot properly close the fist. This may need correction by osteotomy.

Stiffness

Metacarpal fractures invariably unite and, even if angulation persists, malunion is less disabling than stiffness of the hand. The principles of preventive treatment are discussed on page 334.

BENNETT'S FRACTURE–SUBLUXATION

Fracture of the base of the thumb metacarpal with extension into the carpometacarpal joint is an unstable injury. The smaller fragment remains in contact with the trapezium while the major portion of the metacarpal subluxates proximally. The fracture is easy to reduce but difficult to control.

Treatment

Closed reduction is effected by pulling on the thumb, abducting it and extending it. An attempt can be made to hold the position with a plaster cast, which is then worn for 4 weeks. However, if x-ray shows that a perfect position is not maintained, the fracture should be fixed with a small screw or Kirschner wire; the wrist is held in a plaster slab for 4 weeks.

Complications

If the carpometacarpal joint is seriously damaged or subluxed, osteoarthritis may ensue. Treatment is usually conservative, but if pain becomes intolerable an operation may be needed – either arthrodesis of the joint or excision of the trapezium.

METACARPOPHALANGEAL DISLOCATION

Usually the thumb is affected, sometimes the fifth finger and rarely the other fingers. A hyperextension force may dislocate the phalanx backwards, and the capsule and muscle insertions in front of the joint may be torn. If the metacarpal head has been forced like a button through the hole, closed reduction may be impossible.

Closed reduction is attempted by pulling on the thumb and levering the phalanx forwards. If this fails, the joint is exposed from the dorsum and, while strong traction is applied, the metacarpal head is levered into place. The joint is then strapped in the flexed position for 1 week.

TORN COLLATERAL LIGAMENT OF THE THUMB METACARPOPHALANGEAL JOINT

In former years, gamekeepers who twisted the necks of little animals ran the risk of tearing the ulnar collateral ligament of the thumb metacarpophalangeal joint. The injury came to be known as *gamekeeper's thumb*. Nowadays, it is seen in skiers who fall onto the extended thumb, forcing it into hyperabduction. A small flake of bone may be pulled off at the same time.

Special features

The ulnar side of the joint is swollen and very tender, yet the condition is often under-diagnosed as a simple 'sprain'. Before testing the ligament, an x-ray must be obtained to exclude any fracture. A

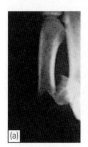 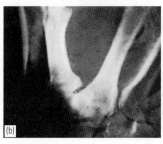 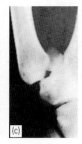 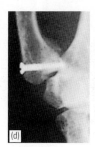 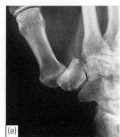

28.8 Injuries of the first metacarpal base A transverse fracture (a) can be reduced and held in plaster (b). Bennett's fracture–dislocation (c) is best held with a small screw (d) or a percutaneous Kirschner wire. (e) Carpometacarpal dislocation resembles a Bennett's fracture. It reduces easily but tends to be unstable and needs to be immobilized in the reduced position for at least 6 weeks.

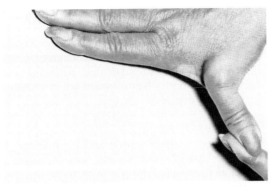

28.9 Gamekeeper's thumb The ulnar collateral ligament of the first metacarpophalangeal joint is completely ruptured; immediate repair is advisable.

local anaesthetic is then injected into the tissues along the inner (adductor) aspect of the joint, and the thumb is stressed in abduction with the metacarpophalangeal joint flexed 30 degrees; if there is no undue laxity (compared with the normal side), a serious injury can be excluded. If there is significant laxity, this is at least a *partial rupture*. The test is then repeated with the thumb fully extended: if there is still significant laxity, it is probably a complete rupture, which will require operative repair.

Treatment

Partial tears can be treated by immobilization of the thumb in a cast or splint for 2 or 3 weeks. This is followed by increasing movement and pinching and gripping exercises.

Complete tears need operative repair. Care should be taken during the exposure not to injure the superficial radial nerve branches. Postoperatively, the joint is immobilized in a thumb spica (leaving the interphalangeal joint free) for 4 weeks, followed by another 2 weeks in a removable splint.

FRACTURED PHALANGES

Phalangeal fractures usually result from direct violence and therefore any part of the bone may be broken; sometimes the flexor tendon sheath is damaged as well.

Treatment

Open wounds should always be treated first. Skin must be preserved and carefully sutured, and wound healing must not be jeopardized by the treatment of the fractures.

Undisplaced fractures

These need the minimum of splintage. Strapping the finger to its uninjured neighbour ('buddy-strapping') will relieve pain and allow movement. After 2 weeks, the strapping can be removed.

Displaced fracture of the proximal or middle phalanx

The bone should be straightened under general anaesthesia, carefully avoiding malrotation; the injured finger is then splinted, leaving the other fingers free. The splint can be discarded after 3 weeks. If reduction cannot be held in this way, fixation with Kirschner wires or a small plate is indicated.

Fractures of the distal phalanx

Distal phalangeal fractures are usually due to crushing injuries or a blow from a hammer. The soft-tissue damage must be treated; the fracture can be ignored.

Note. As in all hand injuries, the danger of stiffness is ever present, and a stiff finger can be worse than no finger. The principles of soft-tissue care should never be neglected: elevate, keep splintage to a minimum, move, exercise.

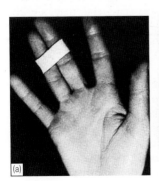
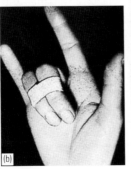
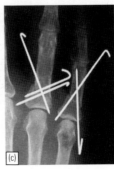

28.10 Fractures of the phalanges (a,b) If the fracture is stable, the finger is strapped to its neighbour for splintage and movement is encouraged. (c) Unstable fractures should be reduced and fixed with percutaneous wires or internal plates and screws. In all cases, movement should be started within a few days of injury or stiffness will ensue.

INTERPHALANGEAL DISLOCATION

Dislocation at the proximal joint is common and is easily reduced by pulling on the finger. Minimal splintage is needed. However, the patient should be warned that swelling and slight loss of movement may persist for months.

SPRAINS OF THE FINGER JOINTS

Partial or complete tears of the ligaments are common and usually due to forced angulation at the joint. Milder injuries require no treatment; with more severe strains, the finger should be splinted for a week or two. However, the patient should be warned that the joint is likely to remain swollen and slightly painful for 6–12 months.

MALLET FINGER

If the fingertip is forcibly bent during active extension, the extensor tendon may rupture or a flake of bone may be avulsed from the base of the distal phalanx. This sometimes occurs when the finger is stubbed when making a bed or catching a ball.

A pure soft-tissue injury can be treated by splinting the distal joint continuously in extension for 8 weeks and then at night only for another 4 weeks. If there is a large flake of bone, a shorter term of splintage will usually suffice; operative fixation is rarely needed.

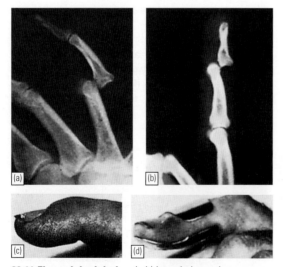

28.11 Finger-joint injuries (a,b) Interphalangeal dislocations. These are easily missed if not x-rayed. Reduction is easily achieved by pulling on the finger. (c,d) Mallet finger deformity, treated by simple splintage.

OPEN INJURIES OF THE HAND

Open injuries range from clean cuts to ragged lacerations, crushing, injection of foreign material, pulp defects and amputations. Knowing the mechanism of injury helps immensely in assessing the type and degree of damage.

Clinical assessment

Examination must be gentle and painstaking. It should be carried out in a clean (and preferably a sterile) environment, and may have to be repeated in the operating theatre when the patient is anaesthetized.

Skin damage is important, but remember that even a tiny, clean cut may conceal nerve or tendon injury. The *circulation* to the hand and fingers must be assessed; *sensation* and *motor activity* are tested in the territory of each nerve.

Tendons are examined with similar care. Note the posture of the hand and fingers; comparison with the opposite hand may show that the normal postural tension in one or other finger is absent, suggesting a tendon injury. If the patient will allow it, active wrist and finger movements are then assessed. *Flexor digitorum profundus* is tested by holding the proximal finger joint straight and instructing the patient to bend the distal joint. *Flexor digitorum superficialis* is tested by asking the patient to flex one finger at a time while the examiner holds the other fingers in full extension; this immobilizes all the deep flexors because they have a common muscle belly, so any active flexion of the injured finger must be performed by the superficial flexor (see Figure 16.2).

X-rays may show fractures or foreign bodies.

Treatment

Preoperative care

The patient may need treatment for pain and shock. If the wound is contaminated, it should be rinsed with sterile crystalloid, and antibiotics should be given as soon as possible. Prophylaxis against tetanus and gas gangrene may also be needed. The hand is lightly splinted and the wound is covered with an iodine-soaked dressing.

Wound exploration

Under general or regional anaesthesia, the wound is cleaned and explored. A pneumatic tourniquet is essential unless there is a crush injury and muscle viability is in doubt. Skin is too precious to waste, and only obviously dead skin should be excised. For adequate exposure, the wound may need enlarging, but *incisions must never cross a skin crease or an interdigital web* because healing will result in a soft-tissue contracture across the crease. Through the enlarged wound, loose debris is picked out, dead muscle is excised and the tissues are thoroughly irrigated with isotonic crystalloid solution. A more thorough assessment of the extent of the injury is then undertaken.

Tissue repair

Fractures are reduced and held with Kirschner wires, unless there is some specific contraindication. *Joint capsule and ligaments* are repaired with fine sutures.

Artery and vein repair (or grafting) may be needed if the hand or finger is ischaemic. *Severed nerves* are sutured with the finest, non-reactive material. If the repair cannot be achieved without tension, a nerve-graft (e.g. from the posterior interosseous nerve at the wrist) should be performed. These procedures are carried out with the aid of an operating microscope.

Extensor tendon repair is usually quite straightforward. *Flexor tendon repair* is more challenging, particularly in the region between the distal palmar crease and the flexor crease of the proximal interphalangeal joint (Zone II), where both the superficial and deep tendons run together in a common sheath. This area has been called – rather portentiously – 'no man's land'. Primary repair with fastidious postoperative supervision gives the best outcome but calls for a high level of expertise and specialized physiotherapy. If the

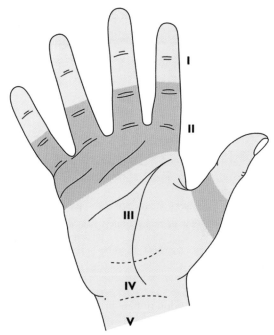

28.13 The zones of injury (I) Distal to the insertion of flexor digitorum superficialis. (II) Between the opening of the flexor sheath (the distal palmar crease) and the insertion of flexor superficialis. (III) Between the end of the carpal tunnel and the beginning of the flexor sheath. (IV) Within the carpal tunnel. (V) Proximal to the carpal tunnel.

necessary facilities are not available, the wound should be washed out and loosely closed, and the patient transferred to a special centre. A delay of several days, with a clean wound, is unlikely to affect the outcome.

Division of the *superficialis tendon alone* should also be repaired. Even though the loss of superficialis action does not altogether prevent finger flexion, it noticeably weakens the hand and may lead to a swan-neck deformity of the finger.

Cuts above the wrist, in the palm or *distal to the superficialis insertion* have a better outcome than injuries in 'no man's land'.

Amputation of a finger as a primary procedure should be avoided unless the damage involves many tissues and is clearly irreparable.

Closure

The tourniquet is deflated and bipolar diathermy is used to stop bleeding; haematoma formation leads to poor healing and tendon adhesions. Unless the wound is contaminated, the skin is closed – either by direct suture without tension or, if there is skin loss, by skin-grafting (skin-grafts are conveniently taken from the inner aspect of the

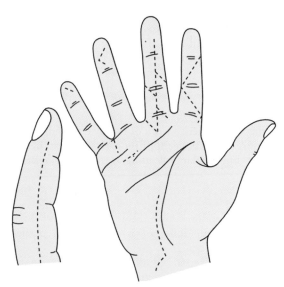

28.12 Hand incisions Permissible incisions in hand surgery. Incisions must not cross a skin crease or an interdigital web. Scarring may cause contracture and deformity.

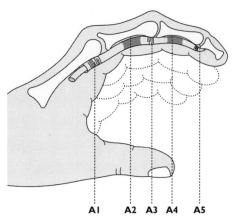

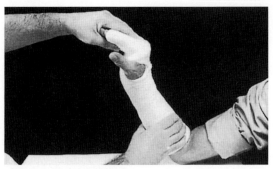

28.15 Postoperative splintage Always splint in the position of safe immobilization.

28.14 Flexor tendon anatomy Fibrous pulleys – designated A1–A5 – hold the flexor tendons to the phalanges and prevent bow-stringing during movement.

upper arm). If tendon or bare bone is exposed, this must be covered by a rotation or pedicled flap. If a severely mutilated finger has to be sacrificed, its skin can be used as a rotation flap to cover an adjacent area of loss.

Dressing and splintage

The wound is covered with a single layer of paraffin gauze and ample wool roll. A light plaster slab holds the wrist and hand in the position of safe immobilization (wrist extended, metacarpophalangeal joints flexed to 90 degrees, interphalangeal joints straight, thumb abducted). This is the position in which the metacarpophalangeal and interphalangeal ligaments are fully stretched and fibrosis therefore least likely to cause contractures. *Failure to appreciate this point is the commonest cause of persistent stiffness after injury.* The rule is slightly modified in two circumstances: (a) after primary flexor tendon suture, the wrist is held in about 20 degrees of flexion to take tension off the repair; and (b) after extensor tendon repair, the meta-carpophalangeal joints are flexed to only about 30 degrees so that there is less tension on the repair.

Postoperative management

The hand is kept elevated in a roller towel or high sling, which can be removed several times a day to exercise the elbow and shoulder.

Rehabilitation

Movements of the hand must be commenced within a few days at most. Splintage should allow as many joints as possible to be exercised,

consistent with protecting the repair. Extensor tendon injuries are splinted for about 4 weeks. Various protocols are followed for flexor tendon injuries, including passive, active or elastic-band-assisted flexion. Early movement promotes tendon healing and excursion. In all cases, the risk of rupture is balanced against the need for early mobilization. Close supervision and attention to detail are essential.

Once the tissues have healed, the hand is increasingly used for more and more complex tasks, especially those that resemble the patient's normal work activities.

Delayed tendon repair

Primary suture may have been contraindicated by wound contamination, undue delay between injury and repair, massive skin loss or inadequate operating facilities. In these circumstances, secondary repair or tendon-grafting may be necessary.

Injury of the profundus tendon with an intact superficialis

Unless the patient's work or hobby demands active flexion of the fingertip, fusion or tenodesis of the distal interphalangeal joint is the most reliable option.

Injury of both the superficialis and profundus tendons

If both tendons have been divided and have retracted, a tendon-graft is needed. Full passive joint movement is a prerequisite. If the pulley system is in good condition and there are no adhesions, the tendons are excised from the flexor sheath and replaced with a tendon-graft (palmaris longus, duplicated extensor digiti minimi, plantaris or a toe extensor). Rehabilitation is the same as for a primary repair. If the pulleys are damaged, the skin cover poor, the passive range of movement limited or the sheath scarred, a two-stage procedure is preferred. The tendons are excised and the pulleys reconstructed with extensor retinaculum or excised tendon. A Silastic rod is sutured to the distal stump of the profundus tendon and rehabilitation is planned to maintain a good passive range of movement. A smooth gliding surface forms around the rod. About 3 months later, the rod is removed through two smaller incisions and a tendon-graft (palmaris longus, plantaris or a lesser toe extensor) is sutured to the proximal and distal stumps of flexor digitorum profundus. Rehabilitation is as for a primary repair.

Pulp and fingertip injuries

In full-thickness wounds without bone exposure, if the open area is greater than 1 cm in diameter, healing will be quicker with a split-skin or full-thickness graft. If bone is exposed and length of the digit is important for the individual patient, then an advancement flap or neurovascular island flap should be considered. If not, primary cover can be achieved by shortening the bone and tailoring the skin flaps ('terminalization'). In young children, the fingertips recover extraordinarily well from injury and they should be treated with dressings rather than grafts or terminalization. Thumb length should never be sacrificed lightly.

Nail-bed injuries

These are often seen in association with fractures of the terminal phalanx. If appearance is important, meticulous repair and split-thickness grafting under magnification will give the best cosmetic result.

CHAPTER 29

INJURIES OF THE SPINE AND THORAX

Spinal injuries are due either to *direct force* (e.g. penetrating wounds form firearms or knives) or, much more commonly, *indirect force* – usually following a fall from a height when the spinal column collapses in its vertical axis, or during violent free movements of the neck or trunk. A variety of mechanisms come into play, often simultaneously: axial compression, flexion, extension, rotation, shear and distraction.

The injury carries a double threat: damage to the vertebral column and damage to the neural tissues. Neurological injury is not always immediate and may occur (or be aggravated) only if and when

29.1 Mechanism of injury The spine is usually injured in one of two ways: (a) a fall onto the head or the back of the neck; or (b) a blow on the forehead which forces the neck into hyperextension. Sudden acceleration, as in a severe rear-end collision, will also result in the head and neck falling into hyperextension.

there is movement and displacement of the vertebral fracture or dislocation. Hence the importance of establishing whether the injury is stable or unstable.

A *stable injury* is one in which the vertebral components will not be displaced by normal movements; an *unstable injury* is one in which there is a significant risk of displacement and consequent damage to the neural tissues. Stability depends on the integrity of the vertebral bodies and the posterior arches as well as the ligaments that link adjacent vertebrae. Generally speaking, it requires damage to both the ligaments and the bony column to produce an unstable spine. Fortunately, only 10 per cent of spinal injuries are unstable and less than 5 per cent are associated with cord damage.

Spinal injuries heal slowly. Non-union is rare but malunion is common and may lead to progressive deformity of the spine.

PRINCIPLES OF DIAGNOSIS AND MANAGEMENT

Diagnosis and management go hand in hand: inappropriate movement during examination can irretrievably change the outcome for the worse. *If there is the slightest possibility of spinal trauma in an injured patient, the spine must be immobilized until the patient has been resuscitated and other life-threatening injuries have been identified and treated.* Immobilization is abandoned only when a serious spinal injury has been excluded by clinical and radiological assessment.

HISTORY

A high index of suspicion is essential; symptoms and signs may be minimal – the history is crucial. Every patient with a blunt injury above the clavicle, a head injury or loss of consciousness should be considered to have a cervical spine injury until proven otherwise. Every patient who is involved in a fall from a height, a crushing accident or a high-speed deceleration accident should similarly be considered to have a thoracolumbar injury. However, lesser injuries also should arouse suspicion if they are followed by pain in the neck or back or neurological symptoms in the limbs.

EXAMINATION

Neck

Look, Feel but do not Move! If there is an unstable injury, movement may imperil the cord. The head and face are thoroughly inspected for bruises or grazes which could indicate indirect trauma to the cervical spine. The neck itself is examined for deformity, bruising or a penetrating injury. The patient may be supporting his or her head with both hands. The bones and soft tissues of the neck are palpated; tenderness, bogginess or an abnormal space between adjacent spinous processes suggests an unstable injury of the posterior part of the cervical spine.

Back

The patient is 'log-rolled' to avoid movement of the thoracolumbar spine. The spine is inspected and palpated as before.

Neurological examination

A full neurological examination should be carried out in every case; this may have to be repeated several times during the first few days. Each dermatome, myotome and reflex is tested.

Tests for nerve root motor function		
Nerve root	**Test**	**Tendon reflex**
C5	Shoulder abduction	Deltoid
C6	Elbow flexion	Biceps
C6	Wrist extension	Brachioradialis
C7	Wrist flexion	Triceps
	Finger extension	
C8	Finger flexion	
T1	Finger abduction	
L1, 2	Thigh abduction	
L3, 4	Knee extension	Quadriceps
L5, S1	Knee flexion	Tendo Achillis
L5	Great toe extension	
S1	Great toe flexion	

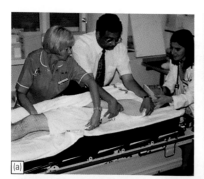
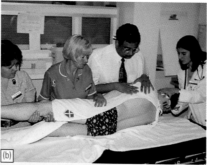
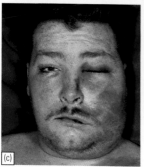
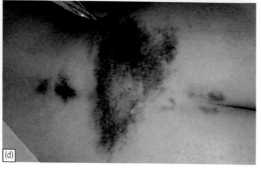

29.2 Examination The neck must be supported throughout the examination, using a semi-rigid collar, sandbags on either side of the head and a tape across the forehead. (a,b) The 'log-rolling' technique is used when turning the patient for examination of the back. Suspicious signs may be noticed immediately: (c) severe facial bruising; (d) bruising over the lower back.

The unconscious patient is difficult to examine; a spinal injury must be assumed until proven otherwise. Features suggesting a spinal cord lesion are a history of a fall or rapid deceleration, a head injury, diaphragmatic breathing, a flaccid anal sphincter, hypotension with bradycardia and a pain response above, but not below, the clavicle.

IMAGING

X-ray examination is mandatory for all accident victims complaining of pain or stiffness in the neck or back, all patients with head injuries or severe facial injuries (cervical spine), patients with rib fractures or severe seat-belt bruising (thoracic spine), and those with severe pelvic or abdominal injuries (thoracolumbar spine). Accident victims who are unconscious should have spine x-rays as part of the routine work-up.

Movement should be kept to a minimum. In the cervical spine, anteroposterior and lateral views (with coverage from C1 to T1) and open-mouth views are needed. 'Difficult' areas, such as the lower cervical and upper thoracic segments, which are often obscured by shoulder and rib images, may require *CT*. CT is also ideal for showing structural damage to individual vertebrae and displacement of bone fragments into the vertebral canal. However, for displaying the intervertebral discs, ligamentum flavum and neural structures, *MRI* is the method of choice.

TREATMENT

The objectives of treatment are:

1. to preserve neurological function;
2. to relieve any reversible neural compression;
3. to restore alignment of the spine;
4. to stabilize the spine;
5. to rehabilitate the patient.

The indications for urgent surgical stabilization are (a) an unstable fracture with progressive neurological deficit and (b) an unstable fracture in a patient with multiple injuries.

Patients with no neurological injury

If the spinal injury is stable, the patient is treated by supporting the spine in a position that will cause no further strain; a firm collar or lumbar brace will usually suffice, but the patient may need to rest in bed until pain and muscle spasm subside.

If the spinal injury is unstable, it should be held secure until the tissues heal and the spine becomes stable. In the cervical spine, this should be done as soon as possible by traction in bed through tongs or a halo device attached to the skull. If the halo is attached to a body cast or a rigid vest, the patient can be got up early and mobilized. Unstable thoracolumbar injuries are more often treated by internal fixation.

Patients with neurological injury

The injury is usually unstable. Conservative treatment is highly demanding and best carried out in a special unit equipped for round-the-clock nursing, 2-hourly turning routines, skin toilet, bladder care and specialized physiotherapy and occupational therapy. After a few weeks, the injury stabilizes spontaneously and the patient can be got out of bed for intensive rehabilitation. The benefit of early surgery to neurological recovery is uncertain. However, if it is incomplete, and especially if neurological loss is progressive, early operative reduction or decompression and stabilization is indicated.

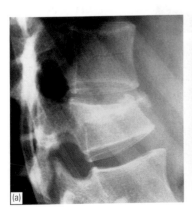

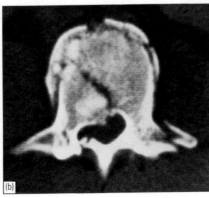

29.3 X-ray diagnosis Plain x-ray alone may be insufficient to show the true state of affairs. (a) This x-ray showed the fracture, but it needed a CT scan (b) to reveal the large fragment encroaching on the spinal canal.

CERVICAL SPINE INJURIES

Clinical features

The patient usually gives a history of a fall from a height, a diving accident or a vehicle accident in which the neck is forcibly moved. In a patient unconscious from a head injury, a fractured cervical spine should be assumed (and acted upon) until proved otherwise.

An abnormal position of the neck is suggestive, and careful palpation may elicit tenderness. Movement is best postponed until the neck has been x-rayed. Pain or paraesthesia in the limbs is significant, and the patient should be examined for evidence of spinal cord or nerve root damage.

Imaging

Plain x-rays must be of high quality and should be examined methodically. In the anteroposterior view, the lateral outlines should be intact, and the spinous processes and tracheal shadow in the midline. An open-mouth view is necessary to show C1 and C2 (for odontoid and lateral mass fractures).

The lateral view must include all seven cervical vertebrae and the upper half of T1, otherwise a serious injury at the cervicothoracic junction will be missed. Four parallel curves should be identified: one running down the front of the vertebral bodies, one down the back of the bodies, one through the posterior borders of the lateral masses and one along the bases of the spinous processes (see Fig. 29.4). Any deviation from this pattern is suggestive of a vertebral fracture or displacement. Do not forget to look at the soft-tissue outlines: the prevertebral soft-tissue shadow should be less than 5 mm in width above the level of the trachea and less than one vertebral body's width below that level; any increase in this space suggests a prevertebral haematoma.

FRACTURE OF C1

Sudden severe load on the top of the head may cause a 'bursting' force which fractures the ring of the atlas *(Jefferson's fracture).* There is no encroachment on the neural canal and, usually, no neurological damage. The fracture is seen on the open-mouth view; the lateral masses are spread away from the odontoid peg. A CT scan is particularly helpful in defining the fracture.

If the fracture is undisplaced, the injury is stable and the patient needs only a rigid collar until the fracture unites. If there is sideways spreading of the lateral masses, the injury is unstable and should be treated either by skull traction or by the application of a halo-body orthosis for 6 weeks, followed by another 6 weeks in a semi-rigid collar.

Fractures of the atlas are associated with injury elsewhere in the cervical spine in up to 50 per cent of cases; odontoid fractures and 'hangman's fractures' in particular should be excluded.

FRACTURED PEDICLE(S) OF C2 ('HANGMAN'S FRACTURE')

In the true judicial 'hangman's fracture', the pedicles of the axis are fractured and the C1/2 disc is torn; the mechanism is extension with distraction. In civilian injuries, the mechanism is more complex, with varying degrees of extension, compression and flexion. This is one cause of death in motor vehicle accidents when the forehead strikes the dashboard. The fracture is potentially unstable.

Undisplaced fractures are treated in a semi-rigid collar or halo-vest until united. Displaced fractures may need reduction before immobilization in a halo-vest for 12 weeks.

FRACTURE OF THE ODONTOID PROCESS

Odontoid fractures are uncommon. They usually occur as flexion injuries in young adults due to high-velocity accidents or severe falls; less often they occur in elderly, osteoporotic people as a

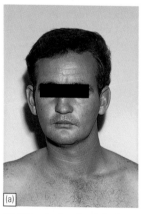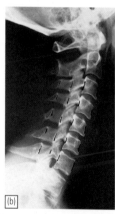

29.4 Cervical spine injuries – clinical and x-ray (a) Look at the position of the neck. This patient complained of neck pain and stiffness after a fall. X-ray showed an odontoid fracture. (b) The lateral x-ray must include all seven cervical vertebrae – nothing less will suffice. Four parallel lines can be traced unbroken from C1 to C7. They are bounded by the anterior surfaces of the vertebral bodies, the posterior surfaces of the bodies, the posterior borders of the lateral masses and the bases of the spinous processes. A segment that is shifted out of line is abnormal.

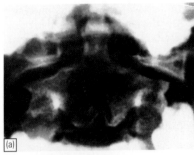

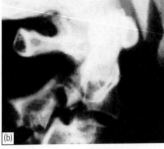

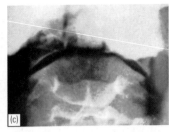

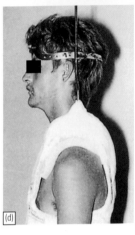

29.5 Fractures of C1 and C2 (a) Jefferson's fracture – bursting apart of the lateral masses of C1. (b) Hangman's fracture – fracture of the pedicle or lateral pillar of C2. (c) Fracture of the base of the odontoid peg of C2. All three fractures can be treated by immobilization of the neck in a 'halo-vest' cast (d).

result of low-energy trauma in which the neck is forced into hyperextension, e.g. a fall onto the face or forehead. Neurological injury occurs in about one quarter of cases.

Plain x-rays usually show the fracture. Three types are recognized: avulsion of the tip (type 1); fracture through the junction of the odontoid peg and body of C2 (type 2); and a fracture through the body of C2 only (type 3).

Type 1 fractures need no more than immobilization in a rigid collar until discomfort subsides.

Type 2 fractures are often unstable and prone to non-union. Undisplaced fractures can be held by fitting a halo-vest, but displaced fractures need to be reduced by traction and then held by operative screw fixation or by a halo-vest.

Type 3 fractures, if undisplaced, are treated in a halo-vest for 8–12 weeks. If displaced, the fracture

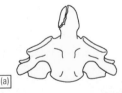

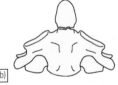

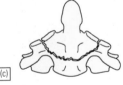

29.6 Fractures of the odontoid process (a) Type 1 – fracture through the tip. (b) Type 2 – fracture at the junction of the odontoid process and the body. (c) Type 3 – fracture through the body of the axis. (d) Lateral x-ray of type 2 fracture.

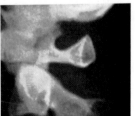

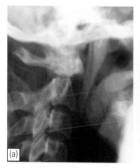
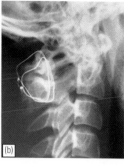
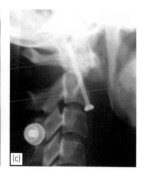
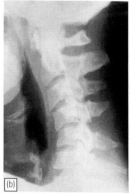

29.7 Odontoid fractures that need fusion (a) Severely displaced fracture which was treated by skull traction and (b) posterior fusion. (c) Unstable type 2 fracture treated by screw fixation.

must first be reduced by traction before immobilization in a halo-vest for 8–12 weeks.

WEDGE-COMPRESSION FRACTURE

This usually occurs in the mid-cervical and lower cervical segments. A pure flexion injury causes compression of the anterior part of the vertebral body (wedge-compression). The injury is stable; all that is needed is a comfortable collar for 6–8 weeks.

BURST FRACTURE

This severe injury results from axial compression of the cervical spine, usually in diving or athletic accidents. Persistent neurological injury is common.

Plain x-rays show a comminuted fracture of the vertebral body. CT or MRI should be performed to look for retropulsion of large fragments into the spinal canal. If there is no neurological deficit, the injury is treated by immobilization in a halo-vest. Neurological deficit calls for urgent anterior decompression followed by immobilization for 6–8 weeks.

CERVICAL SUBLUXATION

This is a pure flexion injury, usually in the lower half of the cervical spine. The bones are intact but the posterior ligaments are torn; the vertebra above tilts forward on the one below, opening up the interspinous space posteriorly. This not always obvious if the routine x-ray shows the spine only in the neutral position. However, on gentle flexion, the gap between the spines is seen to be unusually wide.

Splintage for 6 weeks is usually adequate, but the brace must be sufficiently robust to prevent cervical flexion. If carefully controlled flexion and extension x-rays show persistent instability, a posterior spinal fusion may be necessary.

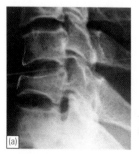
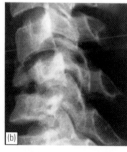
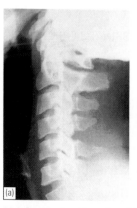

29.8 Cervical compression fractures (a) A simple wedge-compression of a single vertebral body is a stable fracture because the middle and posterior elements remain intact. (b) In this case the middle column is broken and the posterior part of the vertebral body is driven backwards. CT or MRI will show the true state of affairs. The fracture is unstable and the cord is threatened.

29.9 Cervical subluxation (a) The x-ray taken in extension shows no displacement of the vertebral bodies. (b) On carefully controlled flexion there is an unusually wide gap between the spinous processes of C4 and C5.

FRACTURE-DISLOCATIONS BETWEEN C3 AND T1

These are flexion–rotation injuries in which the articular facets ride forward over the facets below. Usually one or both of the articular masses is fractured, but sometimes there is a pure dislocation ('jumped facets'). The posterior ligaments are ruptured and the spine is potentially unstable.

X-rays show the forward displacement of a vertebra on the one below. If the displacement is less than 25 per cent of the vertebral body width, it is probably a *unilateral displacement*. Greater degrees of displacement suggest *bilateral facet dislocation* or *fracture–dislocation;* in these cases, the spine is definitely unstable and cord damage is likely.

Treatment

Unilateral facet displacement

The dislocation is reduced by skull traction until monitoring x-rays show that the upper facet is perched upon the lower; a gentle extension and rotation manoeuvre then completes full reduction. After reduction, the injury is usually stable if there is no fracture. The neck is immobilized in a halo-vest for 6–8 weeks. If there is an associated facet fracture, posterior fusion should be considered.

Bilateral facet dislocation

The displacement must be reduced as a matter of urgency. Skull traction is used, increasing slowly and combining the technique with the use of intravenous muscle relaxants. On reduction, immobilization in a halo-vest for 12 weeks is necessary. If reduction with traction fails, a posterior open reduction and fusion will be required.

AVULSION INJURY OF C7 SPINOUS PROCESS

Fracture of the C7 spinous process may occur with severe voluntary contraction of the muscles at the back of the neck; it has earned the name 'clay-shoveller's fracture'. The injury is painful but harmless. No treatment is required; as soon as symptoms permit, neck exercises are encouraged.

SPRAINED NECK (WHIPLASH INJURY)

Soft-tissue sprains (or wrenching injuries) of the neck are so common after car accidents that they now constitute a veritable epidemic; and the imaginative term 'whiplash injury' has served effectively to enhance public apprehension at its

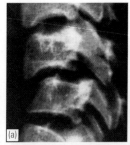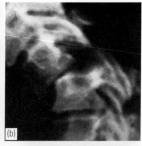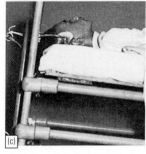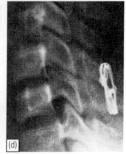

29.10 Fracture–subluxation and fracture-dislocation
(a) A moderate forward slip suggests that this is a rotational injury with unilateral facet displacement. (b) X-ray showing a full-blown fracture-dislocation with severe forward shift; this is an unstable injury with a high incidence of cord damage. The fracture-dislocation was reduced by skull traction (c) followed by posterior wire fixation (d).

occurrence. It usually follows a rear-end collision in which the occupant's body is thrown forwards and the head jerked backwards, with hyperextension of the lower cervical spine; however, it can also occur with flexion and rotation injuries. Women are affected more often than men. There is disagreement about the exact pathology and there is no tidy correlation between the amount of damage to the vehicle and the severity of complaints.

Often the victim is unaware of any abnormality immediately after the collision. Pain and stiffness of the neck usually appear during the next 12–48 hours or, occasionally, only several days later. Pain sometimes radiates to the shoulders. Neck muscles are tender and movements often restricted. X-rays are (excepting any pre-existing degenerative changes) normal.

Simple pain-relieving measures, including analgesic medication, may be needed during the first few weeks. However, the emphasis should be on graded exercises for return of neck movement. The long-term prognosis is variable and a small group of patients appear never to be free of symptoms.

THORACIC SPINE INJURIES

Most thoracic spine injuries result from hyperflexion. Wedge-compressions are relatively common in osteoporotic people; they are usually mechanically stable, but may lead to progressive kyphosis, especially if more than one vertebra is involved.

Severe injuries in younger people carry a high risk of cord damage, particularly those involving T11 and T12 which are not 'splinted' by the rib-cage. If there is any doubt about the presence of fragmentation or displacement of the posterior part of the vertebral body, CT or MRI will be needed to demonstrate the real risk to the spinal cord.

Plain x-rays, whilst showing the lower thoracic spine quite clearly, may be difficult to interpret for the upper thoracic spine because the scapula and shoulders get in the way. Here again, CT or MRI will be helpful.

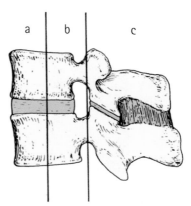

29.11 Structural elements of the lumbar spine The three important structural elements are (a) the anterior column, (b) the middle column and (c) the osseoligamentous complex forming the posterior column.

Treatment

Stable fracture patterns with less than about 30 degrees of kyphosis and without neurological injury are managed symptomatically. If angulation is more marked, bracing or posterior fusion is indicated to avoid an increasing kyphosis.

If there is complete paraplegia and no improvement after 48 hours, conservative management is adequate; the patient can be rested in bed for 5–6 weeks, then gradually mobilized in a brace. However, if there is severe bony injury, with the risk of increasing kyphosis, internal fixation should be considered.

THORACOLUMBAR AND LUMBAR INJURIES

The thoracolumbar junction is particularly prone to injury because it represents a transition zone between the relatively fixed thoracic spine and the relatively mobile lumbar spine. In most cases the injury is sustained in a fall from a height; one can imagine a combination of forces due to axial compression and flexion.

As in the cervical spine, it is important to establish whether the fracture is stable or unstable. A good idea can be formed from studying the lateral x-ray. Stability is provided by three structural elements: the *posterior osseoligamentous complex* (or *posterior column*) consisting of the pedicles, facet joints, posterior bony arch, interspinous and supraspinous ligaments; the *middle column,* comprising the posterior half of the vertebral body, the posterior part of the intervertebral disc and the posterior longitudinal ligament; and the *anterior column,* composed of the anterior half of the vertebral body, the anterior part of the intervertebral disc and the anterior longitudinal ligament. All fractures involving the middle column and at least one other column should be regarded as unstable.

FRACTURES OF THE TRANSVERSE PROCESSES

The transverse processes can be avulsed with sudden muscular activity. Isolated injuries need no more than symptomatic treatment. More ominous than usual is a fracture of the transverse process of L5: this should alert one to the possibility of a vertical shear injury of the pelvis.

WEDGE-COMPRESSION INJURY

This is by far the most common vertebral fracture and is due to spinal flexion with the posterior ligaments remaining intact. In osteoporotic people, fracture may occur with minimal trauma. Pain is usually quite marked, but the fracture is stable (only the anterior column is damaged). Neurological injury is extremely rare.

The patient is kept in bed for a week or two until pain subsides and is then mobilized. Muscle strengthening exercises are important. For minimal wedging, no support is needed. For those with more marked wedging (anterior vertebral body height reduced by 25–50 per cent), a thoracolumbar brace for 3 months is advisable. If

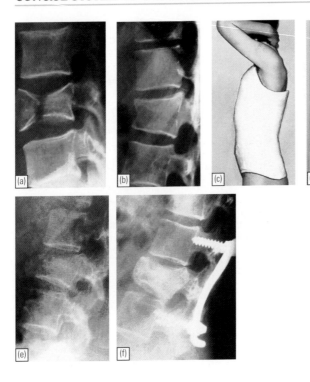

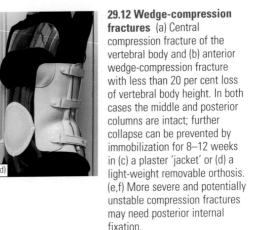

29.12 Wedge-compression fractures (a) Central compression fracture of the vertebral body and (b) anterior wedge-compression fracture with less than 20 per cent loss of vertebral body height. In both cases the middle and posterior columns are intact; further collapse can be prevented by immobilization for 8–12 weeks in (c) a plaster 'jacket' or (d) a light-weight removable orthosis. (e,f) More severe and potentially unstable compression fractures may need posterior internal fixation.

vertebral compression is even more severe than that, posterior spinal fusion should be considered.

BURST INJURY

Severe axial compression may 'explode' the vertebral body, shattering the posterior part and extruding fragments of bone into the spinal canal. The injury is usually unstable. The x-ray appearance may superficially resemble the wedge-compression fracture (see above), but the posterior border of the vertebral body is damaged; this is seen most clearly on CT scans.

If there is minimal retropulsion of bone, no neurological damage and minimal anterior wedging, the patient is kept in bed until the acute symptoms settle and is then mobilized in a thoracolumbar brace, which is discarded at about 12 weeks. Surgery is needed only if there is progressive neurological deterioration.

FRACTURE–DISLOCATION

Segmental displacement may occur with various combinations of flexion, compression, rotation and shear. The spine is grossly unstable. These are the most dangerous injuries and are often associated with neurological damage to the lowermost part of the cord or the cauda equina.

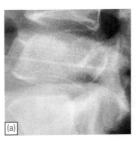
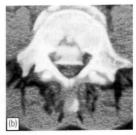

29.13 Lumbar burst fracture Severe compression may cause retropulsion of the vertebral body (a). The extent of spinal canal encroachment is best shown by CT (b).

X-rays may show fractures through the vertebral body, pedicles, articular processes and laminae; there may be varying degrees of subluxation or even bilateral facet dislocation. CT is helpful in demonstrating the degree of spinal canal occlusion.

Most fracture–dislocations will benefit from early surgery. In fracture–dislocation with paraplegia, surgery will facilitate nursing, shorten the hospital stay, help the patient's rehabilitation and reduce the chance of painful deformity. In fracture–dislocation with a partial neurological deficit, surgical stabilization and decompression should provide the best neurological outcome.

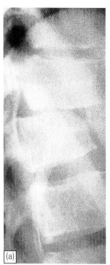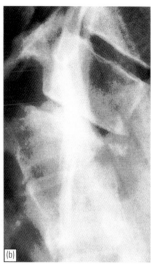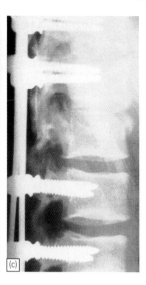

(a) (b) (c)

29.14 Thoracolumbar fracture–dislocation (a) Fracture-dislocation at T11/12 in a 32-year-old woman who was a passenger in a truck that overturned. She was completely paraplegic and operation was not thought worthwhile. (b) Four weeks later the deformity had increased, leaving her with a marked gibbus. (c) Treatment by open reduction and internal fixation.

TRAUMATIC PARAPLEGIA

Injuries of the spine may be complicated by damage to the spinal cord or cauda equina. The injuries most likely to do this are 'burst' fractures and fracture-dislocations of the thoracolumbar region or the lower cervical spine.

Complete transection of the cord results in either paraplegia (thoracic and lumbar lesions) or quadriplegia (cervical lesions). Initially there is complete paralysis and anaesthesia, with loss of the anal reflex (spinal shock). At this stage, and for the first 24 hours, the diagnosis cannot be absolutely certain. However, if the anal reflex returns and the neural deficit persists, the cord lesion must then be assumed complete. Gradually, the features of an upper motor neuron lesion appear, with spastic paralysis and exaggerated reflexes.

Incomplete transection results in partial sensory and motor loss below the level of the lesion. Signs vary according to which part of the cord is damaged.

Cauda equina injury, which is a lower motor neuron lesion, causes flaccid paralysis.

MANAGEMENT

With partial paralysis, decompression and stabilization of the spine offer the best chance of further recovery. With complete paralysis, it is the overall management that is important, especially the early management. The patient must be transported with great care to prevent further damage, and preferably taken directly to a spinal centre. The principles of treatment are outlined below.

Skin

Within a few hours, anaesthetic skin may develop large pressure sores; this can be prevented by meticulous nursing. Immediate fixation of the spine enables these essential nursing procedures to be carried out much more easily and without discomfort to the patient. Creases in the sheets and crumbs in the bed are not permitted. Every 2 hours, the patient is gently rolled onto his or her side and the back is carefully washed (without rubbing), dried and powdered. After a few weeks, the skin becomes a little more tolerant and the patient can turn in bed without assistance. Later the patient should be taught how to relieve skin pressure intermittently during periods of sitting. If sores have been allowed to develop, they may never heal without excision and skin-grafting.

Bladder and bowel

For the first 24 hours the bladder distends only slowly, but, if the distension is allowed to progress, overflow incontinence occurs and infection is probable. In special centres it is usual to manage the patient from the outset by intermittent catheterization under sterile conditions. If early transfer to a paraplegia centre is not possible, continuous closed drainage through a fine Silastic catheter is advised. The disposable bag should be changed twice weekly to prevent blockage. If infection supervenes, antibiotics are given.

As the local reflexes gradually return, automatic emptying of the bladder may occur whenever it becomes distended. If the cauda equina is damaged, this reflex is lost and bladder emptying has to be initiated by manual suprapubic pressure.

Bladder training is begun as early as possible, and patients learn to manage this function themselves.

The bowel is more easily trained, with the help of enemas, aperients and abdominal exercises.

Muscles and joints

The paralysed muscles, if not treated, may develop severe flexion contractures. These are usually preventable by moving the joints passively through their full range twice daily.

With lesions below the cervical cord, the patient should be up within 3 months; standing and walking are valuable in preventing contractures. Calipers are usually necessary to keep the knees straight and the feet plantigrade. The calipers are removed at intervals during the day while the patient lies prone, and while he or she is having physiotherapy. The upper limbs must be trained until they develop sufficient power to enable the patient to use crutches and a wheelchair.

If flexion contractures have been allowed to develop, tenotomies may be necessary. Painful flexor spasms are rare unless skin or bladder infection occurs. They can sometimes be relieved by tenotomies, neurectomies, rhizotomies or the intrathecal injection of alcohol.

Heterotopic ossification is a common and disturbing complication; it is more likely to occur with high lesions and complete lesions. It may restrict or abolish movement, especially at the hip. It is doubtful whether ossification can be prevented, but once the new bone is mature, it can safely be excised.

Morale

The morale of a paraplegic patient is liable to reach a low ebb, and the restoration of his or her self-confidence is an important part of treatment. Constant enthusiasm and encouragement by doctors, physiotherapists and nurses are essential.

Their scrupulous attention to the patient's comfort and toilet is of primary importance: the unpleasant smells associated with skin or urinary infection must be prevented. The earlier the patient gets up the better, and he or she must be trained for a new job as quickly as possible.

FRACTURES OF THE THORACIC CAGE

Complex fractures of the thorax are dealt with in Chapter 22. Isolated fractures of the ribs and sternum are less serious, though it must be remembered that they also may give rise to pneumothorax (sometimes appearing some hours after the initial fracture) or secondary injury to mediastinal structures.

RIB FRACTURES

Rib fractures are almost always due to direct injury. However, in osteoporotic patients, ribs may fracture with minor stresses such as coughing or sneezing.

The patient complains of a sharp pain in the chest. This is markedly aggravated by deep breathing or coughing, or by anteroposterior compression of the chest wall. X-ray shows one or more fractures, usually near the rib angle.

Treatment

In most cases, treatment is needed only for pain; an injection of local anaesthetic will bring immediate relief. Breathing exercises are encouraged.

FRACTURES OF THE STERNUM

The sternum may be fractured by a direct blow to the chest, or indirectly during a flexion injury of the spine.

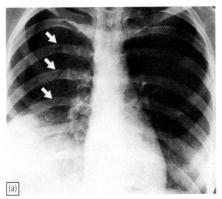

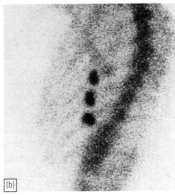

29.15 Fractures of ribs (a) Rib fractures are usually obvious on plain x-ray. (b) Undisplaced fractures are difficult to see; a week later they show up clearly on the radionuclide scan.

The patient complains of severe pain directly over the sternum. X-ray signs are sometimes difficult to discern, particularly if the fracture is undisplaced. *Always x-ray the spine to exclude an associated vertebral compression fracture.*

Treatment

If displacement is minimal, no treatment is needed. If the sternum is severely displaced, it should be lifted forwards (under general anaesthesia) with the aid of a bone-hook.

CHAPTER 30

FRACTURES OF THE PELVIS

Fractures of the pelvis are particularly serious because they are frequently complicated by damage to the soft tissues – urethra, bladder, bowel, and nerves – and this can be fatal. Genitourinary complications occur in about 10 per cent of pelvic fractures and in this group the mortality is in excess of 10 per cent.

Clinical assessment

A fracture of the pelvis should be suspected in every patient with serious abdominal or lower limb injuries. The patient may be severely shocked due to blood loss and visceral damage; resuscitation should be started even before the examination is complete. Local bruising or abrasions may be obvious; ecchymoses often extend into the thigh and perineum, and there may be gross swelling of the labia or scrotum. Bleeding from the urethra or genitalia suggests serious visceral damage. Abdominal tenderness and guarding suggest intraperitoneal bleeding, possibly due to rupture of the spleen or liver.

Pain may be elicited if the pelvic ring is sprung by gentle but firm pressure – first from side to side on the iliac crests, then outwards on the anterior superior iliac spines, and then directly on the symphysis pubis. During rectal examination (which is mandatory), the coccyx and sacrum can be felt; more importantly, the position of the prostate can be gauged: if it is abnormally high, it suggests a urethral injury.

A ruptured bladder should be suspected in patients who do not void or in whom a bladder is not palpable after adequate intravenous fluid replacement.

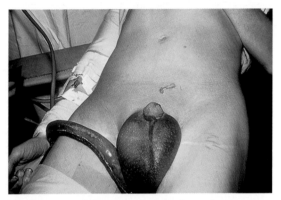

30.1 Fractures of the pelvis – clinical examination This young man crashed on his motorcycle and was brought into the accident and emergency department with a fractured femur. His perineum and scrotum were swollen and bruised; he was unable to pass urine and a streak of blood appeared at the external meatus. X-rays confirmed that he had a fractured pelvis.

Neurological examination is essential. There may be damage to the lumbrosacral plexus.

X-ray

A good anteroposterior view of the pelvis is mandatory, but ideally five views should be obtained: the standard anteroposterior view, an inlet view, an outlet view and two oblique views. A CT scan is invaluable for the diagnosis of sacroiliac disruption and is strongly recommended if surgical stabilization is contemplated.

If there is evidence of abdominal injury, and the patient has haematuria, an intravenous urogram is performed to exclude renal injury. This will also

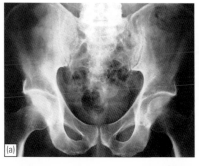

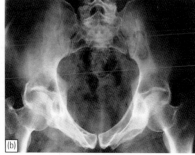

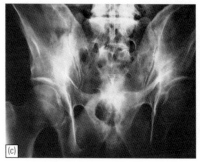

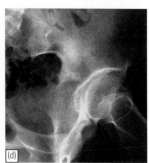

30.2 Pelvic x-rays At least five views are required for diagnosis: (a) anteroposterior; (b) inlet view; (c) outlet view; and (d) right and left oblique views, similar to this view of the left half of the pelvis.

show whether there is any ureteric or major bladder damage.

When a urethral injury is suspected, a urethrogram should be undertaken using 25–30 ml of water-soluble contrast agent with suitable aseptic technique.

Types of fracture

Pelvic fractures fall into four groups: (1) isolated fractures with an intact pelvic ring; (2) fractures with a broken ring – these may be stable or unstable; (3) fractures of the acetabulum: although these are ring fractures, involvement of the joint raises special problems and therefore they are considered separately; and (4) sacrococcygeal fractures.

ISOLATED FRACTURES

Avulsion fractures

A piece of bone is pulled off by violent muscle contraction; this is usually seen in sportsmen and athletes. The sartorius may pull off the anterior superior iliac spine, the rectus femoris the anterior inferior iliac spine, the adductor longus a piece of the pubis, and the hamstrings part of the ischium. All are essentially muscle injuries, needing only rest for a few days and reassurance.

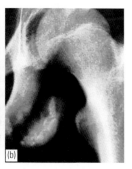

30.3 Avulsion injuries Unusually powerful muscle contraction may tear off a piece of bone at its attachment. Two examples are shown here: (a) avulsion of sartorius attachment; (b) avulsion of hamstring origin.

Direct fractures

A direct blow to the pelvis, usually after a fall from a height, may fracture the ischium or the iliac blade. Bed-rest until pain subsides is usually all that is needed.

Stress fractures

Fractures of the pubic rami are fairly common (and often quite painless) in severely osteoporotic or osteomalacic patients.

FRACTURES OF THE PELVIC RING

The innominate bones and the sacrum form a ring which is held together by the weak symphyseal joint anteriorly and the strong sacroiliac and iliolumbar ligaments posteriorly. Because of the rigidity of the adult pelvis, a break at one point in the ring must be accompanied by disruption at a second point. (Try breaking a ring-shaped biscuit at one point only!) Exceptions are comminuted fractures due to direct blows (including fractures of the acetabular floor), and ring fractures in children, whose symphysis and sacroiliac joints are springy.

Mechanisms of injury

The basic mechanisms of pelvic ring injury are anteroposterior compression, lateral compression, vertical shear and combinations of these. The degree of stability can usually be judged from the fracture pattern.

Anteroposterior compression

The injury is usually caused by a frontal collision between a pedestrian and a car. The pubic rami are fractured or the innominate bones are sprung apart and externally rotated, with disruption of the symphysis – the so-called 'open-book' injury. The sacroiliac ligaments are possibly torn, or there may be a fracture of the posterior part of the ilium. A small separation at the symphysis pubis (usually less than 2 cm) suggests a stable injury; larger separations, especially if a CT scan also shows displacement at a sacroiliac joint, will indicate instability and the need for urgent fixation.

Lateral compression

Side-to-side compression of the pelvis causes the ring to buckle and break. This is usually due to a side-on impact in a road accident or a fall from a height. Anteriorly, the pubic rami on one or both sides are fractured, and posteriorly there is a severe sacroiliac strain or a fracture of the ilium or sacrum. If the sacroiliac injury is much displaced, the pelvis is unstable.

Vertical shear

The innominate bone on one side is displaced vertically, fracturing the pubic rami and disrupting the sacroiliac region on the same side. This occurs typically when someone falls from a height onto one leg. These are usually severe, unstable injuries with gross tearing of the soft tissues and retroperitoneal haemorrhage.

Combination injuries

In severe pelvic injuries there may be a combination of the above.

Clinical features

With isolated fractures and stable injuries the patient is not severely shocked but has pain on attempting to walk. There is localized tenderness but seldom any damage to pelvic viscera.

With unstable injuries the patient is severely shocked, in great pain and unable to stand; he or she may also be unable to pass urine. There may be blood at the external meatus. Tenderness is widespread and attempting to move the ilium is very painful. One leg may be partly anaesthetic because of sciatic nerve injury. These are extremely serious injuries, carrying a high risk of associated visceral damage.

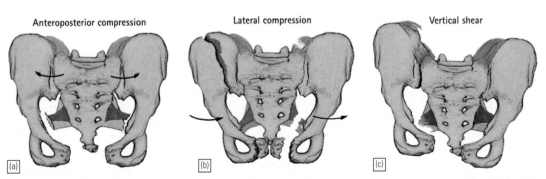

30.4 Fractures of the pelvic ring (a) Anteroposterior compression with lateral rotation causes disruption of the anterior part of the ring – the 'open-book' injury. (b) Lateral compression causes the ring to buckle and break, fracturing the pubic rami on one or both sides; posteriorly the iliac blade may break or the sacrum is crushed. (c) Vertical shear injury, causing disruption of both the sacroiliac and symphyseal regions on one side.

Early management

Treatment should not await full and detailed diagnosis. It is vital in treating any severely injured patient to follow the priorities set out in Chapter 22.

The diagnosis of persistent bleeding is straightforward but it is not always easy to determine the source of the bleeding. *If there is an unstable fracture of the pelvis, haemorrhage will be reduced by rapidly applying a compression belt or an external fixator.* Patients with suspicious abdominal signs should be further investigated by peritoneal aspiration or lavage. If there is a positive diagnostic tap, the abdomen should be explored in an attempt to find and deal with the source of bleeding. If the peritoneal tap is negative, angiography should be performed with a view to embolization of the bleeding vessels.

Urological injury occurs in about 10 per cent of patients with pelvic ring fractures. Patients who cannot pass urine must not be catheterized: gentle retrograde urethrography is harmless and may show a urethral tear. Urogenital damage is particularly likely in bilateral pubic ramus fractures. If the urethra is ruptured, urinary drainage should be provided by suprapubic cystostomy.

Treatment of the fracture

Undisplaced ring fractures

These injuries can be treated by 4 weeks' rest in bed (possibly combined with lower limb traction); the patient is then allowed up, using crutches for another few weeks.

Anterior disruptions without sacroiliac displacement

'Open-book' injuries with a gap of less than 2 cm can usually be treated satisfactorily by bed-rest for about 6 weeks; a posterior sling or an elastic girdle helps to 'close the book'. However, in more severe

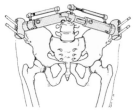
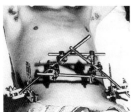

30.5 External pelvic fixation Displaced fractures can often be reduced and held by external fixation.

injuries, whatever the mechanism, the most efficient way of maintaining reduction is by external fixation with pins in both iliac blades connected by an anterior bar. The fixator is retained for 8–12 weeks, but the patient can get up and walk around.

Pubic ramus fractures are usually due to lateral compression, so a sling would be quite inappropriate. If displacement is not severe, bed-rest will suffice.

Displaced fractures with sacroiliac disruption

Severe vertical shear and compression injuries are the most dangerous and the most difficult to treat. The fracture or dislocation must be stabilized. Two techniques are used: (a) anterior external fixation and posterior stabilization using screws across the sacroiliac joint, or (b) plating the symphysis anteriorly and screws across the sacroiliac joint posteriorly. The operation is hazardous (the dangers include massive haemorrhage and infection) and should be attempted only by surgeons with considerable experience in this field.

Complications

Urogenital damage

Compression fractures are the usual cause of urogenital tract damage; but with all pelvic ring disruptions, damage must be excluded. All that

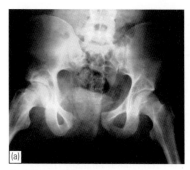
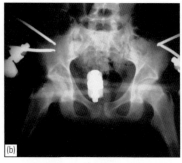
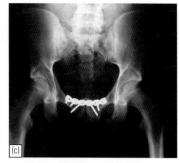

30.6 Internal fixation (a) Severe open-book injury with complete disruption of the symphysis pubis. (b) Reduction and stabilization by external fixator. (c) The symphysis was then firmly held by internal fixation with a plate and screws.

needs to be provided urgently in a seriously ill patient is adequate urinary drainage, which is accomplished by suprapubic cystostomy. Definitive repair can be delayed while the patient's general condition improves and expert urological advice is sought. Late complications include urethral stricture, incontinence and impotence.

Nerve injury

Displacement of the sacroiliac joint or fracture of the sacrum may injure the sciatic nerve or the lumbosacral plexus. Neurapraxia will show signs of recovery within 6 or 8 weeks; otherwise, one must assume that the damage is more severe and some permanent weakness will have to be accepted.

Persistent sacroiliac pain

This is fairly common after unstable pelvic fractures and may occasionally necessitate arthrodesis of the sacroiliac joint.

FRACTURES OF THE ACETABULUM

Fractures of the acetabulum occur when the head of the femur is driven into the pelvis. This is caused either by a blow on the side (as in a fall from a height) or by a blow on the front of the knee, usually in a dashboard injury, when the femur also may be fractured.

Patterns of fracture

There are five main types of acetabular fracture involving (1) the acetabular wall, (2) the anterior column of the acetabulum, (3) the posterior column, (4) the floor of the acetabulum (an uncomminuted transverse fracture), and (5) combinations of the above.

Acetabular wall fractures

Fractures of the anterior or posterior part of the acetabular rim affect the depth of the socket and may lead to hip instability unless they are properly reduced and fixed.

Anterior column fractures

The fracture runs through the anterior part of the acetabulum, separating a segment between the anterior inferior iliac spine and the obturator foramen. It is uncommon, does not involve the weight-bearing area and has a good prognosis.

Posterior column fractures

This fracture runs upwards from the obturator foramen into the sciatic notch, separating the posterior ischiopubic column of bone and breaking the weight-bearing part of the acetabulum. It is usually associated with a posterior dislocation of the hip and may injure the sciatic nerve. Treatment is more urgent and usually involves internal fixation to obtain a stable joint.

Transverse fracture

This is an uncomminuted fracture running transversely through the acetabulum and separating the iliac portion above from the pubic and ischial portions below; sometimes there is also a vertical split into the obturator foramen (a T-fracture). It is usually fairly easy to reduce and to hold reduced.

Complex fractures

Some acetabular fractures are complex injuries which damage various portions of the acetabulum, including the roof and the floor. The articular surface is badly disrupted; the fractures usually need operative reduction and internal fixation and the end result is likely to be less than perfect.

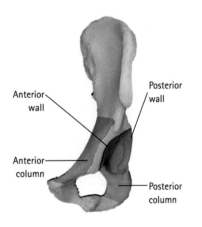

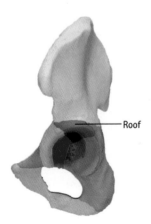

30.7 Acetabular anatomy The important components of the acetabular socket are defined in these illustrations.

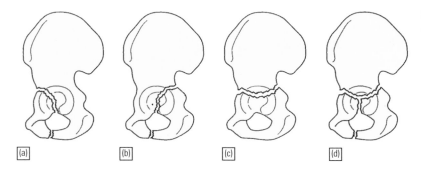

30.8 Tile's classification of acetabular fractures
(a,b) Simple fractures involving either the anterior or the posterior wall or column. (c) Transverse fracture. (d) T-type fracture involving both anterior and posterior columns. There are also composite fractures which severely damage the weight-bearing part of the acetabulum.

Clinical features

There has usually been a severe injury, either a traffic accident or a fall from a height. Associated fractures are not uncommon and, because they may be more obvious, are liable to divert attention from the more urgent pelvic injuries. Whenever a fractured femur, a severe knee injury or a fractured calcaneum is diagnosed, the hips also should be x-rayed.

The patient may be severely shocked, and the complications associated with all pelvic fractures should be sought.. There may be bruising around the hip, and the limb may lie in internal rotation (if the hip is dislocated). No attempt should be made to move the hip.

X-ray

Several views of the hip, and sometimes a CT scan as well, may be needed before the fracture can be accurately visualized.

Treatment

Initial management

Emergency treatment consists of counteracting shock and reducing a dislocation. Traction is then applied to the limb (10 kg will suffice) and during the next 3 or 4 days the patient's general condition is brought under control. Definitive treatment of the fracture is delayed until the patient is fit and operation facilities are optimal. However, the delay should not exceed 7 days, as it becomes increasingly difficult to reduce the fragments accurately.

Conservative treatment

Undisplaced fractures and simple fractures which do not involve the weight-bearing portion (roof) of the acetabulum can often be treated by maintaining traction for 6–8 weeks. If the fracture is significantly displaced, closed reduction can be attempted using a combination of longitudinal

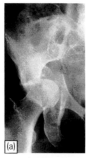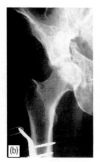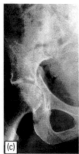

30.9 Conservative treatment This severely displaced acetabular fracture (a) was almost completely reduced by (b) longitudinal and lateral traction. (c) The fracture healed and the patient regained a congruent joint with a fairly good range of movement.

and lateral skeletal traction. If closed reduction fails and adequate surgical expertise is available, operative reduction and internal fixation may be advisable.

Operative treatment

Operative treatment is indicated for all unstable hips and fractures resulting in significant distortion of the ball and socket congruence, as well as for associated fractures of the femoral head and/or retained bone fragments in the joint. The aim should be a perfect anatomical reduction, and the operation is best undertaken in a centre which specializes in this form of treatment.

Complex fractures are difficult to reduce, and in elderly patients operative intervention is not advised unless a persistent posterior dislocation needs to be stabilized. In younger patients, however, the likelihood of osteoarthritis is so great that operative reduction and fixation is justified. However, it should not be attempted in the absence of ideal operating facilities, ample blood for transfusion and a high level of expertise.

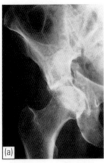
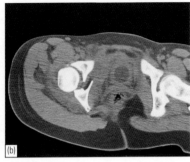
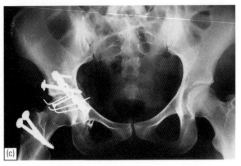

30.10 Internal fixation (a) X-ray shows the fracture, but the degree of displacement is better demonstrated by CT (b). (c) Reduction and fixation with a plate, screws and Kirschner wires.

Complications

Nerve injury

With posterior fractures, the sciatic nerve may be injured. The nerve is usually not severed, so the chances of eventual recovery are good.

Avascular necrosis

As in all severe injuries of the hip, femoral head necrosis may occur. The changes take months or even years to develop. If this progresses to fragmentation and collapse of the head, arthroplasty may be indicated.

Heterotopic bone formation

Heterotopic bone formation is common after severe soft-tissue injury and extended surgical dissections. In cases where this is anticipated, prophylactic indomethacin is useful.

Osteoarthritis

Secondary osteoarthritis of the hip is a common (late) complication, especially if the fracture involves the weight-bearing surface. The fractures must be united before operative treatment is contemplated.

INJURIES OF THE SACRUM AND COCCYX

A blow from behind, or a fall onto the 'tail', may fracture the sacrum or coccyx, or sprain the joint between them.

If the fracture is markedly displaced, reduction is worth attempting. The lower fragment may be pushed backwards by a finger in the rectum. The reduction is stable, which is fortunate. The patient is allowed to resume normal activity, but is advised to use a rubber-ring cushion when sitting.

Persistent pain, especially on sitting, is common after coccygeal injuries. If the pain is not relieved by the use of a cushion or by the injection of local anaesthetic into the tender area, excision of the coccyx may be considered.

CHAPTER 31

INJURIES OF THE HIP AND FEMUR

DISLOCATION OF THE HIP

The incidence of hip dislocation has paralleled the rise in the number of road accidents. The injuries are classified according to the direction of dislocation: posterior (by far the commonest variety), anterior and central.

POSTERIOR DISLOCATION

Usually this occurs in a road accident when someone seated in a truck or car is thrown forwards, striking the knee against the dashboard. The femur is thrust upwards and the femoral head is forced out of its socket; often a piece of bone at the back of the acetabulum is sheared off (fracture–dislocation).

Special features

In a straightforward case the diagnosis is easy: the leg is short and lies adducted, internally rotated and slightly flexed. However, if one of the long bones is fractured – usually the femur – the injury can easily be missed. *The golden rule is to x-ray the pelvis in every case of severe injury* and, with femoral fractures, to insist on x-rays that include the hip and the knee. The lower limb should be examined for signs of sciatic nerve injury.

X-ray

In the anteroposterior film, the femoral head is seen out of its socket and above the acetabulum. Multiple views (and, better still, CT scans) may be needed to exclude a fracture of the acetabular rim or the femoral head.

Treatment

The dislocation must be reduced under general anaesthesia. An assistant steadies the pelvis; the surgeon flexes the patient's hip and knee to 90 degrees and pulls the thigh vertically upwards. X-rays are essential to confirm reduction and to exclude a fracture. If it is suspected that bone fragments have been trapped in the joint, CT is needed.

After reduction, the hip is usually stable, but has been severely injured and needs to be rested. The simplest way is to apply traction and maintain it for 3 weeks. Movement and exercises are begun as soon as pain allows. At the end of 3 weeks the patient is allowed to walk with crutches.

Complications

Sciatic nerve injury

The sciatic nerve is damaged in 10–20 per cent of cases, but fortunately it usually recovers. If, after reducing the dislocation, a sciatic nerve lesion and an unreduced acetabular fracture are diagnosed, the nerve should be explored and the fragment correctly replaced (and screwed in position). Recovery often takes months and in the meantime the limb must be protected from injury and the ankle splinted to overcome the foot-drop.

Avascular necrosis

The blood supply of the femoral head is seriously impaired in at least 10 per cent of traumatic hip

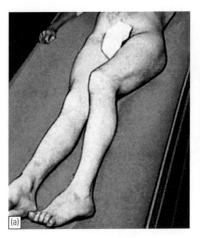

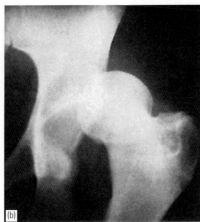

31.1 Posterior dislocation of the hip (a) This patient was brought into hospital following a road accident. It was immediately obvious, from the position of his left lower limb, that he had suffered a posterior dislocation of the hip. This was soon confirmed by the x-ray (b).

dislocations; if reduction is delayed by more than a few hours, the figure rises to 40 per cent. If there is a small necrotic segment, realignment osteotomy is the method of choice. Otherwise, in younger patients, the choice is between femoral head replacement or hip arthrodesis (never an easy procedure). In patients over the age of 50 years a total hip replacement is better.

Osteoarthritis

Secondary osteoarthritis is not uncommon and is due to (1) cartilage damage at the time of the dislocation, (2) the presence of retained fragments in the joint, or (3) ischaemic necrosis of the femoral head. The options are discussed in Chapter 5.

ANTERIOR DISLOCATION

This is rare compared with posterior dislocation. The leg lies externally rotated, abducted and slightly flexed. Seen from the side, the anterior bulge of the dislocated head is unmistakable.

X-ray

In the anteroposterior view the dislocation is usually obvious, but occasionally the head is almost directly in front of its normal position; any doubt is resolved by a lateral film.

Treatment

The manoeuvres employed are almost identical to those used to reduce a posterior dislocation, except that while the flexed thigh is being pulled upwards, it should be adducted; an assistant then helps by applying lateral traction to the thigh. The subsequent treatment is similar to that employed for posterior dislocation. Avascular necrosis is the only complication.

CENTRAL DISLOCATION

A fall on the side, or a blow over the greater trochanter, may force the femoral head medially through the floor of the acetabulum. Although this is called 'central dislocation', it is really a complex fracture of the acetabulum. The condition is dealt with in Chapter 30.

FRACTURE OF THE FEMORAL NECK

The fracture usually results from a fall directly onto the greater trochanter. In younger individuals, the usual cause is a fall from a height or a blow sustained in a road accident; these patients often have multiple injuries and in 20 per cent there is an associated fracture of the femoral shaft. However, this injury is most commonly seen in elderly osteoporotic people; here, less force is required – perhaps no more than catching a toe in the carpet and twisting the hip into external rotation.

In Garden's classification, Stage I is an incomplete impacted fracture, Stage II is a complete but undisplaced fracture, Stage III is a complete fracture with moderate displacement and Stage IV is a severely displaced fracture. Left untreated, a comparatively benign-looking Stage I fracture may rapidly disintegrate to Stage IV.

Special features

There is usually a history of a fall, followed by pain in the hip. If the fracture is displaced, the patient lies with the limb in lateral rotation and the leg looks short.

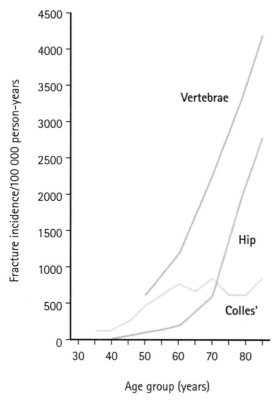

31.2 Incidence of 'osteoporotic' fractures The incidence of brittle fractures in women rises sharply from the menopause onwards.

X-ray

Two questions must be answered: is there a fracture, and is it displaced? Usually the break is obvious, but an impacted fracture can be missed by the unwary. Displacement is judged by the abnormal shape of the bone images and the degree of mismatch of the trabecular lines in the femoral head and neck and the innominate (supra-acetabular) bone. This assessment is important because impacted or undisplaced fractures do well after internal fixation, whereas displaced fractures have a high rate of non-union and avascular necrosis.

Treatment

Operative treatment is almost mandatory. Displaced fractures will not unite without internal fixation, and in any case old people should be got up and active without delay if pulmonary complications and bed sores are to be prevented. Impacted fractures can be left to unite, but there is always a risk that they may become displaced, even while lying in bed, so fixation is safer.

When should the operation be performed? In young patients, operation is urgent: interruption of the blood supply will produce irreversible cellular changes after 12 hours and the way to prevent this is to obtain accurate reduction and internal fixation as soon as possible. In older

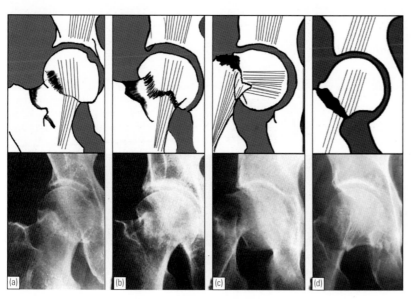

31.3 Garden's classification of femoral neck fractures
(a) *Stage I:* impacted fracture, which in some cases may be an incomplete fracture. (b) *Stage II:* complete but only slightly displaced fracture. The innominate trabeculae are still directly in line with the femoral neck trabeculae. (c) *Stage III:* partially displaced fracture. The femoral head trabeculae are no longer in line with those of the innominate bone. (d) *Stage IV:* complete fracture with full displacement; the proximal fragment appears to be normally aligned with the innominate trabeculae, but that is because the completely detached femoral head has resumed its normal position in the acetabulum.

patients also, the longer the delay the greater is the likelihood of complications; however, here speed is tempered by the need for adequate preparation, especially in the very elderly, who are often ill and debilitated.

What if operation is considered too dangerous? Lying in bed on traction may be even more dangerous! And leaving the fracture untreated too painful. The patient least fit for operation may need it most. Prophylaxis against thromboembolism is very important (see page 134).

The principles are accurate reduction, secure fixation and early activity. Under anaesthesia, the fracture is manipulated and reduction is checked by x-ray. If it is satisfactory, the fracture is securely fixed with cannulated screws, or with a sliding ('dynamic') compression screw which attaches to the femoral shaft. Impacted fractures can be fixed as they lie.

What if the fracture cannot be accurately reduced? In old people the femoral head should be removed and replaced by a metal prosthesis. In patients under 60 it is worth trying open reduction rather than sacrificing the joint.

From the first day, the patient should sit up in bed or in a chair. Walking with crutches is encouraged as soon as possible.

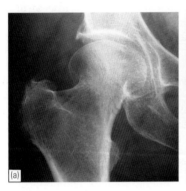
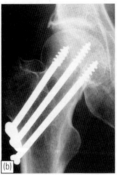
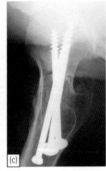

31.4 Femoral neck fracture – treatment (a) This fracture was thought to be securely impacted, but for safety's sake it was fixed with three cannulated screws. (b,c) The postoperative x-rays show that perfect alignment has been maintained in both the anteroposterior and lateral views.

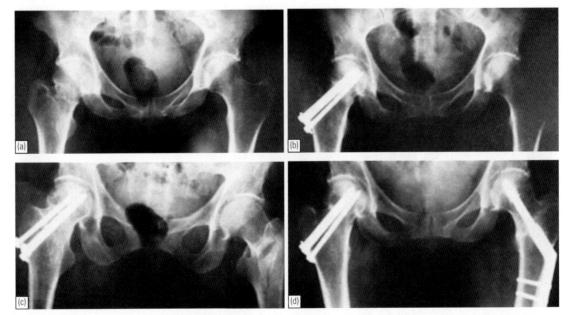

31.5 Bilateral fractures This elderly osteoporotic woman stumbled and fractured (a) her right femoral neck. The fracture was fixed with three long screws (b) and it united soundly. Then, a year later, she tripped and sustained an intertrochanteric fracture on the left side (c). This needed more secure fixation – a large compression screw and plate fixed to the femoral shaft (d).

Fractures in children

If the fracture is undisplaced, it can be held in a plaster cast (a hip spica) until it unites. If it is displaced, it should be reduced and fixed with screws.

Complications

General complications

There is a high incidence of general complications in these elderly and often frail patients. Thromboembolism, pneumonia and bed sores are constant dangers, not to mention the disorders that might have been present before the fracture.

Avascular necrosis

Necrosis of the femoral head occurs in about 30 per cent of patients with displaced fractures and in 10 per cent of those with undisplaced fractures. The reason is simple. The femoral head derives its blood supply from three sources: the nutrient artery, vessels reflected from the capsule, and vessels in the ligamentum teres. When the femoral neck is fractured and severely displaced, the branches from the nutrient artery are severed, the retinacular vessels from the capsule are torn, and the remaining blood supply via the ligamentum teres may be insufficient to prevent ischaemia of the femoral head. The bone dies and eventually collapses. The fracture may still unite but the femoral head becomes distorted and the joint irreversibly damaged.

In patients over 45 years of age, treatment is by total joint replacement. In younger patients, realignment osteotomy may be suitable for small superomedial necrotic segments. Arthrodesis is still favoured by some surgeons, particularly for patients under 30 years; however, the functional outcome is at best unpredictable and at worst unacceptable.

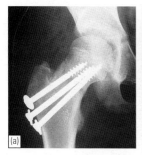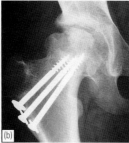

31.6 Femoral neck fracture – avascular necrosis (a) The post-reduction x-ray may look splendid but the blood supply is compromised and 6 months later (b) there is obvious necrosis of the femoral head.

Non-union

More than one-third of all femoral neck fractures fail to unite, and the risk is particularly high in those that are severely displaced. There are many causes: poor blood supply, imperfect reduction, inadequate fixation, and the tardy healing that is characteristic of intra-articular fractures. The bone at the fracture site is ground away, the fragments fall apart and the nail or screw cuts out of the bone or is extruded laterally. The patient complains of pain, shortening of the limb and difficulty with walking. The x-ray shows the sorry outcome.

Treatment of non-union depends on the age of the patient. In those under 50, an attempt may be made to secure union by placing a bone-graft across the fracture and re-inserting a fixation device. In older patients, prosthetic replacement of the femoral head, or total replacement of the joint, must be considered.

Osteoarthritis

Subarticular bone necrosis or femoral head collapse may lead, after several years, to secondary osteoarthritis. If the symptoms warrant it, the joint should be replaced.

INTERTROCHANTERIC (PERTROCHANTERIC) FRACTURES

As with femoral neck fractures, these injuries are common in elderly, osteoporotic women. However, in sharp contrast to the intracapsular neck fractures, the extracapsular intertrochanteric fractures unite very easily and seldom cause avascular necrosis.

Clinical features

Following a fall, the patient is in pain and unable to stand. The limb is shortened and lies in external rotation.

X-ray

The fracture usually runs more or less diagonally from the greater to the lesser trochanter; it may be comminuted and severely displaced, but in some cases the crack can hardly be seen.

Treatment

These fractures are almost always treated by early internal fixation – not because they fail to unite with conservative treatment (they unite quite readily), but (1) to obtain the best possible position and (2) to get the patient up and walking as soon as possible. The fracture is reduced under x-ray control and then fixed with a compression screw

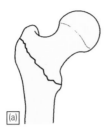
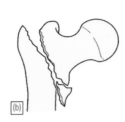
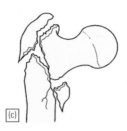
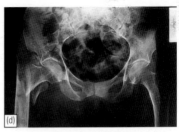

31.7 Intertrochanteric fractures There are several patterns of intertrochanteric fracture, the commonest of which are: (a) undisplaced, (b) displaced but with minimal comminution, and (c) displaced comminuted fracture involving also the greater and lesser trochanters. (d) X-ray of the third type of fracture.

and plate (see Figure 31.5d). The patient is allowed to walk, partially weight-bearing, using crutches until the fracture has united (8–12 weeks).

Complications

General

Early complications are the same as with femoral neck fractures, reflecting the fact that most of these patients are in poor health.

Failure of fixation

Screws may cut out of the osteoporotic bone if reduction is poor or if the fixation device is incorrectly positioned; reduction and fixation may have to be re-done.

Malunion

Varus and external rotation deformities are common. Fortunately they are seldom severe and rarely interfere with function.

SUBTROCHANTERIC FRACTURES

Subtrochanteric fractures may occur at any age if the injury is severe enough, but most occur with relatively trivial injury, in elderly patients with osteoporosis, osteomalacia, Paget's disease or a secondary deposit. Blood loss is greater than with femoral neck or trochanteric fractures.

The leg lies externally rotated and short, and the thigh is markedly swollen. Movement is excruciatingly painful.

X-ray

The fracture is through or below the lesser trochanter and is frequently comminuted.

Treatment

Open reduction and internal fixation is the treatment of choice. Intramedullary nails with

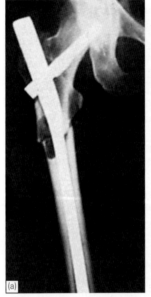
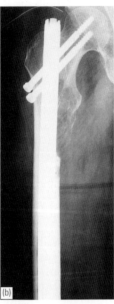

31.8 Subtrochanteric fractures (a) Subtrochanteric fractures are not uncommonly through metastatic tumour deposits; always check for lesions elsewhere. Two methods of internal fixation are shown here and in (b). In both, the stout intramedullary nail bypasses the area of bone lysis.

locking screws into the femoral head or else a compression (dynamic) hip screw and plate will provide satisfactory fixation.

Postoperatively, the patient is allowed partial weight-bearing (with crutches) until union is secure.

Complications

Malunion is fairly common and, if marked, may need operative correction.

FEMORAL SHAFT FRACTURES

The femoral shaft is well padded with muscles – an advantage in protecting the bone from all but the most powerful forces, but a disadvantage in that fractures are often severely displaced by muscle pull, making reduction difficult.

Special features

This is essentially a fracture of young adults and usually results from a high-energy injury. Diaphyseal fractures in elderly patients should be considered 'pathological' until proved otherwise. In children under 4 years of age, the possibility of physical abuse must be kept in mind.

X-ray

Most fractures of the femoral shaft have some degree of comminution, although it is not always apparent on x-ray; it is a reflection of the amount of force involved in these injuries. Displacement may be in any direction. Sometimes there are two fracture lines separated by a unbroken length of bone – the 'segmental fracture'. *The pelvis and knee must always be x-rayed to avoid missing an associated injury.*

Treatment

The risk of systemic complications in these high-energy injuries can be significantly reduced by early stabilization of the fracture. Traction can reduce and hold most fractures in reasonable alignment, and certainly the patient should be transported from the scene of the accident with the limb splinted – many emergency splints

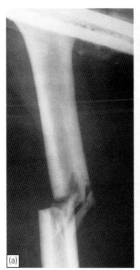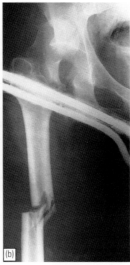

31.9 Femoral shaft fractures – a diagnostic trap (a) Note that the upper fragment is adducted, suggesting that the hip also may be affected. (b) Always x-ray the pelvis; in this case the hip was dislocated.

incorporate a facility to apply traction as well. Definitive treatment will depend on the type of fracture and patient.

Traction and bracing

The main indications for traction are (1) fractures in children, (2) contraindications to anaesthesia, and (3) lack of suitable skill or facilities for internal fixation. It is a poor choice for elderly patients, for pathological fractures and for those with multiple injuries. The chief drawback is the length of time spent in bed (10–14 weeks for adults), with its attendant problems. Some of these difficulties are overcome by reducing the time in traction and then changing to a plaster spica or – in the case of lower-third fractures – functional bracing; this is applicable once the fracture is 'sticky', usually around 6–8 weeks.

While the patient is in traction, joint mobility must be preserved by encouraging movement and exercises. The position of the fragments should be checked repeatedly by x-ray and the system adjusted if necessary.

Open reduction and plating

Fixation with plates and screws was popular at one time but it went out of favour because of the high complication rate, including implant failure. The main indications today are (1) the combination of shaft and femoral neck fractures, and (2) a shaft fracture with an associated vascular injury.

Intramedullary nailing

Intramedullary nailing is the method of choice for most femoral shaft fractures. The basic implant system consists of an intramedullary nail (in a range of sizes) which is perforated near each end so that locking screws can be inserted transversely at the proximal and distal ends; this controls rotation and ensures stability even for subtrochanteric and distal-third fractures.

External fixation

The main indications for external fixation are (1) the treatment of severe open injuries, (2) management of patients with multiple injuries where there is a need to reduce operating time, and (3) dealing with severe bone loss by the technique of bone transport. External fixation is also useful for (4) treating femoral fractures in adolescents.

Open fractures

Open femoral fractures should be carefully assessed for (1) skin loss, (2) wound contami-

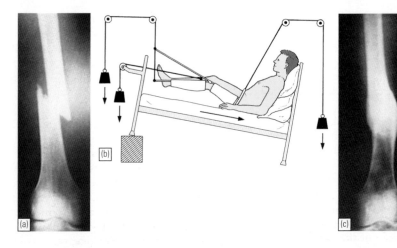

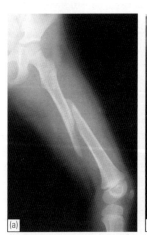

31.10 Femoral shaft fracture – conservative treatment
Conservative treatment is sometimes the best option, though it does call for a long period in bed. (a) Fracture of the femur. (b) Balanced skeletal traction. (c) The fracture has healed in slight angulation.

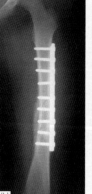

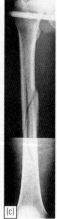

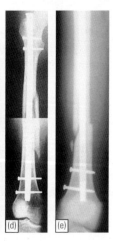

31.11 Femoral shaft fractures – internal fixation
(a) Unstable shaft fractures in children and adolescents, especially those with multiple injuries, can be securely fixed (b) with a plate and screws. In adults, shaft fractures are usually stabilized with a locked intramedullary nail (c,d); this treatment is suitable even for distal-third fractures (e).

nation, (3) muscle ischaemia and (4) injury to vessels and nerves.

The immediate treatment is similar to that of closed fractures. Antibiotics are started and wound cleansing and debridement are carried out with as little delay as possible. The major decision then is how to stabilize the fracture. With small, clean wounds and little delay from the time of injury, the fracture can be treated as for a closed injury, with the addition of prophylactic antibiotics. With large wounds, contaminated wounds, skin loss or tissue destruction, internal fixation should be avoided; after debridement, the wound should be left open and the fracture stabilized by applying an external fixator.

Femoral fractures in children

Infants need no more than 1 or 2 weeks in balanced traction followed by a spica for another 3 or 4 weeks.

Children up to 10 years can be treated in a similar manner, allowing twice as long in traction and then 6 weeks in a spica.

Teenagers may require even longer in traction before changing to a spica. However, if satisfactory reduction cannot be obtained or held, internal fixation with a plate and screws is justified – especially in those with multiple injuries.

Complications

General

Complications such as blood loss, shock, fat embolism and acute respiratory distress are common in high-energy injuries such as this. These conditions are dealt with in Chapter 20.

Vascular injury

The vascular lesion takes priority and the vessel must be repaired or grafted without delay. At the same operation, the fracture is secured by internal fixation.

Thromboembolism

Prolonged traction in bed predisposes to thrombosis. Movement and exercise are important in preventing this; they can be supplemented by foot compression devices or prophylactic doses of anticoagulants. Constant vigilance is needed and full anticoagulant treatment is started immediately if thigh vein or pelvic vein thrombosis is diagnosed.

Infection

In open injuries, and following internal fixation, there is always a risk of infection. Prophylactic antibiotics, and careful attention to the principles of fracture surgery, should keep the incidence below 2 per cent. Management is discussed on page 21.

Delayed union and non-union

It is said that a fractured femur should unite in 100 days plus or minus 20. If union is delayed beyond this time, an exchange nailing is performed using a slightly larger nail; in addition, the fracture may need bone-grafting.

Malunion

Fractures treated by traction and bracing often develop some deformity; no more than 15 degrees of angulation should be accepted.

Until the x-ray shows solid union, the fracture is too insecure to permit weight-bearing; the bone will bend and what previously seemed a satisfactory reduction may end up with lateral or anterior bowing. Shortening is seldom a major problem; if it occurs, and is not too marked, the shoe can be built up.

Joint stiffness

It is surprising how often the knee is affected after a femoral shaft fracture. The joint may be injured at the same time, or it stiffens due to soft-tissue adhesions during treatment; hence the importance of exercise and knee movements.

SUPRACONDYLAR FRACTURES OF THE FEMUR

Supracondylar fractures of the femur are seen (a) in young adults, usually as a result of high-energy trauma, and (b) in elderly, osteoporotic individuals. Direct violence is the usual cause. The fracture line is just above the condyles, but it may branch off distally between them. The pull of the gastrocnemius attachments may tilt the distal fragment backwards.

Special features

The knee is swollen and deformed; movement is too painful to be attempted. The tibial pulses should always be palpated.

X-ray

The fracture is just above the femoral condyles and is transverse or comminuted. The distal fragment is often tilted backwards. The entire femur must be x-rayed so as not to miss a proximal fracture or dislocated hip.

Treatment

If the fracture is only slightly displaced and extra-articular, or if it reduces easily with the knee in flexion, it can be treated quite satisfactorily by skeletal traction through the proximal tibia; the

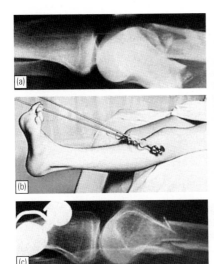
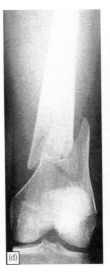
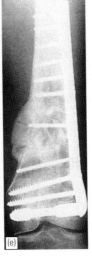

31.12 Supracondylar fractures (a–c) These fractures were, for many years, treated successfully by traction through the upper tibia. (d,e) If the bone is not too osteoporotic, internal fixation with a dynamic condylar screw and plate is a good alternative.

limb is cradled on a Thomas' splint with a knee flexion piece, and movements are encouraged. If the distal fragment is displaced by gastrocnemius pull, a second pin above the knee, and vertical traction, will correct this. At 4–6 weeks, when the fracture is beginning to unite, traction can be replaced by a cast-brace and the patient allowed up and partially weight-bearing with crutches. Non-operative treatment is most likely to be considered if the patient is young and has not suffered multiple injuries.

If closed reduction fails, open reduction and internal fixation with an angled compression device, though difficult, may be successful. This does not necessarily lead to earlier mobilization because the bone is often osteoporotic and the patient may be old and frail, but nursing in bed is easier and knee movements can be started sooner. Unprotected weight-bearing is not permitted until the fracture has consolidated (usually around 12 weeks).

Locked intramedullary nails which are introduced retrograde through the intercondylar notch are also used for these fractures. They provide adequate stability, even in the presence of osteoporotic bone, but (as with compression plates) unprotected weight-bearing is best avoided until union is assured.

Complications

Joint stiffness

Knee stiffness is almost inevitable. A long period of exercise is necessary, but full movement is rarely regained.

Non-union

Knee stiffness increases the likelihood of non-union. This combination is difficult to treat and, unless great care is exercised, the ultimate range of movement at the knee may be less than that at the fracture.

Osteoarthritis

Supracondylar fractures often extend into the joint surface; anatomical restoration by accurate reduction is necessary to reduce the risk of this late complication.

CONDYLAR FRACTURES

One or both femoral condyles may be fractured. The knee is swollen and has the doughy feel of a haemarthrosis.

X-ray

One condyle may be fractured and shifted upwards; occasionally the condyles are split apart and there may also be a supracondylar fracture.

Treatment

The haemarthrosis must be aspirated as soon as possible. Because the articular surface is involved, accurate reduction is important. Open reduction and internal fixation are therefore often employed.

Complications

Stiffness of the knee

This is a common complication. It usually responds to prolonged physiotherapy, although movement may not be fully restored.

Osteoarthritis

As with other intra-articular fractures, secondary osteoarthritis is a late complication.

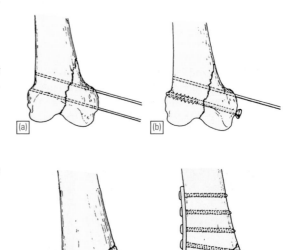

31.13 Femoral condyle fractures (a) A single condylar fracture can be reduced open and held with Kirschner wires preparatory to (b) inserting compression screws. (c,d) More complex fractures are best fixed with a dynamic condylar screw and plate.

CHAPTER 32

INJURIES OF THE KNEE AND LEG

TIBIAL PLATEAU FRACTURES

Fractures of the tibial plateau are caused by a strong bending forces combined with axial loads, e.g. a car striking a pedestrian on the side of the knee (hence the term 'bumper fracture') or a fall from a height in which the knee is forced into valgus or varus. One or both tibial condyles are crushed or split by the opposing femoral condyle.

Special features

The patient is nearly always an adult. The joint is swollen and has the doughy feel of a haemarthrosis. There is diffuse tenderness on the side of the fracture, and also on the opposite side if a ligament is injured.

X-ray

Multiple views (and, sometimes, tomography) are needed to show the true extent of the fracture. Several classifications have been proposed. The one used here is based on Schatzker's classification (Fig 32.1).

Treatment

These fractures all involve the articular surface of the tibia. The guiding principle in their management is straightforward: function is more important than a pretty x-ray. Traction alone often produces a well-functioning knee, though there may be some residual deformity. On the other hand, obsessional surgery to restore a shattered surface can produce a good x-ray appearance – and a stiff knee. Prudence lies somewhere in between.

Undisplaced and minimally displaced fractures of the lateral condyle

These can be treated conservatively. The haemarthrosis is aspirated and a compression bandage is applied. Knee movements are begun and, as soon as the acute pain and swelling have subsided (usually within a week), a hinged cast-

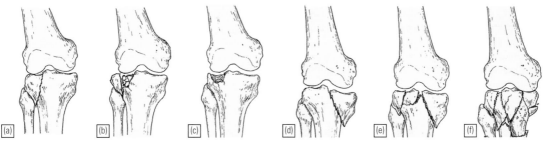

32.1 Tibial plateau fractures (a) Type 1 – simple split of the lateral condyle. (b) Type 2 – a split of the lateral condyle with a more central area of depression. (c) Type 3 – depression of the lateral condyle with an intact rim. (d) Type 4 – a fracture of the medial condyle. (e) Type 5 – fractures of both condyles, but with the central portion of the metaphysis still connected to the tibial shaft. (f) Type 6 – combined condylar and subcondylar fractures.

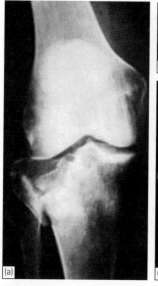
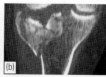
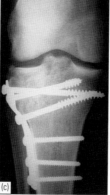

32.2 Comminuted fracture of lateral tibial plateau
(a) There is obviously a fracture of the lateral tibial condyle but the details are hard to make out. (b) Tomography is very helpful; in this case it shows that there is considerable fragmentation. (c) The fracture has been reduced and fixed with a buttress plate and screws.

brace is fitted and the patient is allowed up; however, weight-bearing is not allowed for another 3 weeks. The fracture usually heals by 8–9 weeks. If there is any doubt about the degree of displacement, open reduction and internal fixation with a lag screw would be safer.

Markedly displaced and/or comminuted fractures of the lateral condyle

These should be treated by open reduction and internal fixation. The condylar surface is examined and depressed areas elevated; bone-grafts may be needed to support the reduction. Fixation is usually with lag screws and a buttress plate.

Fractures of the medial condyle

Fractures of the medial tibial condyle are usually more complex than they appear to be at first sight. They are best treated by open reduction and fixation with a buttress plate and screws. Associated lateral ligament damage will need repair.

Bicondylar fractures

These fractures are usually high-energy injuries and do best if reduced and stabilized surgically. Internal fixation with plates and screws is possible, but operative technique needs to be meticulous if wound breakdown problems are to be avoided. A combination of screw fixation and circular external fixation offers satisfactory stabilization with a lower risk of wound complications. *Beware the development of a compartment syndrome.*

Osteoporotic condylar fractures

Elderly individuals with osteoporotic fractures can be treated along the same lines as above. However, if the fracture pattern permits, a total knee replacement (using revision surgery components) may sometimes offer an elegant solution.

Complications

Compartment syndrome

With severe condylar fractures there is a significant risk of developing a compartment syndrome. The leg and foot should be examined repeatedly for suggestive signs (see page 294).

Joint stiffness

Failure to regain full knee bend is an important cause of disability, and is minimized by starting movements early.

Deformity

Some residual valgus or varus deformity is quite common but can be compatible with good

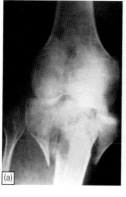
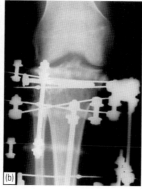
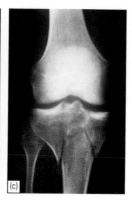

32.3 Bicondylar plateau fractures (a) These injuries are difficult to manage and carry a high risk of soft-tissue complications. If the facilities and expertise are available, they can be treated by a combination of internal and external fixation (b); otherwise non-operative treatment by traction and mobilization may be the better choice, as proved to be the case in this particular patient (c).

function, although constant overloading of one compartment may predispose to osteoarthritis in later life.

Osteoarthritis

If, at the end of treatment, there is marked depression of the plateau, deformity of the knee or ligamentous instability, secondary osteoarthritis is likely to develop after 5 or 10 years. This may eventually require reconstructive surgery.

FRACTURED PATELLA

Three types of fracture are seen: (1) an undisplaced crack across the patella, which is probably due to a direct blow; (2) a comminuted or 'stellate' fracture, due to a fall or a direct blow on the front of the knee; and (3) a transverse fracture with a gap between the fragments – this is an indirect traction injury due to forced, passive flexion of the knee while the quadriceps muscle is contracted; the entire extensor mechanism is torn across and active knee extension is impossible.

Special features

The knee is painful and swollen; sometimes the gap can be felt. Usually there is blood in the joint. It is helpful to establish whether the patient can

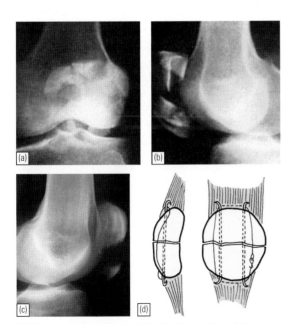

32.4 Fractured patella (a,b) Stellate (comminuted) fracture of the patella. (c,d) Transverse fracture, which is appropriately treated by tension-band wiring and repair of the torn lateral expansions.

actively extend the knee, as this will influence the choice of treatment.

X-ray

The three types of fracture are usually clearly distinguishable, but it is important not to confuse a crack fracture with a congenital bipartite patella in which a smooth line extends obliquely across the superolateral angle of the bone.

Treatment

The key to the management of patellar fractures is the state of the extensor mechanism.

Undisplaced or minimally displaced crack

If there is a haemarthrosis, it is aspirated. The extensor mechanism is intact and treatment is mainly protective. A plaster cylinder holding the knee straight is worn for 4–6 weeks and during this time quadriceps exercises are practised every day.

Comminuted (stellate) fracture

The extensor expansions are intact and the patient may be able to lift the leg. However, the undersurface of the patella is irregular and there is a serious risk of damage to the patellofemoral joint. For this reason, many people advocate patellectomy however slight the displacement. To others it seems reasonable to preserve the patella if the fragments are not severely displaced; a backslab is applied, but removed for daily exercises to mould the fragments into position and to preserve mobility.

Displaced transverse fracture

The lateral expansions are torn and the entire extensor mechanism is disrupted. Operation is essential; the fragments are held apposed by internal fixation (using the tension band principle) and the extensor expansions are repaired. A plaster backslab is worn until active extension of the knee is regained, but flexion and extension exercises are practised each day.

DISLOCATION OF THE PATELLA

Because the knee is normally angled in slight valgus, there is a natural tendency for the patella to pull towards the lateral side when the quadriceps muscle contracts. Traumatic dislocation is due to sudden, severe contraction of the quadriceps muscle while the knee is stretched in valgus and external rotation. Typically this occurs in field sports when a runner dodges to one side. The patella dislocates laterally and the medial retinacular fibres (part of the quadriceps expansion) may be torn.

Clinical features

In a 'first-time' dislocation, the patient may experience a tearing sensation and a feeling that the knee has gone 'out of joint'; when running, he or she may collapse and fall to the ground. Often the patella springs back into position spontaneously; however, if it remains unreduced, there is an obvious (if somewhat misleading) deformity: the displaced patella, seated on the lateral side of the knee, is not easily noticed but the uncovered medial femoral condyle is unduly prominent and may be mistaken for the patella; neither active nor passive movement is possible.

X-ray

In an unreduced dislocation, the patella is seen to be laterally displaced and tilted or rotated. In 5 per cent of cases there is an associated osteochondral fracture.

Treatment

The patella is easily pushed back into place, and anaesthesia is not always necessary. If there is much bruising medially, the quadriceps expansion is torn, and immediate operative repair may prevent later recurrent dislocation.

With the knee straight, a plaster backslab is applied. It is worn for 3 weeks. When the backslab has been removed, flexion is easily regained.

Recurrent dislocation

Patients treated non-operatively for a first-time dislocation have a 15–20 per cent chance of suffering further dislocations. Predisposing factors are generalized joint laxity, marked genu valgum and an unduly high patella.

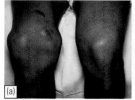
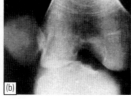

32.5 Dislocation of the patella (a) The right patella has dislocated laterally, giving a broad, flattened appearance to the knee. (b) X-ray showing the patella displaced to the lateral side.

ACUTE KNEE LIGAMENT INJURIES

The bony structure of the knee joint is inherently unstable; were it not for the strong capsule, intra-articular and extra-articular ligaments and controlling muscles, the knee would not be able to function effectively as a mechanism for support, balance and thrust.

Valgus stresses are resisted by the fascia lata, pes anserinus, superficial and deep layers of the medial collateral ligament (MCL) and the tough posteromedial part of the capsule. The main checks to varus angulation are the iliotibial tract and the lateral collateral ligament (LCL). The anterior and posterior cruciate ligaments (ACL and PCL) provide both anteroposterior and rotary stability; they also help to resist excessive valgus and varus angulation.

Injuries of the knee ligaments are common, particularly in sporting pursuits but also in road accidents, where they may be associated with fractures or dislocations. They vary in severity from a simple sprain to complete rupture. It is important to recognize that these injuries are seldom 'unidirectional'; they often involve more than one structure and it is therefore useful to refer to them in functional terms (e.g. anteromedial instability) as well as anatomical terms (e.g. torn MCL and ACL).

Clinical features

The patient gives a history of a twisting or wrenching injury and may even claim to have heard a 'pop' as the tissues snapped. The knee is painful and, in contrast to the story in meniscal injury, swelling appears almost immediately. Tenderness is most acute over the torn ligament, and stressing one or other side of the joint may produce excruciating pain.

Tests for ligamentous stability can be performed if pain allows. Partial tears permit no abnormal movement, but the attempt always causes pain. Complete tears permit abnormal movement, which sometimes causes surprisingly little pain. If there is any doubt about the diagnosis, examination under anaesthesia is mandatory.

Sideways tilting (varus/valgus) is examined, first with the knee at 30 degrees of flexion and then with the knee straight. Movement is compared with the normal side. If the knee angulates only in slight flexion, there is probably an isolated tear of the collateral ligaments; if it angulates in full extension, there is almost certainly rupture of the capsule and cruciate ligaments as well as the collateral ligament.

Anteroposterior stability is assessed first by placing the knees at 90 degrees with the feet resting on the couch and looking from the side for posterior sag of the proximal tibia; when present, this is a reliable sign of PCL instability. Next, the *drawer test* is carried out in the usual way; a positive drawer sign is diagnostic of a tear, but a negative test does not exclude one. The *Lachman test* is more reliable; anteroposterior glide is tested with the knee flexed 15–20 degrees.

X-ray

Stress x-rays of the knee may provide visual evidence of instability. Plain x-rays may show that the ligament has avulsed a small piece of bone – the MCL usually from the femur, the LCL from the fibula, the ACL from the tibial spine and the PCL from the back of the upper tibia.

Treatment

Sprains and partial tears

The intact fibres splint the torn ones and spontaneous healing will occur. The hazard is adhesions, so active exercise is prescribed from the start. Aspirating the haemarthrosis and applying ice-packs intermittently relieves pain. Weight-bearing is allowed, but the knee is protected from rotation or angulation strains by a heavily padded bandage or a functional brace. A complete plaster cast is unnecessary and disadvantageous, as it inhibits movement.

Complete tears

Isolated tears of the MCL or the LCL can be treated as above.

Isolated tears of the ACL may be treated by early operative reconstruction if the individual is a professional sportsman. In all other cases, it is more prudent to follow the conservative regimen described above; the cast-brace is worn only until symptoms subside, and thereafter movement and muscle-strengthening exercises are encouraged. About half of these patients regain sufficiently good function not to need further treatment. The remainder complain of varying degrees of instability; late assessment will identify those who are likely to benefit from ligament reconstruction.

Isolated tears of the PCL are usually treated conservatively.

Avulsion fractures of the tibial intercondylar eminence

Sometimes a severe strain, instead of rupturing a cruciate ligament, results in an avulsion fracture at the insertion of the ligament. The fragment may be only partially displaced and difficult to detect on x-ray. If the fragment can be manipulated back

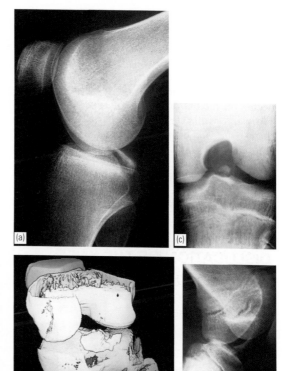

32.7 Cruciate ligament avulsion (a) X-rays showing an avulsion fracture at the insertion of the posterior cruciate ligament. (b) Three-dimensional CT reconstruction, demonstrating the avulsed fragment and its bed. (c,d) Avulsion of the anterior cruciate ligament. In adolescence the avulsed tibial spine seems smaller on x-ray than is actually the case because it is covered by thick articular cartilage.

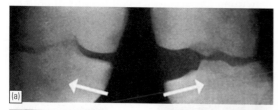

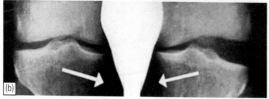

32.6 Ligament injuries Stress x-rays of two different patients showing (a) complete tear of the medial ligament of the left knee and (b) complete tear of the lateral ligament.

into position *and allow full extension of the knee,* immobilization in a plaster cylinder for 6 weeks will suffice. If the fragment cannot be reduced, or if there is a block to full extension, operative reduction and fixation with strong sutures (or with small screws if the physis has closed) will be needed; a plaster cylinder for 6 weeks will still be required. Full movement is usually regained within 3 months.

Combined injuries

With combined ACL and collateral ligament injury, it is wiser to start treatment with joint bracing and physiotherapy in order to restore a good range of movement before following on with ACL reconstruction. The collateral ligament does not usually need reconstruction. A similar approach is adopted for combined injuries involving the PCL, but here all damaged structures will need to be repaired.

Complications
Adhesions

If the knee with a partial ligament tear is not actively exercised, torn fibres stick to intact fibres and to bone. The knee 'gives way' with catches of pain; localized tenderness is present, and pain occurs on medial or lateral rotation. The obvious confusion with a torn meniscus can be resolved by the *grinding test* or by arthroscopy.

Instability

The knee may continue to give way. The instability tends to get worse and predisposes to osteoarthritis. Reconstruction before the onset of degeneration is wise.

DISLOCATION OF THE KNEE

The knee can be dislocated only by considerable violence, as in a road accident. The cruciate ligaments and one or both lateral ligaments are torn.

Clinical features

There is severe bruising, swelling and gross deformity. The circulation in the foot must be examined because the popliteal artery may be torn or obstructed. Distal sensation and movement should be tested to exclude nerve injury.

X-ray

In addition to the dislocation, the films occasionally reveal a fracture of the tibial spine due to ligament avulsion. If there is any doubt about the circulation, an arteriogram should be obtained.

Treatment

Reduction under anaesthesia is urgent. If reduction is achieved, the limb is rested on a backslab with the knee in 15 degrees of flexion; the circulation is checked repeatedly during the next week. Because of swelling, a plaster cylinder is dangerous. If the joint is unstable, an anterior external fixator can be applied. If there is an open wound, or vascular damage which needs operation, the opportunity is taken to repair the ligaments and capsule. Otherwise, these structures are left undisturbed.

When swelling has subsided, a cast is applied and is worn for 12 weeks. Quadriceps muscle exercises are practised from the start. Weight-bearing in the plaster is permitted as soon as the patient can lift the leg. Knee movements are regained when the plaster is removed.

FRACTURES OF THE TIBIA AND FIBULA

A twisting force causes a spiral fracture of both leg bones at different levels; an angulatory force produces short oblique fractures, usually with a separate triangular 'butterfly' fragment.

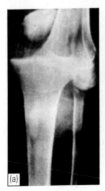 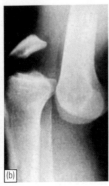 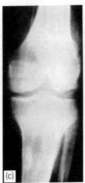 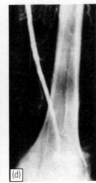

(a)   (b)   (c)   (d)

32.8 Dislocation of the knee
(a,b) This patient was admitted with a dislocated knee. After reduction (c) the x-ray looked satisfactory, but the circulation did not. (d) An arteriogram showed vascular cut-off just above the knee.

Because of its subcutaneous position, the tibia is more commonly fractured, and more commonly sustains an open fracture, than any other long bone. A direct injury may crush or split the skin over the fracture; this is a high-energy fracture and is often from a motorcycle accident. Indirect injuries are low energy; with a spiral or oblique fracture, one of the bone fragments may pierce the skin from within.

Clinical features

The limb should be carefully examined for bruising, severe swelling, crushing or tenting of the skin, an open wound, weak or absent pulses, diminution or loss of sensation and inability to move the toes. Always be on the alert for signs of an impending compartment syndrome.

X-ray

The entire length of both the tibia and fibula, as well as the knee and ankle joints, must be seen.

Management

The main objectives are:

- to limit soft-tissue damage and preserve skin cover,
- to obtain and hold fracture alignment,
- to recognize compartment syndrome,
- to start early weight-bearing (loading promotes healing), and
- to start joint movements as soon as possible.

Treatment of low-energy fractures

Most low-energy fractures, including simple open injuries (Gustilo type I and II injuries after attention to the wounds), can be treated by non-operative methods.

If the fracture is undisplaced or minimally displaced, a full-length cast from upper thigh to metatarsal necks is applied with the knee slightly flexed and the ankle at a right angle. A displaced fracture needs reduction under general anaesthesia with x-ray control before cast application. The limb is elevated and the patient is kept under observation for 48–72 hours. If there is excessive swelling, the cast is split. Patients are usually allowed up (and home) on the second or third day, bearing minimal weight with the aid of crutches. After 2 weeks, the position is checked by x-ray. With stable fractures, the full-length cast may be changed after 4–6 weeks to a functional below-knee cast or brace which is carefully moulded to bear upon the upper tibia and patellar tendon. This liberates the knee and allows full weight-bearing. The cast (or brace) is retained until the fracture unites, which is around 8 weeks in children but seldom under 16 weeks in adults.

Indications for skeletal fixation

In hospitals where experience and facilities for operative skeletal fixation are lacking, non-operative treatment is not only feasible but positively desirable. It allows for a shorter period of hospitalization, but follow-up is more frequent and prolonged. Where appropriate skills and facilities are available, tibial shaft fractures can be surgically fixed. Indeed, many surgeons would hold that unstable fractures, even of low-energy type, are better treated by skeletal fixation from the outset.

- *Locked intramedullary nailing*. This is the method of choice for diaphyseal (shaft) fractures. Union can be expected in more than 95 per cent of cases. However, the method is less suitable for fractures near the bone ends.
- *Plate fixation*. Plating is best for metaphyseal fractures that are unsuitable for nailing. It is also sometimes used for unstable low-energy shaft fractures in children.

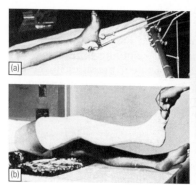
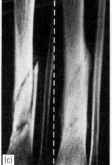
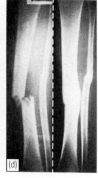

32.9 Fractured tibia and fibula – closed treatment
(a) Skeletal traction is used to reduce any overlap, and also as a provisional treatment when skin viability is doubtful. (b) After 10–14 days, a long-leg plaster cast is applied. This method is generally more suited to low-energy fractures where the initial displacement is slight and the soft tissues are well preserved. (c,d) Two examples, showing the position before and after fracture union, are illustrated.

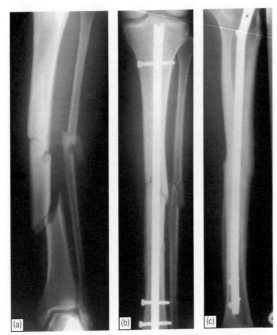

32.10 Fractured tibia and fibula – internal fixation
Closed intramedullary nailing is now the preferred treatment for unstable tibial fractures. (a) Position on admission to hospital. (b,c) Anteroposterior and lateral views after intramedullary nailing. Active movements and partial weight-bearing were started soon after operation.

- *External fixation.* This is an alternative to closed nailing, but postoperative monitoring is demanding. It can be applied for metaphyseal and shaft fractures.

Treatment of high-energy fractures

Initially, the most important consideration is the viability of the damaged soft tissues and underlying bone. Tissues around the fracture should be disturbed as little as possible, and open operations should be avoided unless there is already an open wound. The risk of compartment syndrome prevails in the first 48 hours.

In keeping with the principle of inflicting as little surgical damage as possible to a limb that is already badly injured, external fixation offers several advantages as the method of choice for stabilization. Intramedullary nailing is an alternative, but may be difficult.

Treatment of open fractures

There is a risk of deep infection and chronic osteomyelitis. Gustilo and Anderson's method is popular for classifying these injuries (see Chapter 24, page 289).

A suitable regimen for the treatment of open tibial fractures comprises:

- antibiotics
- debridement
- stabilization
- soft-tissue cover
- rehabilitation.

Antibiotics are started immediately and are continued for a full therapeutic course, which is 3–5 days. A broad-spectrum cephalosporin is suitable for Gustilo grades I–IIIA wounds, but more severe grades benefit from Gram-negative cover using an aminoglycoside such as gentamicin. Metronidazole should be added if soil contamination has occurred.

Full wound assessment is done in the operating theatre and not the emergency department. Ideally, the debridement should be carried out with a plastic surgeon so that wound extensions do not compromise the raising of skin flaps for bone cover. Repeat debridement may be necessary, but exposed bone should preferably be covered within 5 days of the injury. Fracture stabilization may be achieved by several methods depending on the energy of injury; external fixation is favoured for the more severe ones.

Complications

Vascular injury

Fractures of the proximal half of the tibia may damage the popliteal artery. This is an emergency of the first order, requiring angiograms, exploration and repair.

Compartment syndrome

Tibial fractures – both open and closed – and inexpert intramedullary nailing are the commonest causes of compartment syndrome in the leg. Heightened awareness is all! Warning symptoms are increasing pain, a feeling of tightness or 'bursting' in the leg, and numbness in the leg or foot. The diagnosis can be confirmed by measuring the compartment pressures in the leg. Once the diagnosis is made, decompression by open fasciotomy should be carried out with the minimum delay (see page 295).

Infection

Open fractures are always at risk; even a small perforation should be treated with respect, and

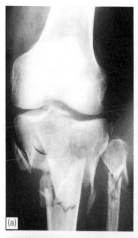
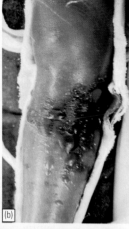
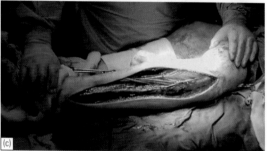

32.11 Compartment syndrome (a) Fractures at this level carry a high risk of causing a compartment syndrome. This patient was initially treated in plaster but he developed intense pain, swelling and blistering (b). Tibial compartment decompression (c) requires two incisions, one medial and one lateral, to reach *all* compartments in the leg.

infection control and fracture union are more likely if fixation is secure. However, if there is a loose implant, it should be removed and replaced by external fixation. Intractable infections also are unlikely to subside unless the implant is replaced by external fixation.

Malunion

Slight shortening (up to 1.5 cm) is usually of little consequence, but angulation should be prevented at all stages; anything more than 7 degrees in either plane is unacceptable. Malunion nearer the ends of the tibia are more likely to lead to early osteoarthritis. Deformity, if marked, should be corrected by tibial osteotomy.

Delayed union and non-union

High-energy fractures and fractures associated with bone loss or deep infection are slow to unite and liable to non-union. Bone-grafting may solve some 'slow' unions; in others, a different mode of fixation may be needed.

Joint stiffness

Prolonged cast immobilization is liable to cause stiffness of the ankle and foot, which may persist for 12 months or longer in spite of active exercises. This can be avoided by changing to a functional brace as soon as it is safe to do so, usually by 4–6 weeks.

Complex regional pain syndrome (algodystrophy)

With distal-third fractures, algodystrophy is not uncommon. Exercises should be encouraged throughout the period of treatment. The management of established algodystrophy is discussed on page 302.

debridement carried out before the wound is closed.

With established infection, skeletal fixation should not be abandoned if the system is stable;

CHAPTER 33

INJURIES OF THE ANKLE AND FOOT

ANKLE LIGAMENT INJURIES

A sudden twist of the ankle momentarily tenses the structures around the joint. This may amount to no more than a painful wrenching of the soft tissues – a sprained ankle. If more severe force is applied, the ligaments may be strained to the point of rupture. If the tear is partial, healing is likely to restore full function to the joint; however, with complete tears, joint instability may persist.

More than 90 per cent of ankle ligament injuries involve the lateral side – usually the anterior talofibular, or both this and the calcaneofibular ligament; only in the most severe injuries is the posterior talofibular ligament torn.

Special features

A history of a twisting injury followed by pain, bruising and swelling is typical. Tenderness is maximal just distal and slightly anterior to the lateral malleolus, and the slightest attempt at passive inversion of the ankle is extremely painful. *It is essential to examine the entire leg and foot: undisplaced fractures of the ankle or the tarsal bones are easily missed.*

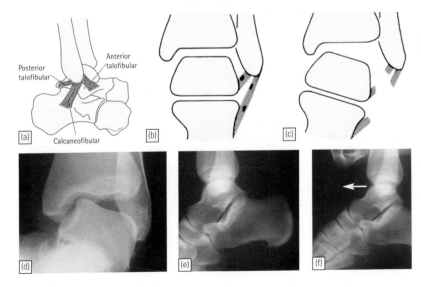

Posterior talofibular — Anterior talofibular — Calcaneofibular

(a) (b) (c) (d) (e) (f)

33.1 Ankle ligament injuries (a) The three components of the lateral collateral ligament of the ankle. (b) The commonest injury is a partial tear of one or other component of the lateral ligament. (c) Following a complete tear of the lateral ligament, the talus may be displaced in the ankle mortise. (d) Stress x-ray showing talar tilt. (e,f) X-rays demonstrating anteroposterior instability. Pulling the foot forward under the tibia causes the talus to shift appreciably at the ankle joint; this is usually seen after recurrent sprains.

Localized soft-tissue swelling and, in some cases, a small avulsion fracture of the tip of the lateral malleolus or the anterolateral surface of the talus are the only corroborative signs of lateral ligament injury. Stress x-rays to demonstrate instability are unnecessary in the acute case unless operative repair is being considered; local or general anaesthesia will be needed.

Treatment

Partial tear

Sprains and strains should be treated by activity. An elastic bandage is applied and active exercises are begun immediately and persevered with until full movement is regained.

Complete tear

Operative repair of acutely ruptured ligaments may be advisable in top-class athletes and dancers. In most patients, however, the injury can be treated by cast immobilization, extending from just below the knee to the toes, with the foot plantigrade. After 6 weeks, the cast can be replaced by a removable brace and physiotherapy is begun. The ligament takes about 10 weeks to heal; at that stage the splint is discarded and the patient is encouraged to return gradually to normal activity.

Complications

Recurrent sprains

Recurrent 'giving way' or a feeling of instability when walking on uneven surfaces is the common complaint. Stress x-rays show either excessive talar tilting in the coronal plane or anterior displacement (an anterior drawer sign) in the sagittal plane.

Recurrent sprains can usually be prevented by raising the outer side of the heel and extending it laterally. A light brace can be worn during stressful activities. If disability is marked, surgical repair or substitution of the torn ligaments is undertaken.

FRACTURES OF THE ANKLE

Fractures and fracture–dislocations of the ankle are common. In the vast majority of cases, the ankle is twisted and the talus tilts and/or rotates forcefully in the tibiofibular mortise, causing a low-energy fracture of one or both malleoli, with or without associated injuries of the ligaments and displacement of the talus. The commonest mechanism is by *abduction and/or lateral rotation of the ankle,* causing the lateral malleolus (or distal end of fibula) to sheer off at an oblique angle,

while the strain on the medial side of the joint may rupture the deltoid ligament or produce a transverse avulsion fracture of the medial malleolus. Similarly, sudden severe *adduction of the ankle* may sheer off the medial malleolus and produce a strain injury or fibular fracture on the lateral side of the joint. Sometimes a forward lunge of the tibia causes the posterior edge of the tibia (the 'posterior malleolus') to fracture as it catches against the dome of the talus. A much less common mechanism of injury is *axial compression of the ankle* (e.g. following a fall from a height), which may shatter the articular plafond of the tibia.

Thus, the diagnosis and treatment of all significant ankle injuries must take account of seven important elements:

- the fibula,
- the tibial malleolus,
- the tibiofibular syndesmosis,
- the medial collateral (deltoid) ligament,
- the lateral collateral ligaments,
- the tibial articular surface, and
- the position of the talus.

Clinical features

Ankle fractures are seen in skiers, footballers and climbers. They also occur, with much lesser force, in osteoporotic postmenopausal women.

A history of a twisting injury followed by intense pain and inability to stand on the leg suggests something more serious than a simple 'sprain'. The ankle is swollen and deformity may be obvious, especially in a fracture–dislocation. The site of tenderness is important: if both the medial and the lateral sides are tender, a double injury (bony or ligamentous) must be suspected.

X-ray

The most obvious change is a fracture of one or both malleoli; however, the 'invisible' part of the injury is just as important – rupture of the collateral and/or distal tibiofibular ligaments. Three views are advisable: anteroposterior, lateral and a 30 degree oblique projection facing the plane of the inferior tibiofibular joint (the 'mortise' view). Fracture lines should be looked for in both the anteroposterior and the lateral x-rays; separation (diastasis) of the tibiofibular joint is best displayed in the 30 degree mortise view. Collateral ligament damage is suggested by displacement or tilting of the talus.

Two different but complementary classifications are employed in assessing these injuries. The

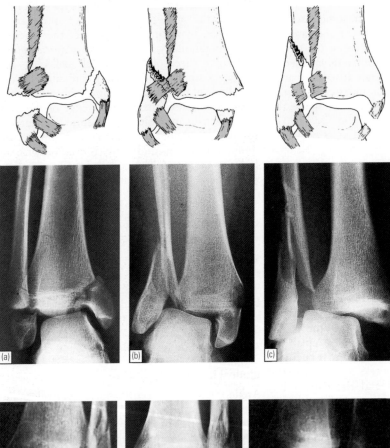

33.2 Ankle fractures – classification The Danis–Weber classification is based on the level of the fibular fracture. (a) *Type A*. A fibular fracture below the tibiofibular syndesmosis and an oblique fracture of the medial malleolus. (b) *Type B*. A fracture at the syndesmosis, often associated with disruption of the anterior fibres of the tibiofibular ligament and fracture of the medial malleolus, or disruption of the medial ligament. (c) *Type C*. A fibular fracture above the syndesmosis; the tibiofibular ligament must be torn, producing an unstable fracture-subluxation of the ankle. Using the Lauge–Hansen classification, (a) would probably have been caused by forced supination and adduction of the foot; (b) by abduction of the ankle; and (c) by severe abduction and external rotation.

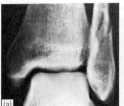
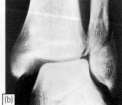
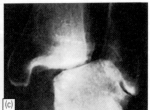

33.3 Stable and unstable ankle fractures It is very important to assess whether the fracture is stable or unstable. (a) This is a stable type B fracture; after reduction, the ankle joint is symmetrically restored and the width of the joint space is regular both superiorly and medially. (b) In this case, although the fracture of the fibula appears to have been reduced, the medial joint space is abnormally widened, the talus is shifted slightly towards the lateral side and is also slightly tilted. The medial ligament must have been torn and may even be trapped in the medial side of the joint, so it is important to explore the medial side, release any obstructing tissue and position the talus correctly before accepting the reduction and immobilizing the ankle. (c) This is an obvious fracture-dislocation with rupture of the tibiofibular syndesmosis and severe damage to the medial collateral ligament. The fibula must be fixed to full length and the tibiofibular joint secured before the ankle can be stabilized.

Lauge–Hansen classification is based on the adduced mechanism of injury, which is useful in planning how to reduce the displaced fragments by reversing the injurious forces during manipulation of the ankle. The *Danis–Weber* classification focuses on the level of the fibular fracture: fractures distal to the tibiofibular joint generally leave the syndesmosis intact, whereas indirect fractures above that level must necessarily have damaged the syndesmotic ligaments. If the mortise becomes

unstable, the talus can be displaced. Thus, careful interpretation of the x-rays is important for both diagnosis and treatment.

Principles of treatment

- Swelling is usually rapid and severe. If the injury is not dealt with within a few hours, definitive treatment may have to be deferred for several days while the leg is elevated so that the swelling can subside.

- As with all fractures involving a joint, the anatomy must be accurately restored and held until healing is complete. Residual displacement or incongruity of the joint will lead to focal stress on the articular surface and the gradual emergence of osteoarthritis.

- The key to congruity and stability of the joint is found in the level of the fibular fracture. If the fracture is below (distal to) the tibiofibular joint, the ankle will be stable once the malleolar fractures are reduced and immobilized; usually a plaster cast will suffice.

- If the fibular fracture is above the level of the tibiofibular joint – even if the fracture appears on x-ray to be undisplaced – one must assume that there is associated damage to the inferior tibiofibular ligaments and the medial components of the ankle joint. If there is no medial malleolar fracture, check carefully for signs of deltoid ligament disruption and displacement of the talus, as well as x-ray features of tibiofibular diastasis. The fibular fracture is best stabilized by internal fixation. Diastasis should be reduced (if necessary under vision) and secured with a screw which transfixes the two bones. Immediate postoperative x-ray examination is essential to ensure that the talus is correctly placed in the mortise; if it is laterally displaced (even slightly), the medial collateral ligament must be explored and any obstructing tissue removed.

- Isolated medial malleolar fractures, if undisplaced, can be managed by plaster immobilization for 4–6 weeks. Displaced fractures should be accurately reduced and fixed with one or two screws. If the talus is shifted laterally, look for an associated fibular fracture; it may even be at the proximal end of the fibula, out of range of the ankle x-ray! Also check for tibiofibular diastasis, which may require open reduction and transverse screw fixation.

- The same principles apply to bi-malleolar fractures and fracture–dislocations. Undisplaced fractures below the tibiofibular joint can be treated by plaster immobilization. Displaced fractures and fracture–dislocations require accurate reduction and internal fixation.

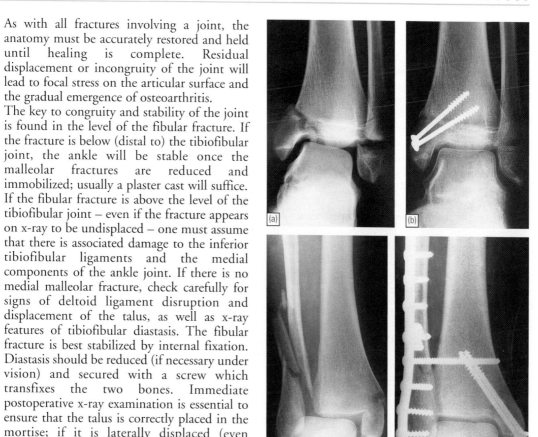

33.4 Ankle fractures – operative treatment (a,b) If the medial malleolar fragment involves a large segment of the articular surface, it is best treated by accurate open reduction and internal fixation with one or two screws. (c,d) An unstable fracture-dislocation almost always needs open reduction and internal fixation. The fibula must be restored to full length and fixed securely; in this case, the medial malleolus also needed internal fixation. Because it is assumed that there was a partial disruption of the distal tibiofibular syndesmosis, a tibiofibular screw has been used to secure the diastasis until the ligaments heal (usually 12 weeks).

Postoperative management

The ankle and foot will be immobilized in a below-knee cast. The patient is allowed walk about, partial weight-bearing with the aid of crutches. For stable, low-level fractures, the cast can usually be discarded after 4 weeks and exercises are then encouraged. For unstable and operatively treated fractures, the cast should be retained for 6–8 weeks. If a tibiofibular transfixing screw has been used, it may need to be retained for somewhat longer.

Complications

Joint stiffness

Swelling and stiffness of the ankle are usually the result of neglect in treatment of the soft tissues.

The patient must walk correctly in plaster and, when the plaster is removed, he or she must, until circulatory control is regained, use a compression stocking and elevate the leg whenever it is not being used actively. Physiotherapy is helpful.

Complex regional pain syndrome

Long-lasting aching, recurrent swelling and regional osteoporosis are fairly common after ankle fractures. The management of this condition is discussed on page 302.

Osteoarthritis

Malunion and/or incomplete reduction will eventually lead to secondary osteoarthritis of the ankle. Symptoms may not become intrusive for 10 or 15 years; however, in some cases (for reasons that are not clear), degenerative changes appear with alarming rapidity and patients may seek treatment within a year or two of the ankle injury.

POSTERIOR MARGINAL FRACTURE OF THE TIBIA

A forward thrust of the leg at the moment of injury may result in a fracture of the posterior margin of the tibial articular surface, either in isolation or in addition to a malleolar fracture. A good lateral x-ray should show both the size of the posterior fragment and whether or not it is displaced.

If the posterior fragment is very small, particularly in the context of more serious associated malleolar fractures, it can be ignored. However, a large posterior fragment, and even more so one that is displaced, should be treated by open reduction and internal fixation with a screw or buttress plate. Unless the articular surface is perfectly restored, secondary osteoarthritis is likely.

Postoperative management is the same as for other ankle fractures.

COMMINUTED FRACTURES OF THE TIBIAL PLAFOND (PILON FRACTURE)

Severe axial compression of the ankle joint (e.g. in a fall from a height) may shatter the tibial plafond. There is considerable damage to the articular cartilage, and the subchondral bone may be broken into several pieces; in severe cases, the comminution extends some way up the shaft of the tibia.

Special features

Swelling is usually severe and fracture blisters are common.

X-rays

This is a comminuted fracture of the distal end of the tibia, extending into the ankle joint. Sometimes the fibula also is fractured. In severe

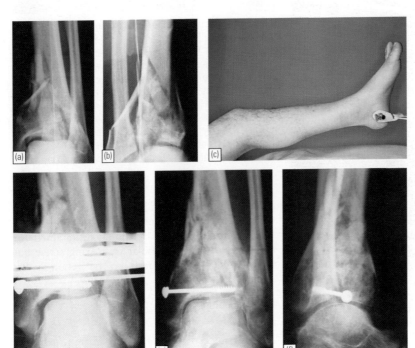

33.5 Pilon fracture of the ankle High-energy pilon fractures (a,b) carry a risk of wound breakdown and infection if treated by wide open reduction and plating. Conservative treatment (c) – traction and movement – is often the best option. If expert facilities are available, open reduction combined with external fixation (d) can be attempted. (e,f) In this case a relatively good result was achieved.

injuries, accurate definition of the fragments is impossible without CT scans.

Treatment

Control of soft-tissue swelling is a priority; this is best achieved either by elevation and calcaneal traction or by applying an external fixator across the ankle joint. It may take 2–3 weeks before the soft tissues improve, by which time surgery may be considered; in most cases, open reduction and fixation will be needed. Postoperatively, physiotherapy is focused on joint movement and reduction of swelling.

Although bony union may be achieved, the fate of the joint is decided by the degree of cartilage injury – the 'invisible' factor on x-rays. Secondary osteoarthritis is a frequent late complication, and symptoms may become severe enough to warrant arthrodesis of the ankle.

ANKLE FRACTURES IN CHILDREN

Physeal injuries are quite common in children and almost a third of these occur around the ankle (see page 273).

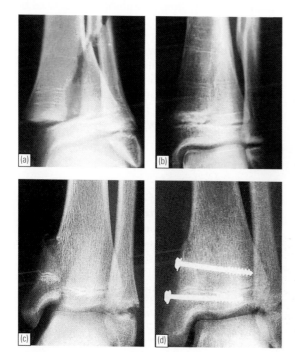

33.6 Physeal injuries (a,b) Type 1 or 2 injuries which do not traverse the width of the physis can be treated conservatively. (c,d) Fractures which disrupt the tibial physis must be treated by accurate open reduction and internal fixation if a good result is to be achieved.

The foot is fixed to the ground or trapped in a crevice and the leg twists to one or other side. The tibial (or fibular) physis is wrenched apart, usually resulting in a Salter–Harris type 1 or 2 fracture. Types 3 and 4 fractures are uncommon but dangerous. The epiphysis is split vertically and one piece of the epiphysis may be displaced; if it is not accurately reduced, it will inevitably result in abnormal growth and deformity of the ankle.

Special features

Following a sprain, the ankle is painful, swollen, bruised and acutely tender.

X-ray

Undisplaced physeal fractures are easily missed. Even a hint of physeal widening should be regarded with great suspicion, and the x-ray examination must be repeated after a week.

Treatment

Salter–Harris types 1 and 2 injuries are treated closed. If it is displaced, the fracture is gently reduced under general anaesthesia. The limb is immobilized in a full-length cast for 3 weeks and then in a below-knee walking cast for a further 3 weeks. Occasionally, surgery is needed to extract a periosteal flap which prevents adequate reduction.

Type 3 or 4 fractures, if undisplaced, can be treated in the same manner, but the ankle must be x-rayed again after 5 days to ensure that the fragments have not slipped. Displaced fractures should be reduced open and fixed with interfragmentary screws which are inserted parallel to the physis. Postoperatively, the leg is immobilized in a below-knee cast for 6 weeks.

Complications

Malunion

Imperfect reduction may result in angular deformity of the ankle – usually valgus. In children under 10 years old, mild deformities may be accommodated by further growth and modelling. In older children the deformity should be corrected by osteotomy.

Asymmetrical growth

Fractures through the epiphysis may result in fusion of the physis. The bony bridge is usually in the medial half of the growth plate; the lateral half goes on growing and the distal tibia gradually veers into varus. CT is helpful in showing where it is. If the bridge is small, it can be excised and replaced by a pad of fat in the hope that physeal growth may be restored. If more than half of the physis is involved, or the child is near the end of the growth period, supramalleolar osteotomy is indicated.

Shortening

Early physeal closure occurs in about 20 per cent of children with distal tibial injuries. Fortunately, the resulting limb length discrepancy is usually mild. If it promises to be more than 2 cm and the child is young enough, proximal tibial epiphysiodesis in the opposite limb may restore equality.

INJURIES OF THE HINDFOOT

Injuries of the foot are apt to be followed by residual symptoms and loss of function which seem out of proportion to the initial trauma. Severe injuries affect the foot as a whole, whatever the particular bone that is fractured. In practice, the entire foot should be examined systematically, no matter that the injury may appear to be localized to one spot. Multiple fractures, or combinations of fractures and dislocations, are easily missed. The circulation and nerve supply must be carefully assessed: a well-reduced fracture is a useless achievement if the foot becomes ischaemic or insensitive.

FRACTURE OF THE TALUS

Talar injuries are rare and due to considerable violence – car accidents or falls from a height. The injuries include fractures of the head, the neck, the body or the bony processes of the talus, dislocations of the talus or the joints around the talus, osteochondral fractures of the superior articular surface and a variety of chip or avulsion fractures.

Clinical features

The foot and ankle are painful and swollen; if the fracture is displaced, there may be an obvious deformity, or the skin may be tented or split. Tenting is a dangerous sign; if the fracture or dislocation is not promptly reduced, the skin may slough and become infected.

X-ray

Undisplaced fractures are not always easy to see, and sometimes even severely displaced fractures are missed because of unfamiliarity with the normal appearance in various x-ray projections. CT can be helpful.

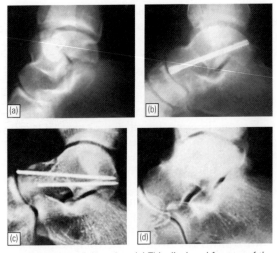

33.7 Fractures of the talus (a) This displaced fracture of the body of the talus was reduced and fixed with a counter-sunk screw (b), giving a perfect result. Fractures of the neck, even if well reduced (c), are still at risk of developing avascular necrosis of the posterior fragment (d).

Treatment

When displacement is no more than trivial, reduction is not needed. A split plaster is applied and, when the swelling has subsided, is replaced by a complete plaster in the plantigrade position. This is worn for 6–8 weeks.

With displaced fractures and fracture–dislocations, reduction is urgent. Closed manipulation is tried first, but should this fail, there must be no hesitation in performing open reduction. The reduced fracture can be stabilized with one or two lag screws. A below-knee plaster is needed for 6–8 weeks.

Complications

Avascular necrosis

Fractures of the neck of the talus often result in avascular necrosis of the body (the posterior fragment). The fracture may fail to unite and the posterior half of the bone eventually collapses. The ankle may need to be arthrodesed.

FRACTURES OF THE CALCANEUM

The patient falls from a height, often from a ladder, onto one or both heels. The calcaneum is driven up against the talus and is split or crushed. More than 20 per cent of these patients suffer associated injuries of the spine, pelvis or hip.

Extra-articular fractures involve the calcaneal processes or the posterior part of the bone. They are easy to manage and have a good prognosis.

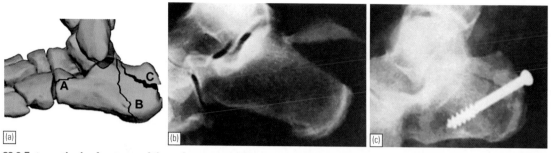

33.8 Extra-articular fractures of the calcaneum (a) Most extra-articular fractures occur through (A) the anterior process, (B) the body of calcaneum or (C) the tuberosity. Sometimes the sustentaculum or the medial tubercle may fracture. (b) Avulsion fracture of the posterosuperior corner, which can be easily fixed by a screw (c).

Treatment is 'closed' unless the fragment is large and badly displaced, in which case it will need to be fixed back in position.

Intra-articular fractures cleave the bone obliquely and run into the superior articular surface; secondary cracks cause further disruption of the bone. The articular facet is split apart and there may be severe comminution.

Special features

The foot is painful, swollen and bruised; the heel may look broad and squat. The tissues are thick and tender, and the normal concavity below the lateral malleolus is lacking. The subtalar joint cannot be moved but ankle movement is possible. Always check for signs of a compartment syndrome of the foot (intense pain, very extensive bruising and diminished sensibility).

X-ray

Extra-articular fractures are usually fairly obvious. Intra-articular fractures, also, can often be identified in the plain films and, if there is displacement of the fragments, the lateral view

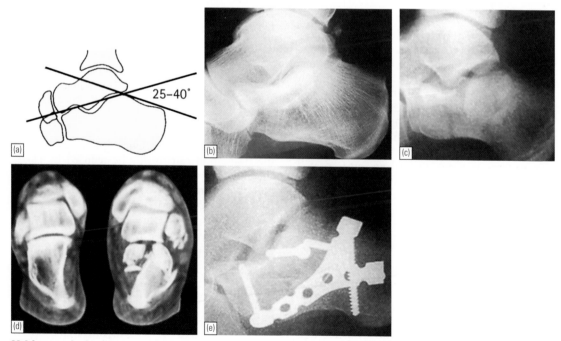

33.9 Intra-articular fractures Fractures involving the talocalcaneal articular surface are serious injuries. (a,b) Normally the lateral x-ray of the calcaneum shows the superior surface raised at an angle under the talus. This is Böhler's angle, normally 25–40 degrees. Fracture of the articular surface may result in flattening of Böhler's angle (c). CT scans (d) provided additional information about the degree of articular fragmentation. (e) With an accurate knowledge of the pathological anatomy, open reduction and internal fixation can be undertaken.

may show flattening of Böhler's angle. However, for accurate definition of intra-articular fractures, CT is essential.

With severe injuries – and especially with bilateral fractures – *it is essential to x-ray the knees, the spine and the pelvis as well.*

Treatment

For all except the most minor injuries, the patient is admitted to hospital so that the leg and foot can be elevated and treated with ice-packs until the swelling subsides. This also gives time to obtain the necessary x-rays and CT scans.

Undisplaced fractures

All undisplaced fractures can be treated closed. Exercises are encouraged from the outset. When the swelling subsides, a firm bandage is applied and the patient is allowed up, non-weight-bearing on crutches for 4–6 weeks.

Displaced avulsion fractures

Displaced fractures of the tuberosity should be reduced and fixed with screws; the foot is then immobilized in slight equinus to relieve tension on the tendo Achillis. Weight-bearing can be permitted after 4–6 weeks.

Displaced intra-articular fractures

These injuries are best treated by open reduction and internal fixation with plates and screws. Bone-grafts are used to fill any defects. If there is much bleeding from the bone, the wound should be drained. This is difficult surgery, which calls for complete familiarity with the local anatomy. Postoperatively, the foot is lightly splinted and elevated. Exercises are begun as soon as pain subsides and, after 2–3 weeks, the patient can be allowed up, non-weight-bearing on crutches. Partial weight-bearing is permitted only when the fracture has healed (seldom before 8 weeks), and full weight-bearing about 4 weeks after that.

Complications

Broadening of the heel

This is quite common and may cause problems with shoe fitting.

Talocalcaneal stiffness and osteoarthritis

Displaced intra-articular fractures may lead to joint stiffness and, eventually, osteoarthritis. This can usually be managed conservatively, but persistent or severe pain may necessitate subtalar arthrodesis. If the calcaneocuboid joint is also involved, a triple arthrodesis is better.

MID-TARSAL INJURIES

Injuries in this area vary from minor sprains, often incorrectly labelled as 'ankle' sprains, to severe fracture–dislocations which can threaten the survival of the foot. Isolated injuries of the navicular, cuneiform or cuboid bones are rare. Fractures in this region should be assumed to be 'combination' fractures or fracture–subluxations until proved otherwise.

Clinical features

The foot is bruised and swollen. Tenderness is usually diffuse across the mid-foot. A medial mid-tarsal dislocation looks like an 'acute club-foot' and a lateral dislocation produces a valgus deformity. It is important to exclude distal ischaemia or a compartment syndrome.

X-ray

Multiple views are necessary to determine the extent of the injury. CT is sometimes needed before a diagnosis can be made.

Treatment

Ligamentous strains

The foot may be bandaged until acute pain subsides. Thereafter, movement is encouraged.

Undisplaced fractures

The foot is elevated to counteract swelling. After 3 or 4 days, a below-knee cast is applied and the patient is allowed up on crutches with limited weight-bearing. The plaster is retained for 4–6 weeks.

Fracture–dislocations

These are severe injuries. Under general anaesthesia, the dislocation can usually be reduced by closed

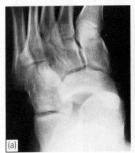 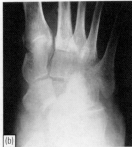

33.10 Mid-tarsal injuries (a) X-ray showing dislocation of the talonavicular joint. (b) X-ray on another patient showing longitudinal compression fracture of the navicular bone and subluxation of the head of the talus. This injury is often difficult to demonstrate accurately on plain x-ray.

manipulation, but holding it is a problem. If there is the least tendency to redisplacement, Kirschner wires are run across the joints to fix them in position. The foot is immobilized in a below-knee cast for 6–8 weeks. Exercises are then begun and should be practised assiduously; it may be 6–8 months before function is regained.

TARSOMETATARSAL INJURIES

Sprains are quite common but dislocation is rare; twisting and crushing injuries are the usual causes. *A fracture–dislocation should always be suspected if the patient has pain, swelling and bruising of the foot after an accident, even if there is no obvious deformity.*

X-rays

A fracture–dislocation is unlikely to be missed on x-ray examination, but the full extent of the injury is seldom clear on the plain x-ray. Multiple views and CT may be needed. Whether or not the talonavicular joint is dislocated, always look carefully for fractures of the navicular or cuneiform bones, which are more difficult to reduce and hold.

Treatment

Undisplaced sprains require cast immobilization for 4–6 weeks. Subluxation or dislocation calls for accurate reduction. Traction and manipulation under anaesthesia achieves reduction (open reduction is rarely needed); the position is then held with Kirschner wires or screws and cast immobilization. A new cast is applied after the swelling has subsided and the patient is instructed to remain non-weight-bearing for 6–8 weeks. The Kirschner wires are then removed and rehabilitation exercises begun.

METATARSAL FRACTURES

Metatarsal fracture may be caused by a direct blow, by a severe twisting injury or by repetitive stress. In the usual case there is a history of injury and the foot is painful and somewhat swollen. X-ray examination will show the fracture.

Treatment

A walking plaster may be applied, mainly for comfort, and is retained for 3 weeks. The fracture unites readily.

In the unlikely event of severe displacement, reduction and Kirschner wire fixation may be justified. In that case, weight-bearing is avoided for 3 weeks and this is followed by a further 3 weeks in a weight-bearing cast.

STRESS INJURY (MARCH FRACTURE)

In a young adult (often a recruit or a nurse), the foot may become painful after over-use. A tender lump is palpable just distal to the mid-shaft of a metatarsal bone, usually the second. The x-ray appearance may at first be normal, but a radioisotope scan will show an area of intense activity in the bone. Later a hairline crack may be visible, and later still a mass of callus or periosteal new bone is seen.

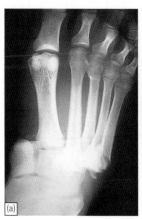 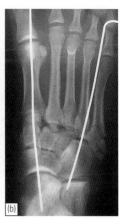 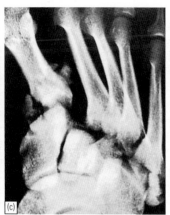 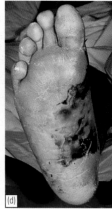

33.11 Tarsometatarsal injuries (a) Dislocation of the tarsometatarsal joints. (b) X-ray after reduction and stabilization with Kirschner wires. (c) X-ray showing a high-energy fracture-dislocation involving the tarsometatarsal joints. These are serious injuries, which may be complicated by (d) compartment syndrome of the foot.

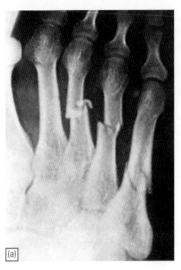

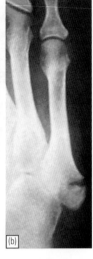

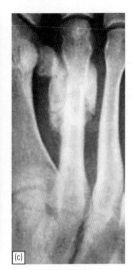

33.12 Metatarsal injuries
(a) Transverse and oblique fractures of three metatarsal shafts. (b) Avulsion fracture of the base of the fifth metatarsal. (c) Florid callus and periosteal new-bone formation around the second metatarsal shaft – the classic sign of a stress fracture.

No displacement occurs and neither reduction nor splintage is necessary. The forefoot may be supported with Elastoplast and normal walking is encouraged.

Note. Similar lesions occur in osteoporotic patients after operations that shorten the big toe, throwing extra stress on the adjacent metatarsals. Elderly patients should be warned about this possibility.

FRACTURED TOES

A heavy object falling on the toes may fracture phalanges. If the skin is broken, it must be covered with a sterile dressing. The fracture is disregarded and the patient encouraged to walk in a suitably adapted boot. However, if pain is marked, the toe can be splinted by strapping it to its neighbour for 2–3 weeks.

FRACTURED SESAMOIDS

One of the sesamoids (usually the medial) may fracture from either a direct injury (landing from a height on the ball of the foot) or sudden traction; chronic, repetitive stress is more often seen in dancers and runners.

The patient complains of pain directly over the sesamoid. There is a tender spot in the same area and sometimes pain can be exacerbated by passively hyperextending the big toe. X-rays will usually show the fracture (which must be distinguished from a smooth-edged bipartite sesamoid).

Treatment is often unnecessary, though a local injection of lignocaine helps for pain. If discomfort is marked, the foot can be immobilized in a short-leg walking cast for 2–3 weeks. Occasionally, intractable symptoms call for excision of the offending ossicle.

INDEX